STRUCTURES

OF THE

Head

and

Neck

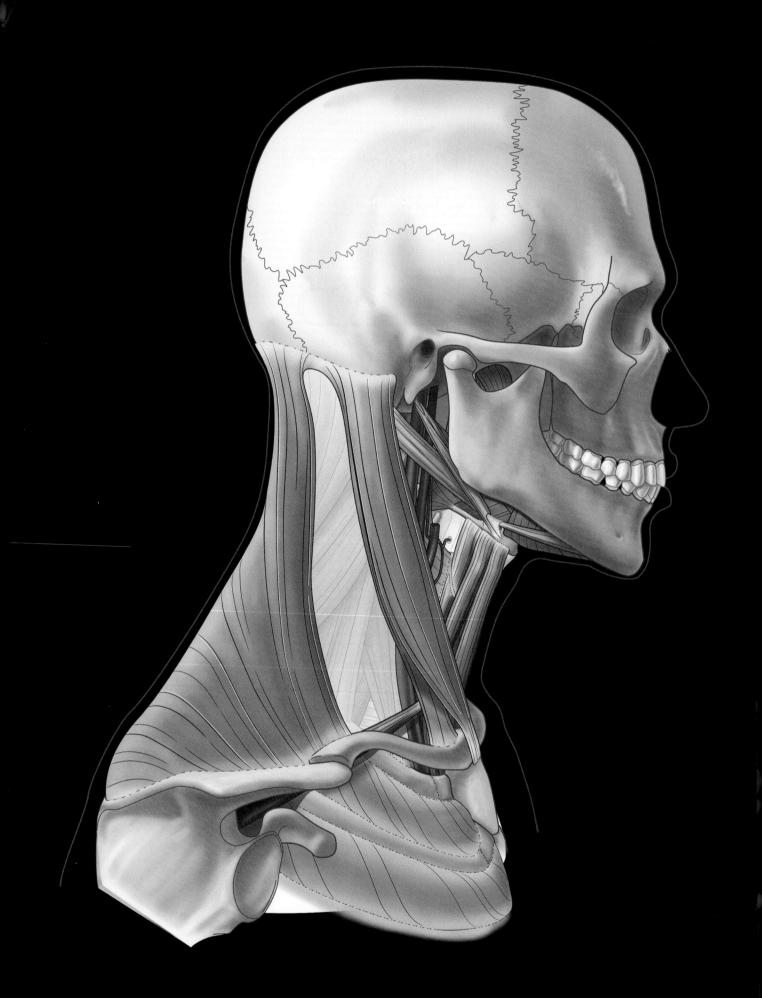

STRUCTURES

OF THE

HEAD
and
NECK

FRANK J. WEAKER, PhD

Professor
Distinguished Teaching Professor
Department of Cellular & Structural Biology
The University of Texas
Health Science Center at San Antonio
San Antonio, Texas

F.A. Davis Company • Philadelphia

F. A. Davis Company
1915 Arch Street
Philadelphia, PA 19103
www.fadavis.com

Copyright © 2014 by F. A. Davis Company

Printed in the United States of America

Last digit indicates print number: 10 9 8 7 6 5 4 3 2 1

Editor-In-Chief: Margaret M. Biblis
Senior Acquisitions Editor: T. Quincy McDonald
Manager of Content Development: George W. Lang
Senior Developmental Editor: Jennifer A. Pine
Art and Design Manager: Carolyn O'Brien

As new scientific information becomes available through basic and clinical research, recommended treatments and drug therapies undergo changes. The author(s) and publisher have done everything possible to make this book accurate, up to date, and in accord with accepted standards at the time of publication. The author(s), editors, and publisher are not responsible for errors or omissions or for consequences from application of the book, and make no warranty, expressed or implied, in regard to the contents of the book. Any practice described in this book should be applied by the reader in accordance with professional standards of care used in regard to the unique circumstances that may apply in each situation. The reader is advised always to check product information (package inserts) for changes and new information regarding dose and contraindications before administering any drug. Caution is especially urged when using new or infrequently ordered drugs.

Library of Congress Cataloging-in-Publication Data

Weaker, Frank J.
    Structures of the head and neck / Frank J. Weaker. — 1st ed.
        p. ; cm.
    Includes index.
    ISBN 978-0-8036-2958-5
    I. Title.
    [DNLM: 1. Head--anatomy & histology. 2. Neck—anatomy & histology. 3. Central Nervous System—anatomy & histology. 4. Dental Hygienists. 5. Stomatognathic System—anatomy & histology. WE 705]
    QM535
    611'.91—dc23
                                    2013016352

PREFACE

The complexity of the head and neck can be overwhelming for the novice dental hygiene student who is in the initial stages of learning anatomy.

This book was written to assist novice students in learning and understanding the complex regional anatomy that will form the foundation of their careers in dental hygiene. The book is written in a student-friendly style, with over 400 vividly colored and labeled illustrations, tables, and flowcharts. Each chapter begins with a set of objectives to help the student focus on what should be learned by the completion of the chapter. The objectives are followed by a brief overview that explains the topic of the chapter and why it is relevant to the student. Review questions follow the major subdivisions of the chapter; these questions allow the student to reflect on the subject matter before continuing on to new material. Major features of each chapter are the specialty boxes that contain additional information regarding structure and function, clinical correlates, and developmental anatomy. Each chapter contains tables or flowcharts to help the student organize the information to study. In addition to the chapter summary, each chapter ends with a Learning Lab, a unique feature that offers the student the opportunity to experience hands-on learning and problem solving through two types of exercises. The Laboratory Activities encourage students to explore anatomy through palpation of their own bodies and through creation of models and simple sketches. Students will create a model of the muscles of the neck, and palpate skeletal features, muscles, and lymph nodes as well as examine surface features of the face and oral cavity. The Learning Activities help reinforce students' recognition of anatomical structures by presenting detailed diagrams from the text for labeling, self-testing, and study. Other Learning Lab exercises include clinical vignettes in which students must apply their knowledge of anatomy to solve a clinical problem.

This book is organized in a blended regional and systemic approach to studying the structures of the head and neck. It begins with a chapter on anatomical terminology and introduction to the study of the head and neck. The second chapter focuses on the structure of the skull and vertebrae. In Chapter 3, the muscles of the head and neck are presented in a regional approach that includes the neck, pharynx and larynx, face, and mouth (Chapters 4–9), followed by Chapter 10 on the fascial spaces of the mouth and neck, which are clinically relevant to the spread of infection from the teeth to the neck. The blood vessels and lymphatic structures are presented as a system (Chapters 11 and 12), but are also related to their regional locations. The concluding chapters discuss neuroanatomy, and include many features that are clinically relevant to patient care and to the understanding of medical histories related to neurological disorders. Chapter 13 on the brain and spinal cord is a concise overview of the organization and function of the central nervous system. Chapter 14 on sensory and motor pathways is generally not included in an anatomy text, but is important to understanding pain and motor function. Chapter 15 on the autonomic nervous system presents a brief description of the structure and function of the sympathetic and parasympathetic nervous systems, which can be affected by pharmacological drugs used in a dental practice. Chapter 16 offers an overview of cranial nerve function, with an emphasis on those nerves related to the dental profession. The discussion of the trigeminal nerve in Chapter 17 is a comprehensive presentation of the branches and functions of the nerve, and is followed by Chapter 18 on intraoral injections. In this chapter, the pertinent branches of the trigeminal nerve and their distribution are reviewed, injection techniques are compared, and the hazards presented by the surrounding structures around the injection sites are discussed. The final chapter, Chapter 19, is a unique discussion of orofacial reflexes, which can be invoked during a dental examination. In addition, the chapter allows the student to incorporate nerves, muscles, and nerve pathways presented in previous chapters into a functional unit.

I have attempted to write this book similar to the way I teach anatomy in the classroom. It is my hope that you will find anatomy a rewarding learning experience and understand its revelence to clinical practice and body functions.

Frank J. Weaker, PhD

REVIEWERS

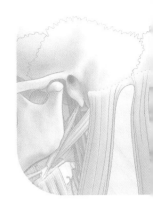

Suzanne M. Edenfield, EdD RDH
Department Head
Department of Dental Hygiene
Armstrong Atlantic State University
Savannah, Georgia

Christine Fambely, DH, Cert. in Health Ed, BA, MEd
Instructor
Dental Hygiene
John Abbott College
Ste. Anne, Quebec

Tracy Gift, RDH, MS
Director
Dental Programs
Mohave Community College
Bullhead City, Arizona

Wanda C. Hayes, BSDH, RSH, CDA
Instructor
Dental Health Professions
York Technical College
Rock Hill, South Carolina

Linda Hecker, CDA, RDH, BS, MA
Professor and Director of Dental Hygiene
Dental Hygiene
Burlington County College
Pemberton, New Jersey

Shahnaz Kanani, DDS
Professor
Science Division and Dental Hygiene Department
Valencia College
Orlando, Florida

Elaine Hopkins Madden, RDH, BS, MEd
Professor, Dental Hygiene
Health Sciences
Cape Cod Community College
West Barnstable, Massachusetts

Paula Malcomson, RDH, BA, BEd
Professor
Health Sciences-Dental Programs
Fanshawe College of Applied Arts and Technology
London, Ontario, CANADA

Patricia Mannie, RDH, MS
Instructor and Director of Hygiene
Dental Hygiene
St. Cloud Technical and Community College
St. Cloud, Minnesota

Martha McCaslin, CDA, MA
Professor and Program Director
Health and Public Services
Dona Ana Community College
Las Cruces, New Mexico

Frances McConaughy, RDH, MS
Professor
Dental Hygiene
Weber State University
Ogden, Utah

Kathleen Feres Patry, RHD
Instructor
Dental Hygiene
Canadian National Institute of Health Inc.
Ottawa, Ontario

Sandra Pence, RDH, MS
Program Director
Dental Hygiene Program
University of Alaska, Anchorage
Anchorage, Alaska

Constance Baker Phillips, DDS, MA
Assistant Professor
Dental Hygiene
Farmingdale State College
Farmingdale, New York

Tammy Morgan-Schubert, RDH
Professor
Health Sciences-Dental Programs
Cambrian College
Sudbury, Ontario

Anne Uncapher, RDH, MA
Associate Professor
Dental Hygiene Department
Broome Community College
Binghamton, New York

Helen Symons, CDA, RDH, BS, MA
Professor
School of Health Sciences, Dental Hygiene Program
Fanshawe College
London, Ontario

Janette Whisenhunt, CDA, RDH, BS, MEd, PhD
Department Chair
Dental Education
Forsyth Technical Community College
Winston-Salem, North Carolina

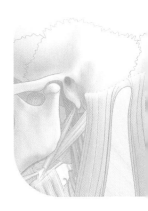

ACKNOWLEDGMENTS

First, I would like to thank the staff at F.A. Davis who allowed me the opportunity to write this textbook in the manner in which I teach my students. I am particularly grateful to Quincy McDonald, Acquisition Editor, and to Jennifer Pine, Senior Developmental Editor, who encouraged and guided me through writing and organization of this textbook.

No anatomical textbook would be complete without vivid illustrations. I would like to acknowledge David F. Baker, Supervisor of Medical Illustrations, of the Academic Technology Services of The University of Texas Health Science Center at San Antonio, for the wonderful illustrations in the book. I would like to thank two of my colleagues, Drs. Earlanda L. Williams and Damon C. Herbert for their support and suggestions while writing this book. I would like to also thank Dr. Archie Jones of the Department of Periodontology who helped me with the photographing of the structures of the oral cavity.

Finally, I would like to thank my family and students: the students for their encouragement and suggestions, and my wife and family for their patience and support throughout the completion of this textbook.

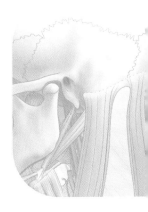

BRIEF CONTENTS

TABLE OF CONTENTS

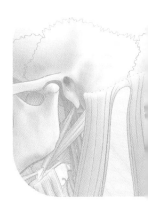

Structures of the

Head
and
Neck

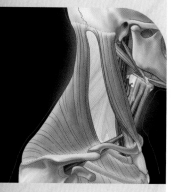

chapter 1

Essentials of Anatomy

1. Explain why the study of head and neck anatomy supports the role of a dental hygienist.
2. Use correct terminology to describe planes, direction, and relationships of structures within the body relative to the anatomical position.
3. Illustrate the structure of a neuron and describe how the neuron contributes to the structure of peripheral nerves and the nervous system.
4. Discuss the organization of the nervous system and discuss how information is transferred between the central nervous system and peripheral structures.
5. Describe the compartmentalization of the neck and the regional divisions of the head.

WHY STUDY ANATOMY?

Anatomy is the foundation of all clinical sciences, which includes dentistry. The technological advances in patient care over the century have been dependent on the knowledge of the structure and function of the human body. It is almost inconceivable that anyone would be allowed to clinically treat patients without foundational knowledge of human anatomy. Yet, some students entering the field of dental hygiene question the need to study anatomy. After all, a hygienist takes radiographs and cleans teeth; the dentist and the physician treat the patient. Although that sentiment may have been partially true in the past, the role of a dental hygienist as a member of the dental health-care team has greatly changed and continues to expand. In many respects, the dental

hygienist is the public relations spokesperson for a dental practice. Unless there is a dental emergency, the hygienist is the first to render treatment, and first impressions are very important in patient retention. One of your first duties as a dental hygienist will be to relax the patient and assure the patient that he or she is receiving the best dental care. Of course, your hand skills are of utmost importance; however, a patient is more secure when you are able to explain the technical procedures, the significance of examining the oral cavity and related structures, and the assessment of the health of the oral cavity (triage). A patient who does not have confidence in the dental hygienist may choose not to return to that dental practice.

The dental hygienist must be aware that systemic diseases can affect the oral cavity, and, conversely, that disease in the oral cavity can affect other parts of the body. As an example, infection from an abscessed tooth can travel into the neck, and, if not controlled, can enter the thoracic region, which contains the heart. In addition to localized swelling of the oral cavity, the floor of the mouth, and the neck, the patient may experience difficulty in swallowing and breathing as the infection spreads, and if it is not treated, death may occur.

Roles of the dental hygienist are expanding. In many states, dental hygienists are allowed to administer intraoral injections. This not only requires anatomical knowledge of the injection sites but also awareness of structures that might be endangered by the aberrant placement of the needle of a syringe. The dental hygienist must also know what nerves innervate the teeth and surrounding tissues in order to deliver the anesthetic to achieve proper anesthesia (that is, to block pain) for a dental procedure. Some small rural communities do not have a resident dentist. Dental clinics are staffed by dental hygienists who must triage the patient for proper dental care, recognize systemic disease observable in the oral cavity, and refer patients to dental and medical health-care professionals. In such cases, a strong foundational knowledge of the anatomy of the human body is critical to the practicing dental hygienist.

How Is Anatomy Taught?

There are two basic approaches to teaching gross anatomy: by systems or by regions. Both have their own advantages and disadvantages. The regional approach is generally associated with courses that involve dissection. This approach allows the student to appreciate the structural relationships of the various systems—that is, skeletal, cardiovascular, nervous, and muscular—in specific regions such as the oral cavity or the neck. The disadvantage is that structures are uncovered in layers, so that finding the root structure of nerves and vessels not only takes time to uncover but also takes time to draw a mental picture of how the more peripheral structures sequentially branch from their origin. The systems approach is more easily taught in courses that do not have laboratory dissection. The advantage of the systems approach is just the opposite. Vessels and nerves can be followed from their origin to their peripheral distribution and the entire skeletal and muscular systems can be studied at the same time. In this book, the two approaches have been merged. In some chapters, the muscles of the region may be highlighted; however, relationships of other major structures in the region are introduced. In chapters that are more systems oriented, the regional location is also presented. The teaching concept is to understand the global organization of a system and to visualize the location of specific components in various regions.

How to Study Anatomy

The human body is a complex structure capable of movement, independent thought, speech, and interaction with the environment. At the beginning, you may feel overwhelmed by the countless number of named structures and the basic functioning of the nervous system. Answering the review questions within the chapter and completing the exercises at the end of each chapter will guide you with your study of the structures of the head and neck.

Although memorization is the first step of learning, understanding anatomy also requires visualization of structural relationships and knowing the blood supply, innervation, and function of the systems of the body. A very effective way to achieve visual learning is to label diagrams, or, even better, to draw, color, and label your own diagrams. You do not need to be an artist; the diagram is a way for you to create a mental image by imprinting an image into your brain. Creating flowcharts and tables will also serve as a way to organize and reduce your notes to better manage your study. Examples of flowcharts and tables are presented in the textbook. Do not try just to memorize their content; just try to re-create the charts and tables as a means of testing your knowledge of the subject. Whenever possible, personalize these charts and tables by adding additional information that you feel will help you study.

ANATOMICAL TERMINOLOGY

To communicate with one another, either verbally or in writing on paper or electronic devices, we must share a common language. The same holds true in the study of anatomy. Consider scientific terminology as a second (foreign) language. To communicate properly with other health-care professionals, you must speak the language, which requires learning a new vocabulary and the definition of terms.

In the discipline of anatomy, all terminology is based on the **anatomical position**, in which an individual is standing erect with head, eyes, and toes directed forward and upper limbs hanging at the sides with the palms facing forward (Fig. 1–1). The *right* side versus the *left* side refers to the individual's (your patient's) body and not your own. Relationships of structures are frequently described relative to planes drawn through the body. A **median plane** divides the body into equal right and left halves (Figs. 1–1 and 1–2). A **sagittal plane** is a vertical plane passing through the body parallel to the median plane but does not divide the body into equal right and left parts (Fig. 1–2). A **frontal** or **coronal plane** divides the body into front and back parts. A **transverse** or **horizontal plane** divides the body into upper and lower parts (Fig. 1–2). Radiologists commonly refer to the transverse plane as **axial**.

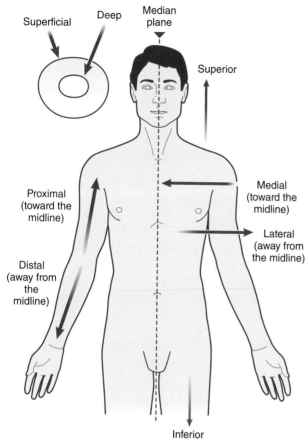

Figure 1–1 In the anatomical position, the palms of the hand are facing forward. Opposing terms are indicated by the arrows.

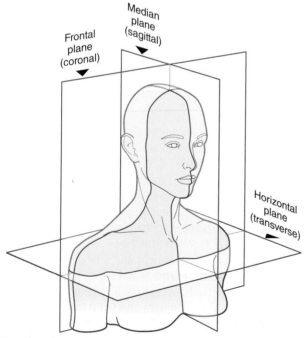

Figure 1–2 The frontal plane divides the body in anterior and posterior parts; the horizontal plane divides the body into superior and inferior parts. The median plane is a sagittal plane that divides the body into equal right and left parts.

Other terms are used to designate the position of one structure either to another or to a surface (Fig. 1–1). These terms are presented as opposing pairs according to their usage. **Superior** and **cranial** are used to describe a structure that is located toward the head, whereas **inferior** and **caudal** describe position relative to the feet. In quadrupeds (animals that walk on four legs), **anterior** is a positional term meaning toward the head, and **dorsal** refers to a structure's position to the tail. In the study of the human body, anterior is synonymous with **ventral**, which refers to the abdominal/thoracic area or the front of the body. Dorsal can be used interchangeably with **posterior** to reference the back. Structures are frequently discussed in relation to the median plane of the body. **Medial** describes proximity to the median plane, whereas **lateral** describes distance away from the median plane. The terms **proximal** (near) and **distal** (far) are used in comparing structures to a fixed point. As an example, the elbow is proximal to the shoulder joint, while the wrist is distal to the same joint. **Superficial** and **deep** are generally used in reference to distance from the surface of, or to, a reference point. For example, the skin is superficial to the sternum, or the heart is deep to the sternum. The body lying with the face downward is in the **prone position**, in contrast to the **supine position** in which the body is facing upward. Although generally used in describing nerve fibers, **afferent** and **efferent** are also used to describe the flow of lymph. Afferent means going toward a structure, whereas efferent describes going away from a structure. Thus, afferent vessels carry lymph to lymph nodes to be filtered, and the filtered lymph leaves the lymph nodes via efferent vessels (Fig. 1–3). Another set of terms is used to refer to organs as **visceral** or **splanchnic** and the body wall as **parietal** or **somatic**.

Review Question Box 1-1

1. Can a person lying in the supine position also be in the anatomical position? If so, why?
2. If you are lying in the prone position, is your heart deep or posterior to the vertebral column? If so, why?
3. Is a midsagittal plane through the body the same as the median plane? If so, why?

BASIC STRUCTURE AND FUNCTION OF THE NERVOUS SYSTEM

The **nervous system** coordinates and regulates bodily activities such as movement, respiratory rate, and cardiac rate. Additionally, the nervous system is responsible for such noncognitive activities as emotion, personality, memory, judgment, critical thinking, and reasoning. It also

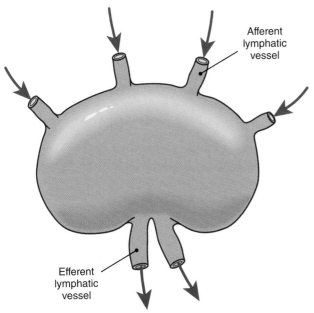

Figure 1–3 A lymph node is used to illustrate afferent (toward the structure) and efferent (away from the structure).

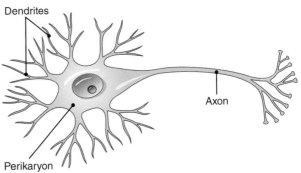

Figure 1–4 Multipolar neurons have numerous dendrites and a single axon attached to the perikaryon.

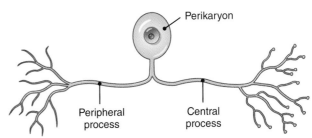

Figure 1–5 Pseudounipolar neurons have a central process and peripheral process attached to the perikaryon by a common stem.

allows us to sample our environment and distinguish the general sensations of pain, temperature, touch, pressure, proprioception (movement), and tickle as well as the special senses of taste, smell, vision, hearing, and equilibrium.

The Neuron

Although other cell types are present, the **neuron** is the basic unit of structure and function of the nervous system. Unlike other cell types, the neuron is able to respond and transmit a stimulus along its plasma membrane. Various types of stimuli (i.e., mechanical, temperature, and chemical) are transduced into electrical impulses that travel along the membrane and can be transferred to another cell. Impulses initiated in the brain are transferred to muscles, and these impulses result in movement. Impulses from receptors in the periphery are transferred to neurons, which allow the body to recognize changes in the environment.

The neuron is composed of a cell body, which is also called the **perikaryon**, and nerve processes. One type of cell process, the **dendrite**, receives the stimulus and carries the information toward (afferent) the perikaryon, whereas the **axon** carries the stimulus away (efferent) from the cell body (Fig. 1–4). Neurons are classified by the number of cell processes, the size of the cell, the speed of conduction, and their modality. As an example, a **motor** neuron carries information from the central nervous system (efferent) to peripheral muscles, and this information causes their contraction. **Sensory** nerves, on the other hand, carry sensations such as pain and temperature to the central nervous system (afferent).

Two examples of neurons that are important in understanding the nervous system are the multipolar neuron and the pseudounipolar neuron. The **multipolar** neurons are the most numerous and receive this name because they are characterized by multiple dendrites (Fig. 1–4). The **pseudounipolar** neuron appears to have one process but actually has a peripheral process and a central process that divides from a common stem (Fig. 1–5). Multipolar neurons can be motor or sensory, but pseudounipolar neurons are sensory only.

Peripheral Nerves

Unlike wireless communication, analog telephones use wires to carry information from one destination to another. The nervous system operates the same way. The telephone cables that connect the central nervous system to the peripheral structures (i.e., muscles, glands, and viscera) are called **nerves**.

Individual nerve processes are referred to as **nerve fibers**. Bundles of nerve fibers are surrounded by layers of connective tissue to form a **fascicle**. Several fascicles are surrounded by additional connective tissue to form a **peripheral nerve**, which is frequently called a *nerve* (Fig. 1–6). Nerves can contain both motor and sensory fibers. Axons can be myelinated or unmyelinated. **Myelinated** axons are surrounded by concentric whorls of cell membranes characteristic of specialized cells in the nervous system (Fig. 1–7). In the peripheral nervous system,

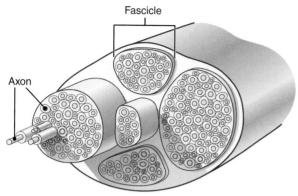

Figure 1–6 Cross section through a nerve. A fascicle is formed by numerous axons enclosed by a sheath of connective tissue. Multiple fascicles are organized into a nerve by additional layers of connective tissue.

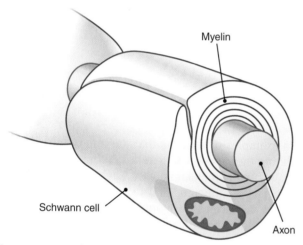

Figure 1–7 Myelinated nerve fibers are surrounded by whorls of membranes that act as an insulator.

several Schwann cells wrap their membranes around the axon to form myelin (Fig. 1–8). The more heavily myelinated the nerve fiber, the faster the nerve impulse is transmitted. **Unmyelinated** nerve fibers are surrounded by a single membranous layer, and multiple fibers appear to be embedded in one cell (Fig. 1–9). Impulses transmitted in unmyelinated fibers move relatively slowly.

Review Question Box 1-2

1. Why is the neuron considered the basic structural and functional unit of the nervous system?
2. What is the structural and functional difference between multipolar and pseudounipolar neurons?
3. Do all nerve fibers in a peripheral nerve have the same structure and function?

Major Divisions of the Nervous System

The nervous system is composed of two major subdivisions, the **central nervous system (CNS)** and the **peripheral nervous system (PNS)**. The **CNS** is composed of the **brain** and **spinal cord**, whereas the **PNS** is composed of *nerves* that carry information to and from the CNS to reach the peripheral structures of the body (muscles, glands, and sensory receptors). The PNS is further divided into afferent and efferent divisions. The *afferent* division is **s**ensory; that is, sensory nerves carry information (i.e., pain and temperature) from peripheral receptors to the brain and spinal cord. The *efferent* division is *motor*; motor nerves carry

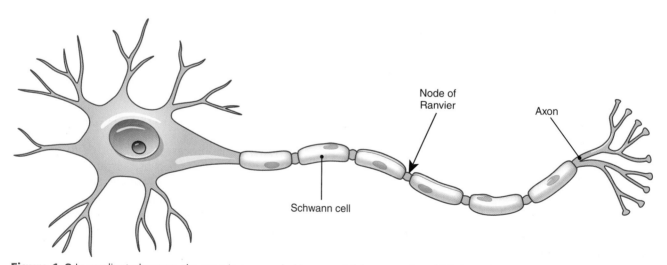

Figure 1–8 In myelinated nerves, the axon in surrounded by several Schwann cells, which form the myelin.

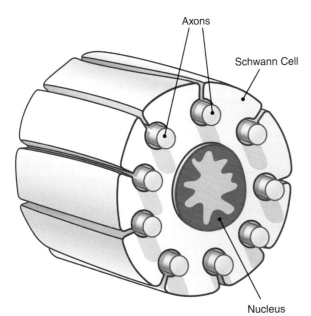

Figure 1–9 The unmyelinated axon is surrounded by a single layer of membranes. Unlike the myelinated axon, several unmyelinated axons are embedded in a single cell.

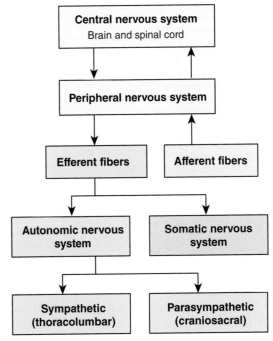

Figure 1–10 Divisions of the nervous system.

information away from the CNS and are involved in muscle contraction. The efferent division is further subdivided into the **somatomotor nervous system** (voluntary) and **autonomic nervous system** (involuntary) (Fig. 1–10). The somatomotor nerves innervate skeletal muscle, whereas the autonomic nerves innervate cardiac muscle, smooth muscle, and glands. Sensory and motor fibers from both somatomotor and autonomic nervous systems travel through either spinal or cranial nerves to innervate their target tissues and organs.

Review Question Box 1-3

1. Compare the structure and function of the central nervous system to the peripheral nervous system.
2. Compare the functions of the somatomotor and autonomic nervous systems.

 Box 1-1 Somatomotor Versus Autonomic Nervous Systems

The somatomotor system innervates skeletal muscle, whereas the autonomic nervous system innervates smooth muscle, cardiac muscles, and glands. In the somatomotor system, only one neuron is required to convey a stimulus from the spinal cord to the skeletal muscle. In contrast, the autonomic nervous system requires two neurons to stimulate the target tissue. The nerve cell body of the first neuron is located in either the spinal cord or the brain stem. The second neuron is located in a peripheral ganglion that is distant from the spinal cord and brain stem. The first neuron is designated as the **preganglionic neuron**, whereas the neuron whose cell body is located in a ganglion is referred to as the **postganglionic neuron**. The axons arising from the neurons are referred to as **preganglionic fibers** and **postganglionic fibers**, respectively.

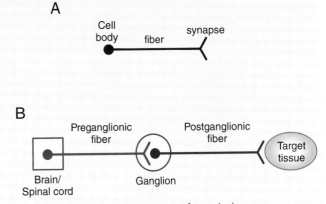

(A) Schematic of the components of a typical nerve.
(B) The two-neuron chain of the autonomic nervous system is composed of a preganglionic neuron and a postganglionic neuron. The preganglionic nerve fiber synapses on the cell body of a postganglionic neuron in a ganglion.

Spinal Nerves

A **spinal nerve** is a peripheral extension from the *spinal cord*, which innervates the skin and muscles of the body wall, with the exception of the head, which is mostly innervated by cranial nerves. The neck is unusual in that it contains muscles that are innervated by either spinal or cranial nerves. Understanding the origin, fiber content, and function of spinal nerves will aid in the comprehension of the more complex cranial nerves, which are clinically important to the dental profession.

Spinal Cord

To understand the concept of spinal nerves, it is necessary to visualize the internal organization of the spinal cord. A cross section through the spinal cord demonstrates several important surface and internal features. On the dorsal surface, there is a narrow midline cleft called the **dorsal median sulcus**. The ventral surface features a much broader midline cleft called the **ventral median fissure** (Fig. 1–11). Internally, the spinal cord contains neurons and nerve cell processes. The *perikarya* (singular: *perikaryon*) are clustered in an H-shaped structure called the **gray matter**. The "upper arms" of the H- are referred to as the **dorsal horns** (Fig. 1–11). This area contains the perikarya (nerve cell bodies) of sensory nerves, which relay information to the brain. The "lower arms" are called the **ventral horns** (Fig. 1–11), which contain the perikarya of the **alpha motor neurons.** The axons of these neurons innervate the skeletal muscles in the trunk and extremities. In the thoracic (T) and upper lumbar (L) regions of the spinal cord between T1 and L2 there is a triangular-shaped extension of the gray matter known as the **intermediolateral cell column** (Fig. 1–11), which contains the perikarya of sympathetic nerves of the autonomic nervous system (to be discussed later). The gray matter is surrounded by bundles of *myelinated* nerve fibers that convey messages to and from the brain. Because of the whitish appearance of myelinated nerves in fresh tissue, this area is referred to as the **white matter** (Fig. 1–11).

Roots of Spinal Nerves

The spinal nerves are attached to the spinal cord by a series of two pairs of rootlets designated as the **dorsal root** and the **ventral root** because of their respective attachments to the spinal cord. The ventral root is the motor component of the spinal nerve. The ventral root contains *axons* of the alpha motor neurons that are located within the *ventral horn* and the autonomic neurons, which lie within the *intermediolateral cell column* of the spinal cord. The dorsal root is the sensory component of the spinal nerve. It contains the processes of a specialized neuron, referred to as a pseudounipolar neuron. The cell bodies are located in a swelling on the dorsal root known as the **dorsal root ganglion**. The term **ganglion** refers to an aggregation of nerve cell bodies located outside the brain or spinal cord (Fig. 1–12).

Branches (Rami) of Spinal Nerves

All spinal nerves have at least four branches or **rami** (singular: **ramus**) (Fig. 1–13) and are listed according to their branching from the spinal nerve.

1. **Meningeal ramus**—This small branch supplies the protective coverings of the spinal cord and contains sensory nerve fibers. Although it has an important sensory function in the perception of pain, the hygienist is generally not concerned with this nerve in clinical practice.
2. **Ventral primary ramus**—This is the larger of two terminal branches of the spinal nerve. The ventral primary ramus supplies the skin and muscle of the anterior body wall, anterior neck, legs, and arms. Most of the trunk muscles and neck muscles discussed in this book are innervated by the ventral primary rami of spinal nerves. An individual ramus is designated by the first letter of the region of the spinal cord (cervical, thoracic, lumbar, and sacral) followed by a number representing the exact exit point from the spinal cord. Rami of several spinal nerves can form a plexus, which in turn forms multiple nerves that innervate the skin and muscles. An example is the cervical plexus, which is composed of rami from C1 to C4. Ventral primary rami contain sensory fibers and motor fibers to skeletal muscle, smooth muscle, cardiac muscle, and glands (Fig. 1–14).
3. **Dorsal primary ramus**—This is the smaller of the two terminal branches that supply the skin and

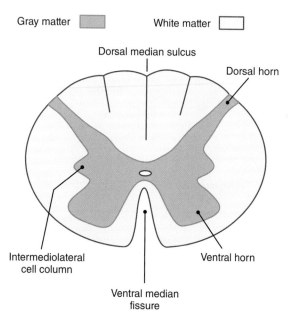

Gray matter ▢   White matter ▢

Dorsal median sulcus

Dorsal horn

Intermediolateral cell column

Ventral horn

Ventral median fissure

Figure 1–11 The spinal cord contains a central core of gray matter that is H- or butterfly-shaped surrounded by white matter. The dorsal horns are sensory and the ventral horns are motor.

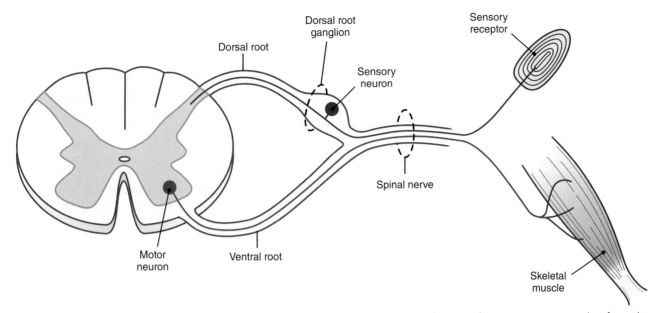

Figure 1–12 A spinal nerve is formed by the merging of a dorsal or sensory root and a ventral or motor root emerging from the dorsal and ventral horns, respectively. The dorsal root ganglion contains the nerve cell bodies of the sensory nerve that receive stimuli from a peripheral receptor. The axon of a motor nerve courses through the ventral root to enter the spinal nerve to reach skeletal muscle.

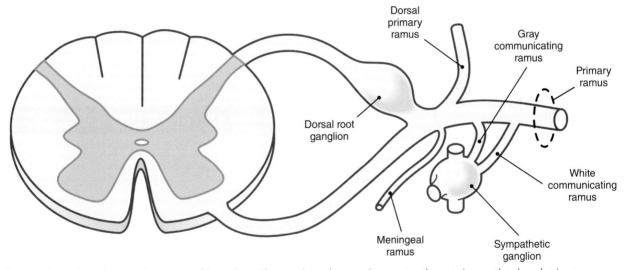

Figure 1–13 Spinal nerves have several branches. The meningeal ramus innervates the meninges; the dorsal primary ramus supplies the skin and muscles of the back. The white and gray communicating rami connect to the sympathetic ganglion. The ventral primary ramus forms the nerves of the anterior portion of the body.

muscle of the trunk. The dorsal primary ramus supplies the back and contains sensory fibers as well as motor fibers to skeletal muscle, smooth muscle, and glands. The dorsal primary ramus will not be discussed, because the back muscles are not in the scope of this textbook.

4. **Gray communicating rami**—One of two branches that join sympathetic ganglia to the spinal nerve and that contain motor fibers to smooth muscle, cardiac muscles, and glandular secretion. These nerve fibers

are important to the dental hygienist and are discussed in Chapter 15.

5. **White communicating rami**—Second of two branches that join spinal nerves to the sympathetic ganglia at the levels of T1 to L2 and also contain motor fibers to smooth muscle, cardiac muscle, and glands as well as sensory fibers from the viscera. As for the gray communicating rami, these nerve fibers are important to the dental hygienist and are discussed in Chapter 15.

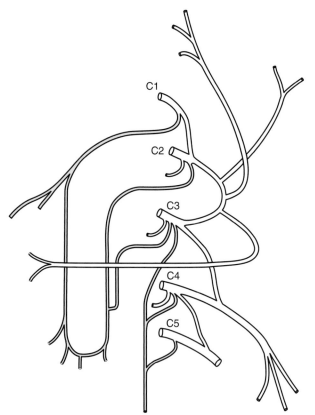

Figure 1–14 The cervical plexus is an example of how several primary rami of adjacent spinal cord segments form larger nerves. The motor branches of the plexus are yellow, and the sensory branches are white.

As a general rule, nerve branches of the ventral and dorsal primary rami that innervate skeletal muscles contain three fiber types, namely *efferent fibers to skeletal muscle*, *afferent fibers* to receptors in the muscle, and *efferent sympathetic fibers* that supply smooth muscles of blood vessels within the skeletal muscle. On the other hand, cutaneous (to the skin) branches from these rami are composed of *efferent sympathetic fibers* to glands, smooth muscle in the skin, and blood vessels and *afferent fibers* to receptors that perceive pain, temperature, conscious touch, and pressure.

Review Question Box 1-4

1. How is the spinal cord organized?
2. What is the significance of the horns of the gray matter of the spinal cord?
3. What is the effect when the following structures are severed?
   a. ventral root
   b. dorsal root
   c. spinal nerve

Cranial Nerves

Understanding the fiber composition and the function of cranial nerves is important to the dental hygienist because most of the structures of the head and neck are innervated by cranial nerves. Some of the structures that are innervated by these nerves include the skin of the face and neck, the muscles of facial expression, the muscles of mastication, the salivary glands, the teeth and their surrounding supporting tissues, and the tongue.

The **cranial nerves** are 12 pairs of peripheral nerves that mostly arise from the brain and brain stem. Each pair of nerves has a designated name and can alternatively be referred to by a Roman numeral (Table 1–1). Cranial nerves are similar to spinal nerves in that they supply motor fibers to muscle and sensory fibers to the skin, but in addition they contain fibers for the five special senses so that one can *see, taste, smell, hear, and maintain equilibrium*. They comprise the source of the nerves for the **parasympathetic nervous system**. Unlike spinal nerves, each cranial nerve has a specific function and can contain one or more fiber type(s). As an example, the olfactory nerve (cranial nerve I) only contains fibers for the special sensation of smell. The facial nerve (cranial nerve VII) contains parasympathetic fibers, taste fibers, and motor fibers to skeletal muscle. Details of the cranial nerves will be discussed later (Chapters 15 to 17).

Review Question Box 1-5

1. Why are the cranial nerves considered components of the peripheral nervous system?
2. What makes cranial nerves different from spinal nerves?
3. What fiber types are found only in cranial nerves?

OVERVIEW OF THE HEAD AND NECK

Although knowledge of the structure and function of the entire body will help the dental hygienist understand a patient's medical history, this textbook is limited to structures of the head and neck that have a direct impact on treating the patient's oral health needs. Most sources recognize a minimum of 10 body systems. Only the reproductive and urinary systems are not represented in the head and neck. Thus, the oral cavity has direct structural and functional relationships to structures in the head and an indirect relationship to the body systems of the trunk via the neck (Fig. 1–15).

TABLE 1–1	Cranial Nerves and Their Basic Functions	
Number	**Nerve**	**General Functions (Not Inclusive)**
I	Olfactory	Smell
II	Optic	Vision
III	Oculomotor	Eye movement; pupillary constriction; rounding of the lens
IV	Trochlear	Eye movement
V	Trigeminal	Motor to muscles of mastication; general sensory to the face, mouth, and teeth; and anterior two-thirds of the tongue
VI	Abducens	Eye movement
VII	Facial	Motor to muscles of facial expression; taste to the anterior two-thirds of tongue and soft palate; visceral motor to submandibular and sublingual salivary glands
VIII	Vestibulocochlear	Hearing, equilibrium, and balance
IX	Glossopharyngeal	Motor to a muscle of the pharynx; general sensation to the pharyngeal wall; general sensation and taste to the posterior one-third of the tongue; visceral motor fibers to parotid gland
X	Vagus	Motor to muscles of larynx, pharynx, and palate; visceral sensation; visceral motor organs of thorax and abdomen
XI	Accessory	Motor to two muscles in the neck
XII	Hypoglossal	Motor to muscles of the tongue

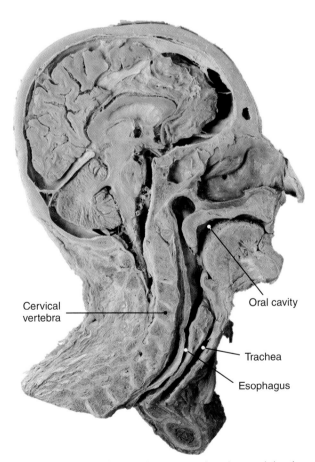

Figure 1–15 The oral cavity is connected to the trunk by the neck. The esophagus connects the food passageways of the head to the stomach, whereas the trachea connects the air passages of the head to the lungs.

Organization of the Head

The **head** is the location of the command center of the body and is very complex. It is composed of the skull, visceral organs that are vital to the functioning of the body, and muscles necessary for mastication and facial expression. Cavities within the skull contain organs that control all body functions, as well as special sense organs that allow us to see, taste, smell, hear, and maintain equilibrium. These cavities also serve as the entryways to the respiratory and the digestive systems.

The skull or cranium is divided into a **cranial vault**, which encases the brain, and the **facial skeleton**, which serves as the attachment site for the muscles of facial expression and the muscles of mastication. In addition to protecting the brain, other cavities within the bones of the skull serve as protective compartments and functional spaces for several organ systems. The **nasal cavity** contains structures that humidify and cleanse the air that we breathe and contains the receptors for the special sense of smell or olfaction (Fig. 1–16). The **paranasal sinuses**, which are extensions of the respiratory system, decrease the weight of the skull and increase the resonance of our voice. The **orbit** contains the eyes (vision), whereas the **tympanic cavity** contains the cochlear (hearing) and the vestibular apparatus (equilibrium). And, of course, the **oral cavity**, which contains the teeth and their supporting apparatus, is of special interest to the dental hygienist (Fig. 1–16).

The facial skeleton is covered superficially by skin and muscle; this region is referred to as the **superficial face**. The combination of these structures accounts for our

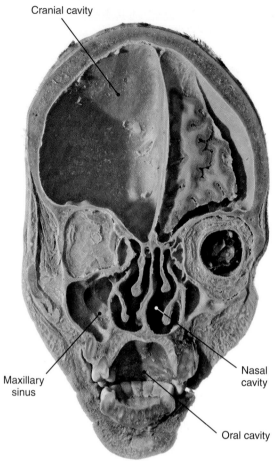

Figure 1–16 The skull contains cavities to protect vital and sensory organs. These spaces include the cranial cavity, nasal cavity, orbit, tympanic cavity and ear canal, paranasal sinuses, and oral cavity.

individual appearance. Between the cheek bone and the ear lies a bony arch known as the *zygomatic arch*. This arch separates the **temporal fossa** (Fig. 1–17A) above from the **infratemporal fossa** (Fig. 1–17B), which is inferior to the arch and medial to the ramus of the mandible. The infratemporal fossa contains structures of particular interest to the dental profession, such as the muscles of mastication and the blood vessels and nerves that supply the tongue, teeth, and other structures within the oral cavity.

Organization of the Neck

The **neck** is a tubular constriction that connects the head to the trunk of the body. Its functions are to move the head and to serve as a conduit for structures passing to and from the head and the trunk. The air passageways of the head are connected to the lungs in the trunk by the trachea (Fig. 1–15). Food and fluids ingested into the oral cavity are transferred by the esophagus (Fig. 1–15) to the stomach to continue the process of digestion. Blood vessels, nerves, and lymphatic structures must pass through the neck to circulate nutrients and gases, innervate and receive commands from structures in the head, and protect via immune responses. In addition, the neck contains endocrine organs that regulate the metabolic rate and the storage of calcium.

The neck is surrounded by a layer of skin that protects its internal structures from the environment. Internally, it is divided into compartments by sheets of connective tissue called **fascia**. The outermost sheath, which is called the **investing fascia**, encloses two superficial muscles of

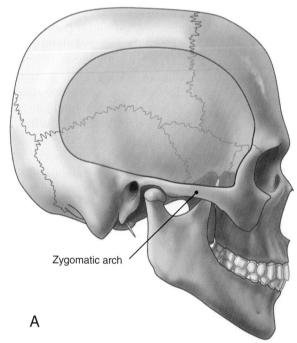

A

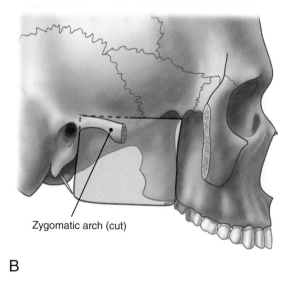

B

Figure 1–17 **(A)** The temporal fossa is the shallow depression that is shaded superior to the zygomatic arch. **(B)** The zygomatic arch has been cut to reveal the infratemporal fossa, which is an irregularly shaped space inferomedial to the zygomatic arch.

the neck. These muscles and the investing fascia form a **musculofascial collar** that is involved in the rotation of the head (Fig. 1–18). Deeper layers of fascia surround the muscular and visceral compartments. The **muscular compartment** contains muscles that elevate and depress the hyoid bone when swallowing and speaking, whereas the **visceral compartment** contains the pharynx, larynx, esophagus, trachea, and thyroid and parathyroid glands (Fig. 1–18). A **neurovascular compartment**, which is surrounded by a tubular sheath of fascia, is located lateral to the visceral compartment (Fig. 1–18). The neurovascular compartment contains the major arteries and veins of the neck as well as lymphatic vessels and nerves. The neck is supported posteriorly and articulates with the base of the skull via the **cervical vertebrae.** The cervical vertebrae and the intrinsic muscles of the neck are encased by the **prevertebral fascia** to form the **vertebral compartment** (Fig. 1–18). Muscles in this compartment are involved in

flexion, extension, and rotation of the neck, which ultimately affects the position of the head.

Review Question Box 1-6

1. What sensory organs are found only in the head?
2. What is the role of the skull regarding the functions of the head?
3. What is the significance of the compartmentalization of the neck?

SUMMARY

Anatomy is the building block of all clinical sciences, and knowledge of head and neck anatomy will carry over into your clinical practice. The head and neck is a very complex region of the body. By merging systemic anatomy and regional anatomy, the structural relationships and functional concepts should be easier to learn. Learning anatomical terminology and understanding the fiber content of spinal nerves are two of the most important concepts for the novice in anatomy. Learning anatomical terminology is similar to studying a foreign language; the terms must be practiced by verbal pronunciation, translated by pointing to structures, and used when describing structural relationships.

One of the reasons most patients go to any clinician is pain. Understanding how pain is initiated and the types of pain will help you in your diagnosis of a patient. Motor fibers are also clinically relevant because they control the muscles that open and close the mouth. In addition, they regulate the secretions of organs, such as the salivary glands, that are very important to oral health. They also innervate the heart and arteries and thus regulate blood pressure, which can be affected by intraoral injections of anesthesia. Combining the regional and system approaches will help you understand the three-dimensional structure of the head and neck.

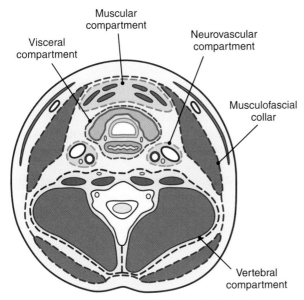

Figure 1–18 A transverse section through the neck demonstrates the fascial compartments.

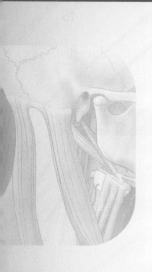

LEARNING LAB
Exercises for review, practice, and study

Laboratory Activity 1-1

Using Anatomical Terminology

Learning and understanding anatomical terminology is like studying a second language. A good learning technique is to practice verbalizing the terms and to associate the terms to an object or an activity.

Objective: In this exercise, you will practice the anatomical terms introduced in this chapter by saying the terms out loud and demonstrating the meaning of the terms on yourself or your partner.

Materials Needed: A ruler, pencil, or other suitable straight edge

Step 1: Stand in the *anatomical position*. Your eyes, legs, and toes should be pointed forward, while your arms should be lying at your side with the palms of your hands directed to the front of your body. Realize that the palms of your hands are directed to the *anterior* or *ventral* surface of your body, whereas the back of your hand is facing the *posterior* or *dorsal* surface of your body.

Step 2: With a ruler, pencil, or other suitable straight edge, demonstrate the four planes that can be drawn through the body. The *median plane* is equivalent to a line drawn vertically through the midline of the body, which divides it into equal right and left parts. A line parallel to the median plane is a *sagittal plane* and divides the body into unequal right and left parts. The *horizontal* or *transverse plane* divides the body into upper and lower parts. The *frontal* or *coronal plane* is at right angles to both the sagittal and horizontal planes and divides the body into front and back parts.

Step 3: Practice using the terms that are used to denote direction. *Superior* refers to a structure positioned toward the head, whereas *inferior* is directed toward the feet. Is your heart superior or inferior to your stomach? Distal and proximal are used to reference the location of a structure to a fixed point. *Distal* means away from, whereas *proximal* is close to a reference point. Which joint, the wrist or the elbow, is proximal to the shoulder? Structures or movements are described in reference to the median plane. The arm is *lateral* to the median plane, whereas the heart is in a more *medial* position.

Afferent and efferent are also terms of direction. *Afferent* is used to describe movement toward a structure, whereas *efferent* denotes movement away from a structure. In the nervous system, *motor fibers* are also called *efferent fibers* because they convey a stimulus away from the central nervous system; *sensory fibers* are *afferent* because they carry a stimulus to the central nervous system.

For Discussion or Thought:

1. What is the purpose of using standardized anatomical terminology in dentistry?

Laboratory Activity 1-2

Draw and Label a Spinal Nerve

Drawing diagrams creates mental images of complex structures and relationships. Understanding the structure and composition of spinal nerves is an important concept in anatomy that will help you understand the innervations of muscles, viscera, and glands.

Objective: In this exercise, you will draw and label structures in the spinal cord and neurons that contribute to the formation of spinal nerves.

Materials Needed: Drawing paper and colored pens or pencils. *Optional:* A photocopy of Figures 1–12 and 1–13 from this chapter for easy reference.

Step 1: The shape of the spinal cord actually varies, but this is not important at this time. Using Figures 1–12 and 1–13 as a guide, draw a flattened oval to represent the spinal cord. On the surface, label the *dorsal median sulcus*, which is a slight depression on the dorsal surface. On the ventral surface, label the *ventral median fissure*, which is a deeper furrow.

● Recognition of these two surface features helps determine the proper orientation of the spinal cord. Within the cord, draw and label the H (butterfly)-shaped *gray matter* to include the *dorsal*, *ventral*, and *lateral horns*. The *lateral horn* is a pyramid-shaped projection between the dorsal and ventral horns that contains the *intermediolateral cell column*. Shade the white and gray matter using two different colors. Which horn is motor? Which is sensory?

Step 2: The *spinal nerve* is formed by the convergence of the dorsal and ventral roots.

● Draw and label the *ventral root* that is attached to the spinal cord near the ventral horn.
● Draw and label the *dorsal root*, which is attached to the spinal cord near the dorsal horn.
● Draw and label the *dorsal root ganglion* on the dorsal root proximal to the union of the dorsal and ventral roots as they form the spinal nerve.
● Draw and label the division of the spinal nerve into *dorsal, meningeal, ventral*, and *gray* and *white communicating rami*.
● Draw and label the *spinal* (autonomic) *ganglion* that is connected to the ventral primary ramus by the *white* and *gray* communicating rami.

Step 3: The spinal nerve contains *efferent (motor) fibers* to *skeletal muscle* and *afferent (sensory) fibers* to *sensory receptors*.

● Draw and label symbols that indicate a sensory receptor and skeletal muscle. Return to the spinal cord and with a colored pencil, draw and label a small solid circle in the ventral horn to represent the *perikaryon* (cell body) of a motor neuron. Extend a line representing a *nerve fiber* into the ventral root and continue the line through the ventral primary ramus to reach the skeletal muscle. Draw an arrow toward the skeletal muscle to indicate the direction of the nerve impulse.
● Next, with a different colored pencil, draw and label a similar circle in the dorsal root ganglion that represents the perikaryon of a sensory neuron. Indicate the uniqueness of the pseudounipolar neuron by extending a line (representing the nerve fiber) a short distance from the perikaryon (it should look like a lollipop) that divides with branches coursing in opposite directions. Now continue the line in the direction of the ventral primary ramus to reach the sensory receptor. Return to the dorsal root ganglion and extend the line toward the dorsal horn. Draw an arrow that indicates the direction of a nerve stimulus toward the spinal cord.

The final diagram should look like a composite of Figures 1–12 and 1–13.

For Discussion or Thought:

1. *The perikaryon of the motor neuron is located in the spinal cord, which is considered a component of the central nervous system. Why is the motor neuron of the ventral horn considered a part of the peripheral nervous system?*

Learning Activity 1-1

Learning Terminology

Match the numbered structures with the correct terms listed below.

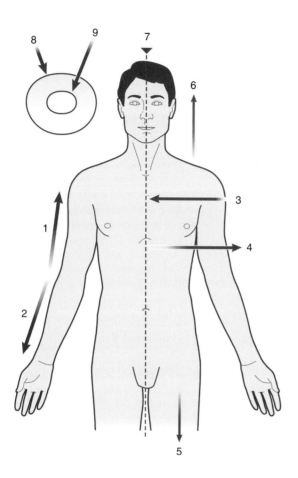

_____ Deep		_____ Median plane	
_____ Distal		_____ Proximal	
_____ Inferior		_____ Superficial	
_____ Lateral		_____ Superior	
_____ Medial			

Learning Activity 1-2

Identifying the Structure of the Spinal Cord

Match the numbered structures with the correct terms listed to the right.

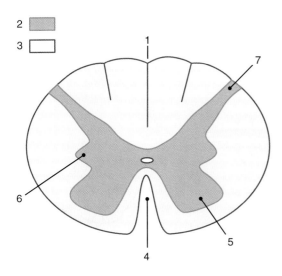

_____ Dorsal horn

_____ Dorsal median sulcus

_____ Gray matter

_____ Intermediolateral cell column

_____ Ventral horn

_____ Ventral median fissure

_____ White matter

Learning Activity 1-3

Identifying Components of the Spinal Nerve

Match the numbered structures with the correct terms listed below.

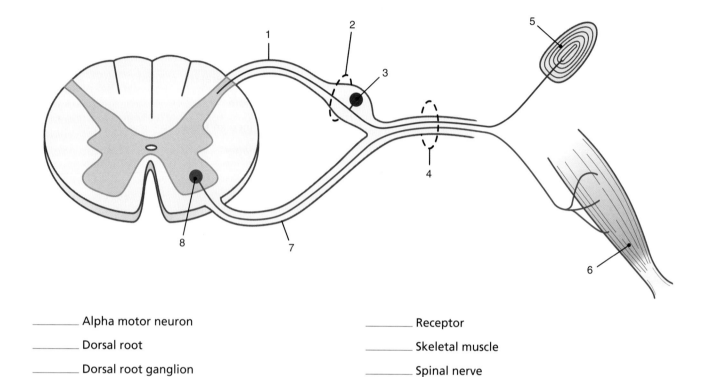

_____ Alpha motor neuron

_____ Dorsal root

_____ Dorsal root ganglion

_____ Pseudounipolar nerve

_____ Receptor

_____ Skeletal muscle

_____ Spinal nerve

_____ Ventral root

Learning Activity 1-4

Transverse Section of the Neck

Match the numbered structures with the correct terms listed below.

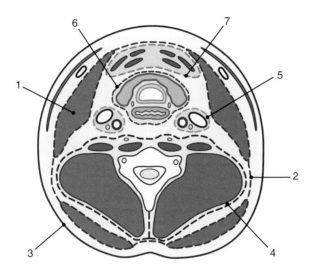

_____ Investing fascia

_____ Muscular compartment

_____ Musculofascial collar

_____ Neurovascular compartment

_____ Skin

_____ Vertebral compartment

_____ Visceral compartment

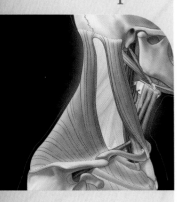

2

Skull and Cervical Vertebrae

Objectives

1. Compare the structure of cartilage and bone and discuss the functions of bones and the physiological forces that affect bone that are important to the dental hygienist.
2. Describe the articulation between bones and give examples of each.
3. Distinguish the difference between the neurocranium and the viscerocranium and identify the bones from these divisions of the skull.
4. Identify the bones of the skull, the features of each bone, and the major apertures of the skull and name the structures that pass through these openings.
5. Identify the general features of the cervical vertebrae and identify features that are specific to the atlas and axis.

Overview

Have you ever thought what you would look like without a skeleton? Certainly, you would look nothing like you look right now. The rigidity of bone gives the body form and structure. Without bones, you would be a shapeless mass, probably very low to the ground because there would be no structural girders to resist the force of gravity. Humans comprise an advanced group of animals that are classified as vertebrates, which possess a backbone. The backbone gives us form and symmetry. The bodies of vertebrates tend to be tubular and elongated. The backbone courses along the length of the body and contains a canal that surrounds the spinal cord, an extension of the nervous system. The digestive system, which is also tubular, lies anterior to the backbone. The digestive tube begins as the mouth cranially (toward the head) and terminates caudally (toward the tail) as the anus.

Most of us take our skeleton for granted until we fracture a bone and become immobilized or suffer bone loss because of disease. This is especially true in the oral cavity. Patients suffering from periodontal disease demonstrate bone loss over a period of time, which can result in the loss of teeth.

   In this chapter, we explore the structure of the skull and vertebral column. The clinical relevance of the relationship of teeth to the jaw bones is obvious; however, the dental hygienist needs to be aware of other features of the skull. Protection of the brain is an important function; in addition, the skull has many openings for the passage of blood vessels and nerves that supply not only the teeth but also the muscles of the face, the muscles of mastication, and the glands of the head and neck. Also, the location and content of the foramina are very important in the administration of intraoral injections for many dental procedures.

INTRODUCTION TO THE SKELETAL SYSTEM

The **skeletal system** is formed by bone and cartilage. Bones provide a framework to support and give shape to the body. In addition, the bones protect visceral organs and provide for movement and lifting of objects. Cartilage has limited weight-bearing ability but in many joints forms a protective cover over the articular surfaces of bone that allows smooth movement. Loss of articular cartilage is one cause of joint pain.

General Characteristics of Bone

Bone is a mineralized connective tissue; though it appears rigid and hard, it is a living tissue capable of changing shape according to environmental conditions. Bone is resorbed either with the application of pressure or during inflammatory responses, such as in periodontal disease. In fact, the orthodontist uses pressure to move teeth by reshaping the bony socket but is mindful that too much pressure applied too quickly can cause permanent bone loss.

Functions of Bone

Bones have several functions that are important to the dental hygienist. First, by virtue of the *attachment* of muscles to the skeleton, bones serve as the mechanical basis of movement. The temporomandibular joint is a good example. Movement of this joint between the temporal bone and the mandible allows us to open and close the jaw while eating or speaking. Bones *protect* the vital organs such as the brain and the viscera of the thorax, abdomen, and pelvis. Bones provide *support* for the body, and, of particular interest to the dental hygienist, alveolar bone supports the teeth. Bones also serve as a *storage site* for calcium, and its marrow is a continuing source of blood cells. The dental hygienist must realize that the amount of calcium is dependent on diet, hormonal regulation, and age. Osteoporosis, which is a loss of bone

mass, affects the bony sockets of the teeth, as well as the entire body.

Classification of Bone According to Shape

Bones are classified according to their shape. **Long bones**, such as the bones of the upper and lower extremities, hands, and feet, have an elongated tubular shape (Fig. 2–1). The distal ends of these bone flare to form the **epiphysis** or head of the bone. The tubular shaft is

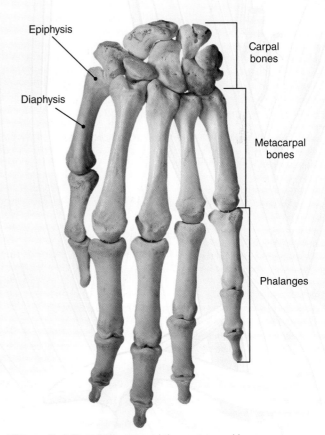

Figure 2–1 The phalanges and the metacarpal bones are examples of long bones, whereas the carpal bones are short bones.

referred to as the **diaphysis**. Long bones serve as levers and aid in movement. **Short bones** are more cuboidal in shape and are found in the ankle and wrist (Fig. 2–1). **Flat bones**, exemplified by the bones that form the brain case, have a protective function (Fig. 2–2). **Irregular bones** (Fig. 2–2), such as the facial bones, vary in shape and protect visceral structures such as the eyes and lacrimal gland. In addition, the facial bones provide a stationary surface for the attachment of muscles.

General Composition of Bone

Regardless of their anatomical designation, all bones are made of **compact** and **spongy bone**. Compact bone is formed by dense layers or **lamellae** of bone cells and a mineralized matrix that surrounds small blood vessels. On the other hand, spongy bone is composed of thin plates or **trabeculae** of bone cells and matrix. Compact bone forms the outer weight-bearing **cortical bone**, whereas the spongy bone forms the central **medullary region** of the gross bone (Fig. 2–3). The spaces between the trabeculae are filled with varying amounts of fat and blood-forming tissue, which is

referred to as **bone marrow**. In the skull and face, the compact bone forms flattened plates of bone that are referred to as **outer** and **inner cortical plates**. The spongy bone in between these cortical plates is called the **diploë** (Fig. 2–4).

General Characteristics of Cartilage

Cartilage is a semirigid connective tissue, but, unlike bone, cartilage is not mineralized. The firmness of cartilage is maintained by binding water to the matrix that surrounds the **chondrocytes**, which are the cells of the cartilage. There are three types of cartilage: hyaline, elastic, and fibrocartilage. Cartilage has several functions in addition to being a component of the skeleton. This tissue forms a supportive structure for the viscera by preventing the collapse of airways (i.e., the larynx and trachea) as well as the auditory tube that connects the middle ear to the nasopharynx. In regard to the skeleton, cartilage is a shock absorber and is found on the articular surface of bones of cartilaginous (Fig. 2–5) and synovial joints

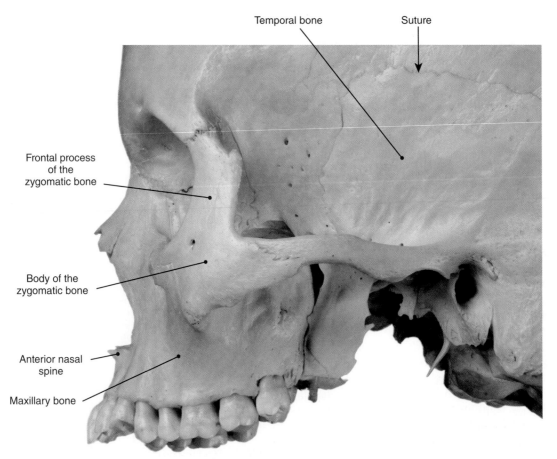

Temporal bone   Suture

Frontal process
of the
zygomatic bone

Body of the
zygomatic bone

Anterior nasal
spine

Maxillary bone

Figure 2–2 The temporal bone is one of the flat bones of the skull, whereas the zygomatic and maxillary bones are examples of the irregular bones of the skull. Many facial bones have a central body with extensions or processes. Small thornlike projections are called *spines*. Most bones of the skull are held together by sutures.

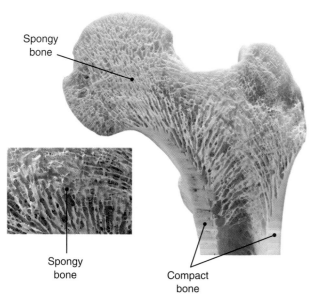

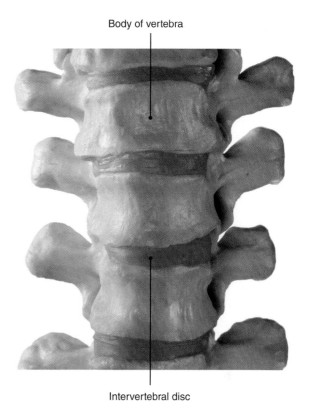

Figure 2–3 Compact bone is the dense outer layer of gross bones. The medullary region of bones is characterized by thin plates of spongy bone.

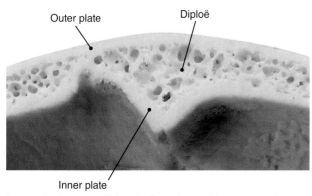

Figure 2–4 Bones of the skull are formed by inner and outer plates of compact bone separated by the trabecular bone of the diploë.

Figure 2–5 The cartilaginous joint between the intervertebral disc and the bodies of the vertebrae is an example of a symphysis. The disc is composed of fibrocartilage.

(Fig. 2–6). With age, the articular cartilage loses the ability to bind water and can degenerate from the wear and tear on a joint, thus making movement of the joint very painful. The epiphyseal cartilage (or the growth plate) is an important joint that can be used by the orthodontist to predict potential growth of the mandible required for the proper spacing of the developing molar teeth.

Review Question Box 2-1

1. What functions of bone are of clinical interest to the dental hygienist? Why?
2. What is the relationship between bone and cartilage?
3. What is the difference between compact bone and spongy bone? Where are they found in gross bones?

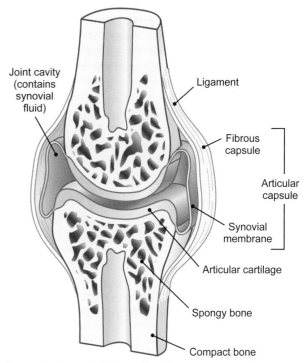

Figure 2–6 Synovial joints allow free movement. The joint is enclosed by a fibrous capsule that is lined by a synovial membrane. Synovial fluid is secreted into the synovial cavity, which allows the articular cartilage on the epiphyses of the bone to glide smoothly over each other during movement.

Joints

Joints are the contact points or **articulations** between bones. Some joints allow movement, as when you open and close your lower jaw (mandible). Other joints firmly bind one bone to another, such as the bones that enclose the cranial cavity (which surrounds the brain). Joints are classified according to the way the bones are united.

Fibrous Joint

Fibrous joints are held together by fibrous connective tissue. Examples of fibrous joints that are of interest to the dental hygienist are the sutures of the skull and the gomphosis. **Sutures** tightly bind the bones of the skull by means of a thin layer of connective tissue (Fig. 2–2). The **gomphosis** is a specialized joint of the oral cavity by which the peglike roots of the teeth are attached to the bony sockets of the alveolar process (Fig. 2–7). The connective tissue that binds the teeth to the bone is called the *periodontal ligament*.

Cartilaginous Joint

Cartilaginous joints are held together by cartilage. Two subtypes of this joint are important to the dental hygienist. First is the **synchondrosis**, which is represented by the epiphyseal plate or growth plate that is responsible for the growth in length of developing long bones. Although the epiphyseal plates associated with bones of the extremities are classic examples, the spheno-occipital synchondrosis (growth plate between the sphenoid and occipital bones) is a comparable example in the skull. As we undergo puberty, the bones of the epiphyses and the diaphysis fuse, and growth can no longer take place. This articulation is referred to as a **synostosis** and frequently can be visualized as a thin plate of bone at the location of the epiphyseal plate (Fig. 2–8). The **symphysis** represents the second type of cartilaginous joint. The fibrocartilage between the adjacent bodies of the vertebrae holds the bones together and acts as a shock absorber for the vertebral column (Fig. 2–5). Many older patients suffer from neck and back pain because of degenerating or bulging discs pinching on spinal nerves.

Synovial Joints

Synovial joints form the fully moveable joints of the body (Fig. 2–6). The bones are held together by a fluid-filled **fibrous capsule**, which is usually reinforced by ligaments. The articular surface of each bone is covered by a layer of hyaline cartilage that is referred to as **articular cartilage**. The fibrous capsule is lined internally by a **synovial membrane** that secretes a viscous lubricant known as **synovial fluid**. This fluid prevents friction as the articular surfaces slide over each other during movement. In individuals with osteoarthritis,

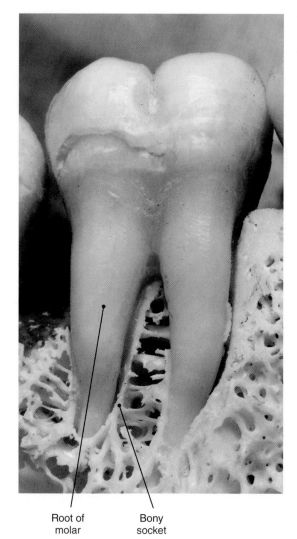

Root of molar   Bony socket

Figure 2–7 The articulation of the root of a tooth with its socket of bone is a gomphosis.

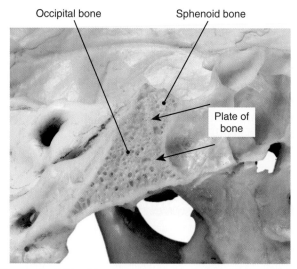

Occipital bone   Sphenoid bone

Plate of bone

Figure 2–8 The thin plate of bone is the spheno-occipital synostosis, which indicates the location of the growth plate (synchondrosis) of cartilage that was active during the growth of the bones.

the articular cartilage degenerates, allowing the bones to rub on each other. This causes pain and inflammation in the joint. The **temporomandibular joint (TMJ)** is a very important synovial joint to the dental hygienist because many patients suffer from TMJ disorders. The structure and movements of the TMJ will be discussed in Chapter 7.

Review Question Box 2-2

1. Give examples of the type of joints that can be found in the head and neck.

STRUCTURE OF THE SKULL

The **skull** or **cranium** is composed of 22 bones that are joined together by sutures (Figs. 2–9 through 2–13). The skull consists of the **cranial vault** or **neurocranium** that surrounds the brain and the **facial skeleton** or **viscerocranium** that defines our facial appearance. The following is a summary of the bones of the cranial vault and the facial skeleton.

Cranial Vault

The cranial vault (brain case) or *neurocranium* is formed by four single and two pairs of named bones that surround and protect the brain (Figs. 2–9 through 2–13).

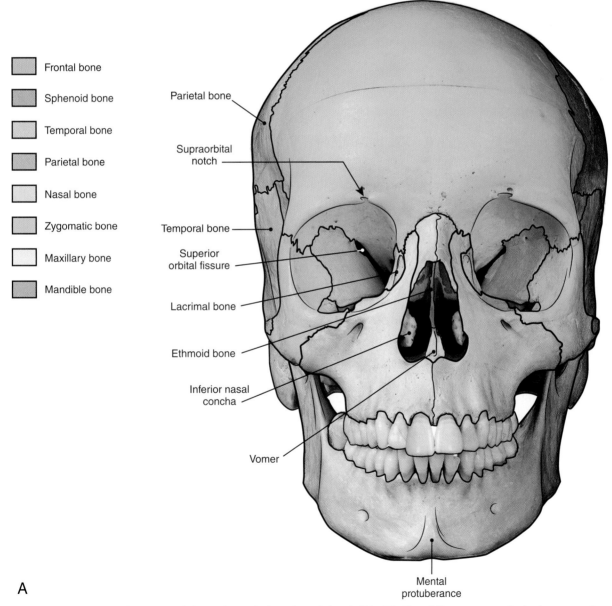

A

Figure 2–9 Frontal view of the skull. **(A)** A color-coded version of the skull in **(B)**. The piriform aperture is the large opening enclosed by the maxillary and nasal bones.

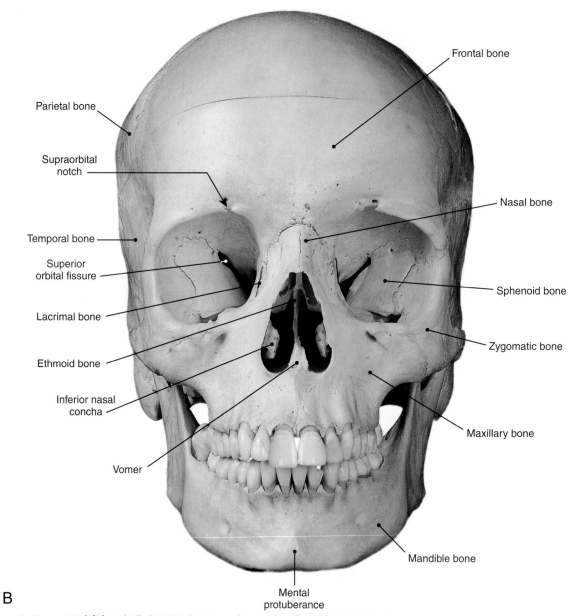

Frontal bone

Parietal bone

Supraorbital notch

Nasal bone

Temporal bone

Superior orbital fissure

Lacrimal bone

Sphenoid bone

Ethmoid bone

Zygomatic bone

Inferior nasal concha

Maxillary bone

Vomer

Mandible bone

B

Mental protuberance

Figure 2–9—cont'd (B) A skull showing bones and several surface features.

The characteristics of the following bones are discussed in this chapter:

a. Frontal bone
b. Parietal bones (2)
c. Occipital bone
d. Temporal bones (2)
e. Sphenoid bone
f. Ethmoid bone

The neurocranium is divided into two parts. The **calvaria** or skullcap is the dome-shaped structure that covers the superior surface of the brain. This is equivalent to the structure that is removed to expose the brain. The **cranial base** is the floor of the neurocranium on which the brain rests (Fig. 2–13).

Facial Skeleton

In addition to determining our facial features, the facial skeleton or *viscerocranium* serves as an attachment site for muscles; contributes to the formation of the orbit, the nasal cavity, and the oral cavity; and supports the teeth. There are eight named bones, two of which are not paired (Fig. 2–9).

a. Nasal bones (2)
b. Maxillae (2)
c. Lacrimal bones (2)
d. Zygomatic bones (2)
e. Mandible
f. Inferior nasal conchae (2)
g. Palatine bones (2)
h. Vomer

In this chapter, the major features of the bones of the skull are described. Other pertinent features are added in subsequent chapters.

GENERAL SURFACE FEATURES OF BONE

Many bones of the skull exhibit a central mass or **body** (Fig. 2–2) with extensions that are referred to as **processes.** An example of this is the anterior nasal spine of the maxilla (Fig. 2–2). The surfaces of bones exhibit

numerous markings produced by the insertion of ligaments and tendons or by the passageways of blood vessels and nerves. These surface features can be in the form of elevations, roughened surfaces, depressions, grooves, canals, or foramina.

Linear Elevations

Linear elevations can be either raised **lines** (Fig. 2–11) on the surface of the bone for the attachment of muscles, or **crests** (Fig. 2–13A), which are roughened

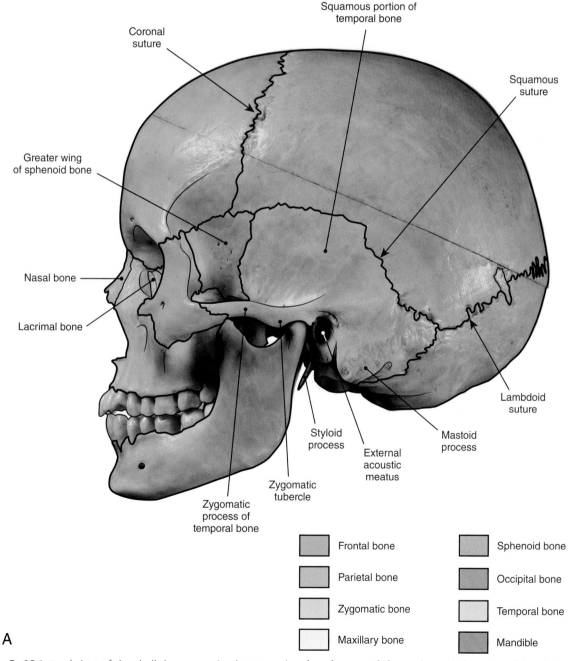

Frontal bone

Parietal bone

Zygomatic bone

Maxillary bone

Sphenoid bone

Occipital bone

Temporal bone

Mandible

A

Figure 2–10 Lateral view of the skull demonstrating bones and surface features. **(A)** A color-coded version of the skull in **(B)**.

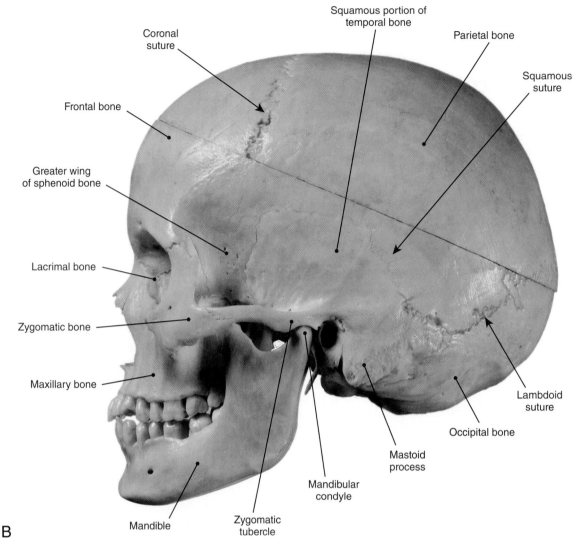

Coronal suture

Squamous portion of temporal bone

Parietal bone

Frontal bone

Squamous suture

Greater wing of sphenoid bone

Lacrimal bone

Zygomatic bone

Maxillary bone

Lambdoid suture

Occipital bone

Mastoid process

Mandibular condyle

Mandible

Zygomatic tubercle

B

Figure 2–10—cont'd

ridges on the surface of bone. These ridges can serve as attachment for muscles or the dura mater that covers the brain.

Rounded Elevations

Rounded elevations also demonstrate a variety in size and shape. As an example, a **protuberance** (Figs. 2–9 and 2–11) is a bulge on the surface of the bone. A smaller raised eminence (round elevation) is called a **tubercle** (Fig. 2–10). Some elevations are oval-shaped projections, such as the **condyles** (Fig. 2–12) located at articulations between bones.

Sharp Elevations

Elevations can also have a sharp appearance. A **process** (Fig. 2–10A) is a relatively large extension of bone, whereas a **spine** (Fig. 2–2) is a small thornlike projection.

Depressions

Depressions on the surface of bones vary in shape and depth. A **fossa** (Figs. 2–13B and 2–23A) designates a relatively large depressed area, whereas a **fovea** (Fig. 2–23B) is a smaller, shallow pit. Some bones demonstrate long, shallow indentations that are called **grooves** (Fig. 2–13A), which transmit blood vessels and nerves.

Openings

Bones also demonstrate holes of varying shape and size for the passage of vessels, nerves, and other structures. An **aperture** (Figs. 2–9 and 2–17) is a large opening; on the other hand, a **foramen** (Fig. 2–17) is a circular to oval-shaped opening. Other openings include narrow, cleftlike slits called **fissures** (Figs. 2–9 and 2–19). Some structures travel through long, narrow, tubelike channels in the bone called **canals** (Figs. 2–13A and 2–14). A **meatus** (Fig. 2–10A) is similar to a canal, but generally has a wide

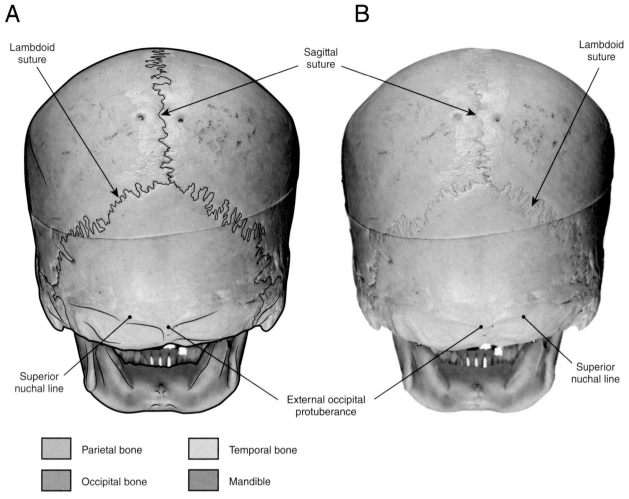

A

Lambdoid
suture

Sagittal
suture

Lambdoid
suture

Superior
nuchal line

External occipital
protuberance

B

Superior
nuchal line

Parietal bone   Temporal bone

Occipital bone   Mandible

Figure 2–11 Posterior view of the skull. **(A)** A color-coded illustration of the skull in **(B)**. The occipital bone is characterized by the external occipital protuberance and superior nuchal lines. The parietal bones are joined by the sagittal suture, whereas the occipital and parietal bones are connected by the lambdoid suture.

opening toward the surface. Structures that pass through the major openings are summarized in Table 2–1.

 Review Question Box 2-3

1. What is the difference between the viscerocranium and the neurocranium?
2. What is the significance of the various surface elevations, depressions, and openings of the bones of the skull?

BONES OF THE CRANIAL VAULT (NEUROCRANIUM)

Parietal Bones

The **parietal bones** form the roof and lateral wall of the cranium (Figs. 2–10 and 2–11). There are no named foramina associated with these bones that are of significant interest to the dental hygienist.

Occipital Bone

The **occipital bone** forms the posteroinferior portion of the cranium. The **external occipital protuberance** is a very easily identifiable feature on the external surface of the bone (Fig. 2–11). Extending laterally from the protuberance are two prominent lines, the **superior nuchal lines**, which are the sites of attachment for muscles and fascia to the back of the head (Fig. 2–11). Another prominent feature on both the external and internal surfaces is the large opening known as the **foramen magnum** that surrounds the brain stem (Figs. 2–12, 2–13A, and 2–14). Externally, on each side of this opening are two raised knuckle-shaped structures that are called the **occipital condyles** (Fig. 2–12). The condyles articulate with the first cervical vertebra. The **hypoglossal canal**, which is located along the internal walls of the foramen magnum (Figs. 2–13A and 2–14), forms a channel through the occipital bone that opens onto the outer surface at the base of the condyles. This canal is the passageway for the **hypoglossal nerve** to exit the skull and innervate the tongue (Table 2–1).

Frontal Bone

The **frontal bone** forms the anterosuperior portion of the neurocranium (Figs. 2–9 and 2–10). Its external feature is the forehead, whereas internally the frontal bone forms the roof of the orbit (Fig. 2–13A) and nasal cavity.

The **supraorbital notch** is a shallow indentation located on the superior margin of the orbit just inferior to the eyebrows (Figs. 2–9 and 2–17). In some skulls, the notch is totally enclosed by bone and is called the *supraorbital foramen*. The notch (foramen) forms a passageway for blood vessels and nerves that supply the forehead and

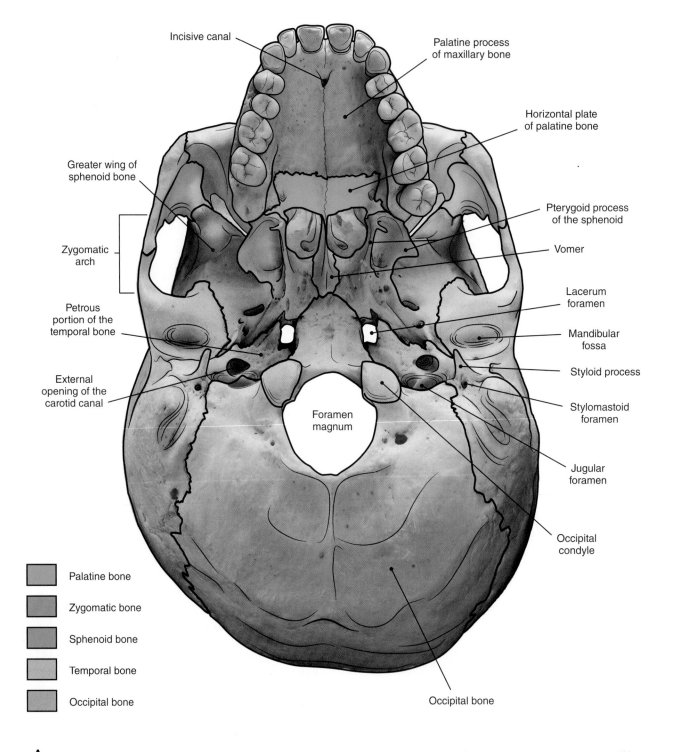

Incisive canal

Palatine process of maxillary bone

Greater wing of sphenoid bone

Horizontal plate of palatine bone

Zygomatic arch

Pterygoid process of the sphenoid

Vomer

Petrous portion of the temporal bone

Lacerum foramen

Mandibular fossa

External opening of the carotid canal

Styloid process

Stylomastoid foramen

Foramen magnum

Jugular foramen

Occipital condyle

Palatine bone

Zygomatic bone

Sphenoid bone

Temporal bone

Occipital bone

Occipital bone

A

Figure 2–12 Inferior view of the skull. **(A)** A color-coded illustration of the skull in **(B)**. In addition to numerous openings, the bones display various processes for the attachment of muscles and connective tissue.

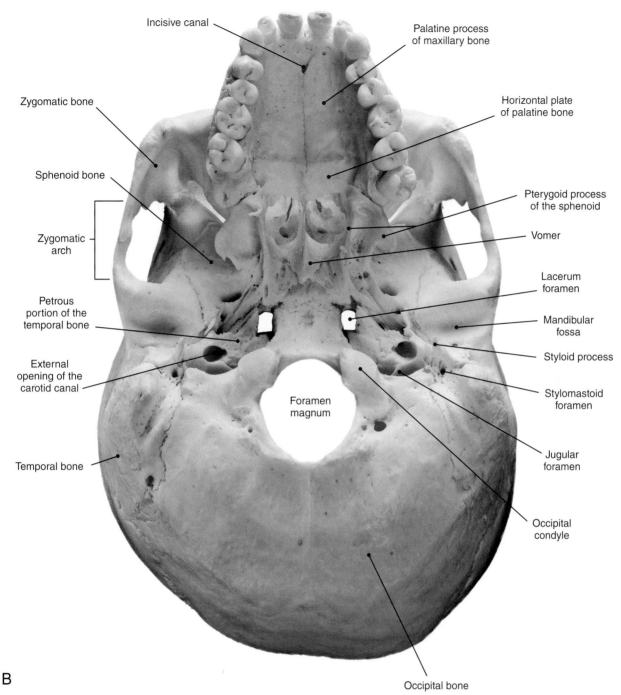

Incisive canal

Palatine process
of maxillary bone

Zygomatic bone

Horizontal plate
of palatine bone

Sphenoid bone

Pterygoid process
of the sphenoid

Zygomatic
arch

Vomer

Lacerum
foramen

Petrous
portion of the
temporal bone

Mandibular
fossa

External
opening of the
carotid canal

Styloid process

Stylomastoid
foramen

Foramen
magnum

Jugular
foramen

Temporal bone

Occipital
condyle

B

Occipital bone

Figure 2–12—cont'd

upper eyelid (Table 2–1). Internally, the **orbital plate** forms the roof of the orbit, and anteriorly a thin midline ridge called the **frontal crest** serves as the attachment of the dura mater of the brain (Fig. 2–13A).

Temporal Bones

The **temporal bones** are located inferior to the parietal bones (Fig. 2–10). These bones have several important features. The **squamous** portion is the flattened part of a temporal bone just inferior to the squamous suture (Fig. 2–10). This surface serves as an attachment site for the temporalis muscle, which is one of the muscles of mastication. Three processes extend from the central mass or body of the bone. The **zygomatic process** (Fig. 2–10A), the most lateral of these processes, joins anteriorly to the zygomatic bone to form the zygomatic arch (Fig. 2–12). Near the base of the process is a depression in the bone known as the **mandibular fossa** (Fig. 2–12). The fossa accommodates the *condyle* of the

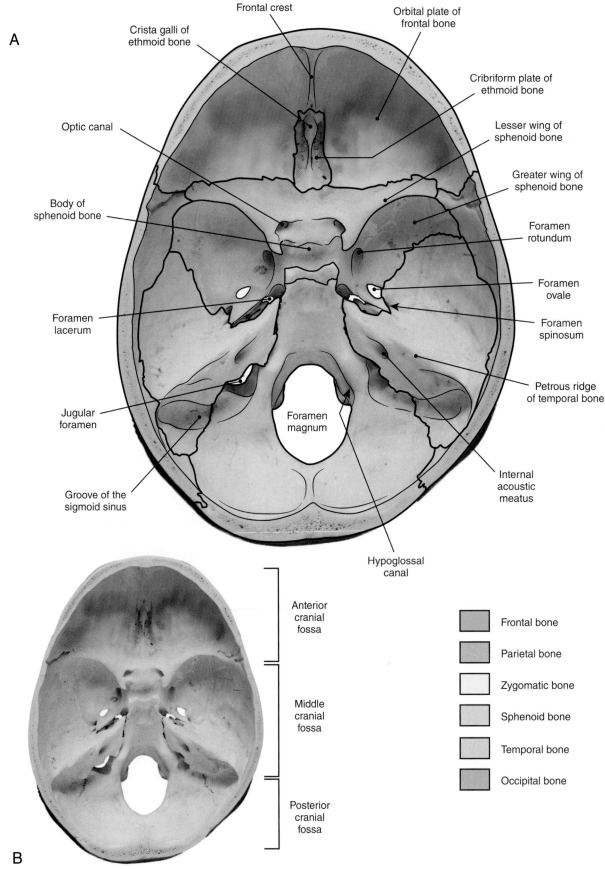

Figure 2–13 The bones of the cranial base support the brain. **(A)** A color-coded skull demonstrates the bones and surface features of the cranial fossa. The bones display a variety of openings for the passage of blood vessels and nerves. **(B)** The cranial base is divided into anterior, middle, and posterior cranial fossae, which contain lobes of the brain.

mandibular bone (Fig. 2–10B). This articulation is the *temporomandibular joint*, which is clinically important and is discussed in more detail in Chapter 7. Just posterior to the zygomatic process is the **tympanic portion** of the temporal bone, which is easily recognized by the **external acoustic meatus** (Fig. 2–10A) leading to the middle ear. Posterior to the meatus is a bulge projecting inferiorly called the **mastoid process** (Fig. 2–10), which contains the mastoid air cells. The air cells play a role in hearing. The **styloid process** is located on the inferior surface of the temporal bone (Figs. 2–10A and 2–12) and is an attachment site for muscles. A small opening, the **stylomastoid foramen,** is located between these two processes (Fig. 2–12) and is the point of exit of the **facial nerve** to reach the face (Table 2–1). Two relatively large foramina are located medial to the styloid process. The **jugular foramen** is located just medial to the styloid process at the junction between the occipital bone and the temporal bone (Figs. 2–12 through 2–14). This allows the passage of the **glossopharyngeal nerve (IX), vagus nerve (X), accessory nerve (XI),** and **internal jugular vein** outside the cranial cavity (Table 2–1). The **external opening of the carotid canal** is located just

anterior to the jugular foramen (Fig. 2–12) and is the pathway in which the **internal carotid artery** reaches the brain (Table 2–1).

On the floor of the cranial base inside of the skull, the **petrous portion** of the temporal bone forms a bulge in the middle of the cavity (Figs. 2–13A and 2–14). This portion of the temporal bone contains the inner ear (cochlea and semicircular canals). The **jugular foramen** is located posteromedially to the petrous bone, near its junction with the occipital bone, whereas the *internal opening of the carotid canal* is located anteriorly, at the apex of the petrous ridge near the junction of the temporal bone to the sphenoid bone (Fig. 2–14). **The internal acoustic meatus** is located on the posteromedial slope of the petrous bone (Figs. 2–13A and 2–14). In life, it contains the **facial nerve** and the **vestibulocochlear nerve** (Table 2–1).

Sphenoid Bone

The **sphenoid bone** is a wedge-shaped or butterfly-shaped bone situated between the frontal and temporal bones. This complex bone also has contacts with the ethmoid, occipital, vomer, parietal, and zygomatic bones (Figs. 2–12 and 2–13A). There are four main components of the sphenoid bone: the **body**, the **greater wing**, the **lesser wing**, and the **pterygoid process**. Three of these features are located on the floor of the cranial fossa (Figs. 2–13A and 2–14). The central portion of the body forms a saddle-shaped depression called the **sella turcica** (Turkish saddle) (Fig. 2–14), which contains the **pituitary gland**. The *lesser wing* forms the posterior portion of the orbit and contains the **optic canal** (Figs. 2–13A and 2–14), through which the **optic nerve** (II) passes (Table 2–1). The *greater wing* spreads laterally from the base and can be seen on the lateral exterior of the skull between the frontal, parietal, and temporal bones (Fig. 2–10). The greater wing of the sphenoid bone exhibits four paired openings in a slightly curved line. From anterior to posterior, they are the **superior orbital fissure** (Fig. 2–14), the **foramen rotundum**, the **foramen ovale,** and the **foramen spinosum** (Figs. 2–13A and 2–14). The superior orbital fissure contains the **oculomotor nerve (III)**, the **trochlear nerve (IV)**, the **abducens nerve (VI)**, the **opthalmic division (V1)** of the trigeminal nerve, and the **supraorbital vein** (Table 2–1). The **maxillary division (V2)** of the trigeminal nerve passes through the foramen rotundum (Table 2–1), whereas the **mandibular division (V3)** of the trigeminal nerve courses through the foramen ovale (Table 2–1). The **middle meningeal artery** enters the skull through the foramen spinosum (Table 2–1).

The *pterygoid process* is located on the inferior surface (Fig. 2–12) and is composed of the **medial** and **lateral pterygoid plates** (Fig. 2–18). A small projection of bone, the **pterygoid hamulus,** extends from the medial pterygoid plate (Fig. 2–18). These structures are important

TABLE 2–1	Summary of Important Apertures and Their Contents*	
Foramina or Openings	**Content**
Foramina in cribriform plate	Olfactory nerves
Optic canal	Optic nerve
Superior orbital fissure	Oculomotor, trochlear, abducens, and ophthalmic nerves; supraorbital vein
Inferior orbital fissure	Infraorbital and zygomatic nerves
Foramen rotundum	Maxillary nerve
Foramen ovale	Mandibular nerve
Foramen spinosum	Middle meningeal artery
Foramen magnum	Medulla
Jugular foramen	Glossopharyngeal, vagus, and accessory nerves; internal jugular vein
Hypoglossal canal	Hypoglossal nerve
Internal acoustic meatus	Facial and vestibulocochlear nerves
Stylomastoid foramen	Facial nerve
Transverse foramen	Vertebral artery
Vertebral canal	Spinal cord
Intervertebral foramen	Spinal nerves
Carotid canal	Internal carotid artery

*The table does not represent all of the apertures of the skull and their contents.

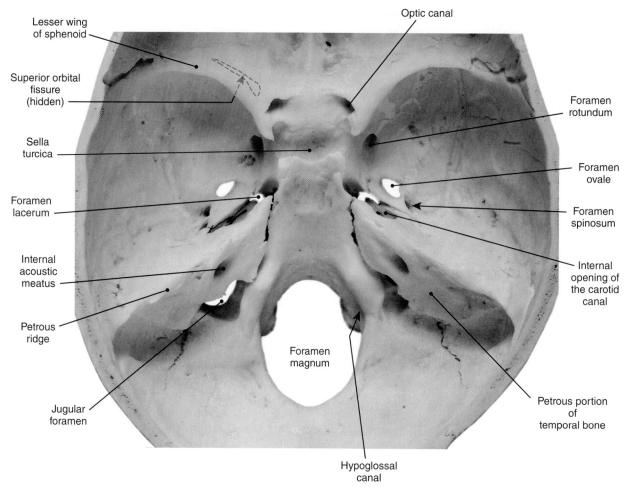

Figure 2–14 Middle and posterior cranial fossae display a number of surface features, including several foramina for passage of blood vessels and nerves.

attachment sites for several muscles of the pharynx and palate and are described in Chapter 4.

Ethmoid Bone

The **ethmoid bone** is a difficult bone to visualize in an intact skull. It contributes to the formation of the roof, septum, and superolateral wall of the nasal cavity and to the medial wall of the orbit. In the anterior portion of the cranial cavity, the **cribriform plate** of the ethmoid bone (Fig. 2–13A) contains many small foramina for the passage of the tiny **olfactory nerves** (Table 2–1). A small crest of bone, known as the **crista galli,** is located in the middle of the cribriform plate (Fig. 2–13A). This structure serves as a point of attachment of the membranous coverings of the brain. In the midline of the nasal cavity, its **perpendicular plate** contributes to the anterosuperior portion of the nasal septum (Fig. 2–15). The superolateral wall of the nasal cavity is formed by two extensions of the ethmoid bone called the **superior** and **middle conchae** (Fig. 2–16). The middle nasal concha can be viewed by looking through the **piriform aperture** (external pear-shaped opening) of the nasal cavity (Fig. 2–17).

STRUCTURAL ORGANIZATION OF THE NEUROCRANIUM

Calvaria

The **calvaria**, or skullcap, is formed by portions of the *frontal, parietal, temporal,* and *occipital bones,* which are firmly joined by sutures. Recall that a suture is a fibrous, immoveable joint. The contact points between the bone form irregular interdigitating edges that bind the bones. Starting anteriorly, the **coronal suture** joins the frontal bone to the two parietal bones (Fig. 2–10). On the lateral surface, the **squamous suture** binds the parietal bone to the temporal bone (Fig. 2–10). On the superior surface, the **sagittal suture** unites the two parietal bones in the median plane (Fig. 2–11). Posteriorly, the **lambdoid suture** joins the occipital bone to the two parietal bones (Fig. 2–11).

Cranial Base

The **cranial base** of the skull is that portion of the neurocranium on which the brain lies. The **cranial cavity** is the actual space that contains the brain and

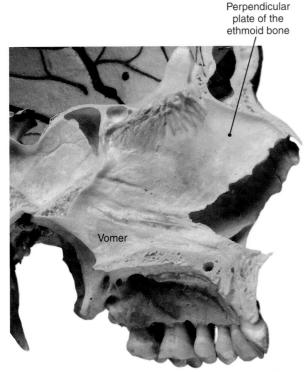

Figure 2–15 A portion of the nasal septum is formed by the perpendicular plate of the ethmoid bone and the vomer. The orange filaments are the position of the olfactory nerves on the superior portion of the nasal septum.

is surrounded by the calvaria and cranial base. The cranial base is formed by the sphenoid and ethmoid bones as well as portions of the frontal, parietal, temporal, and occipital bones (Fig. 2–13A). Portions of the brain occupy three depressions of the cranial base, which are referred to as the **cranial fossae** (singular: **fossa**). The cranial base is subdivided anteriorly by the lesser wing of the sphenoid bone and posteriorly by the petrous ridge of the temporal bone into the anterior, middle, and posterior cranial fossae (Fig. 2–13B). Each fossa contains important anatomical features such as foramina for the passage of the cranial nerves leaving the skull and grooves for the dural venous sinuses.

Anterior Cranial Fossa

Portions of the frontal, ethmoid, and sphenoid bones form the **anterior cranial fossa**, which houses the frontal lobe of the brain. The most predominant features of the fossa are the *orbital plates* and *frontal crest of the frontal bone* and the *crista galli* and *cribriform plate of the ethmoid bone*. The frontal crest and the crista galli are attachment sites for the cranial dura, whereas the openings of the cribriform plate (Fig. 2–13A) contain sensory fibers of the olfactory nerve (Table 2–1).

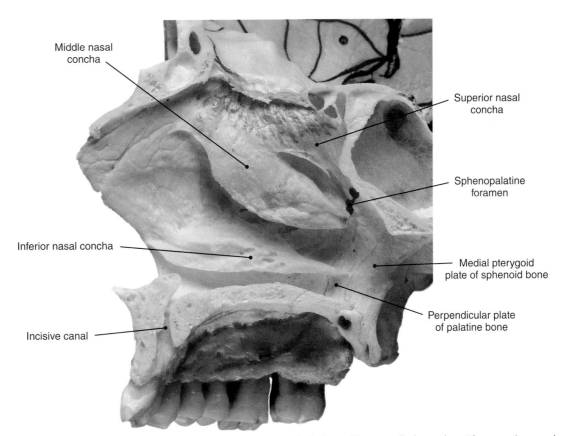

Figure 2–16 The lateral wall of the nasal cavity generally displays three shell-shaped bones called *conchae*. The superior nasal conchae and the middle nasal conchae are processes of the ethmoid bone. The orange filaments are branches of the olfactory nerve on the superior nasal concha. The larger inferior nasal concha is a separate bone.

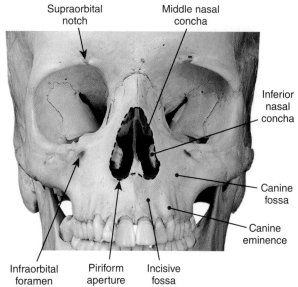

Supraorbital notch

Middle nasal concha

Inferior nasal concha

Canine fossa

Canine eminence

Infraorbital foramen

Piriform aperture

Incisive fossa

Figure 2–17 Frontal view of the skull. The piriform aperture (dashed line) is a large opening in the skull leading into the nasal cavities. The inferior and middle nasal conchae can be seen through the piriform aperture. The infraorbital foramen is a smaller-caliber passageway for blood vessels and nerves. Features of the maxillary bone are also shown.

Box 2-1 Fontanels

The skull of a newborn baby has "soft spots" on its surface in the areas of the lambdoid and coronal sutures. These "soft spots" are called **fontanels** and result from the incomplete closure of the sutures between the bones to allow flexibility of the skull as the baby passes through the birth canal. Fontanels are made of the connective tissue in which the bone forms. The posterior fontanel is smaller and "closes" within months of childbirth. The anterior fontanel is much larger, and it takes at least 2 years for bone growth to be completed. Clinicians can monitor the closure of the anterior fontanel for the proper growth and development of a child.

Middle Cranial Fossa

The floor of the **middle cranial fossa**, which houses the temporal lobe of the brain, is made of portions of the sphenoid and temporal bones. The fossa is bounded anteriorly by a ridge formed by the *lesser wing of the sphenoid bone* and posteriorly by the *petrous ridge of the temporal bone* (Fig. 2–13A). Some of the more important landmarks of this fossa include the *sella turcica* (Turkish saddle), which houses the pituitary gland and several openings associated with the cranial nerves and blood vessels that include the *foramen spinosum*, the *foramen ovale*, the *foramen rotundum*, and the *superior orbital fissure* (Figs. 2–13A and 2–14). Toward the apex of the petrous ridge there is a large jagged-edged opening called

the **foramen lacerum**, which is filled with cartilage in real life (Figs. 2–13A and 2–14).

Posterior Cranial Fossa

The **posterior cranial fossa** is formed mostly by the occipital bone and houses the cerebellum and occipital lobe of the brain. One of the most noticeable features is the large *foramen magnum,* which accommodates the attachment of the spinal cord to the brain stem (Figs. 2–13 and 2–14). Three other openings are associated with the cranial nerves. The *hypoglossal canal,* which is located superolateral in the bone surrounding the foramen magnum (Figs. 2–13A and 2–14), is the passageway of the hypoglossal nerve (XII) out of the skull. The *jugular foramen,* which is situated between the occipital and temporal bones (Figs. 2–13A and 2–14), is the exit point for the glossopharyngeal (IX), vagus (X), and spinal accessory (XI) nerves. The *internal acoustic meatus* on the posteromedial surface of the petrous ridge (Figs. 2–13A and 2–14) contains the outgoing fibers of the facial (VII) and vestibulocochlear (VIII) nerves (Table 2–1).

Review Question Box 2-4

1. What is the difference between the calvaria and the cranial base?
2. What do you think is the most important bone of the neurocranium? Why?
3. What are the boundaries of the cranial fossae?
4. Name the openings that are found in each cranial fossa.

BONES OF THE FACIAL SKELETON (VISCEROCRANIUM)

The face is formed by the following paired bones: maxilla, palatine, zygomatic, lacrimal, nasal, and inferior nasal concha, and the following single bones: vomer and mandible (Fig. 2–9).

Maxillae or Maxillary Bones

The **maxillae** (singular: **maxilla**) form the upper jaw and a large portion of the face between the orbit and upper teeth (Fig. 2–9). The maxillary bone is important to the dental hygienist because it supports the teeth and its foramina are sites of intraoral injections for dental procedures of the maxillary teeth. The maxillae articulate with the nasal, frontal, and zygomatic bones to form a portion of the floor of the orbit (Fig. 2–19). The **alveolar process** is the portion of the maxilla in which the teeth are attached. Each tooth occupies an **alveolus** or socket. On the outer surface, there is an elevation of the bone appropriately referred to as the **canine eminence** (Fig. 2–17). Medial to this eminence is a shallow fossa called the **incisive fossa**, which lies between the roots of the central and lateral incisors. Superolateral to the canine eminence there is a deeper depression referred to as the **canine fossa** (Fig. 2–17). Posterior to the second or third molar (if present), there is a rounded eminence known as the **maxillary tuberosity** (Fig. 2–20). This structure is an important attachment site for one of the muscles of mastication. Internally, the **palatine processes** form the anterior portion of the hard palate. The **incisive canals** are located at the anterior tip of the hard palate. The canals contain blood vessels and nerves that supply the palate and the anterior portion of the nasal cavity (Figs. 2–12, 2–16, and 2–18). The **infraorbital foramen**, which is located on the external surface inferior to the orbit, contains blood vessels and nerves that supply that area of the face (Fig. 2–17).

Palatine Bones

The **palatine bones** can best be seen from an inferior view (Figs. 2–12 and 2–18). Their **horizontal plate** forms most of the posterior portion of the hard palate. On the lateral edge of the palatine bone, there are two small openings, the **greater** and **lesser palatine foramina** (Fig. 2–18), which contain blood vessels and nerves that supply the

hard and soft palate. The **perpendicular plate** of the palatine bone forms a portion of the posterior lateral wall of the nasal cavity. It is characterized by the **sphenopalatine foramen** (Fig. 2–16), which transmits blood vessels and nerves that supply the nasal cavity.

Clinical Correlation Box 2-1

Le Fort Fractures and Osteotomy

Some individuals have distorted facial features caused by the extension of the maxillary bone too anterior to the mandible or the mandible's extending anterior to the maxilla. Oral surgeons can surgically repair the position of the maxilla by orthognathic (jaw) surgery (osteotomy) based on the patterns of the Le Fort fractures. Trauma to the face can cause three predictable fracture patterns called **Le Fort fractures**, named after René Le Fort, a French physician who described them in 1901. Le Fort I fractures extend from the nasal septum anteriorly and course posteriorly in a horizontal plane above the apices of the maxillary teeth toward the pterygoid plates. This fracture detaches the hard palate from the base of the skull. Oral surgeons can re-create the fracture, which allows the surgeon to raise, lower, or move forward the upper jaw (maxilla).

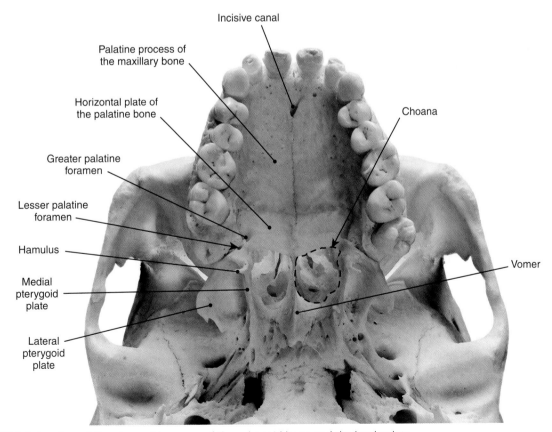

Figure 2–18 Inferior view of the pterygoid process of the sphenoid bone and the hard palate.

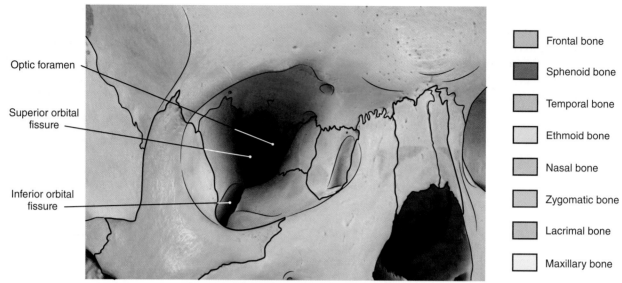

Optic foramen

Superior orbital fissure

Inferior orbital fissure

Frontal bone

Sphenoid bone

Temporal bone

Ethmoid bone

Nasal bone

Zygomatic bone

Lacrimal bone

Maxillary bone

Figure 2–19 Frontal view of the bones that form the orbit.

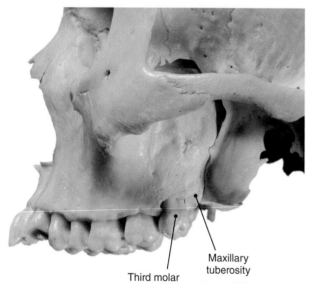

Maxillary tuberosity

Third molar

Figure 2–20 Lateral view of the maxilla showing the maxillary tuberosity posterior to the third molar.

Zygomatic Bones

The **zygomatic bones** form the cheek bones (Figs. 2–2 and 2–10). The bones have two processes: the **frontal process**, which articulates with the frontal bone, and the **temporal process**, which joins with the temporal bone. The zygomatic process of the temporal bone and the temporal process of the zygomatic bone form the **zygomatic arch** (Figs. 2–2 and 2–10).

Lacrimal Bones

The **lacrimal bones** are very small bones that contribute to the formation of the medial wall of the orbit (Figs. 2–9 and 2–19). They are located between the maxillary and the ethmoid bones. Each bone has a small groove for the lacrimal sac and the nasolacrimal duct that carries tears from the eyes to the nose.

Nasal Bones

The **nasal bones** form the bridge of the nose and the superior border of the **piriform aperture** (the pear-shaped anterior openings into the nasal cavities) (Figs. 2–9 and 2–17). The lateral and inferior border of the aperture is formed by the maxillary bone.

Vomer

The **vomer** is a thin midline bone within the nasal cavity that contributes to the posteroinferior portion of the nasal septum. It is located inferior to the perpendicular plate of the ethmoid bone (Fig. 2–15). The vomer, along with the horizontal plate of the palatine bone and the pterygoid process of the sphenoid bone, forms the posterior openings of the nasal cavity called the **choana** (Figs. 2–12 and 2–18).

Inferior Nasal Conchae

The **inferior nasal concha** is located on the lateral wall of the nasal cavity inferior to the middle nasal concha (Figs. 2–16 and 2–17).

Mandible

The **mandible** is important to the dental hygienist because it supports the teeth and its foramina are sites of intraoral injections for dental procedures of the lower jaw. The mandible consists of a horseshoe-shaped bone (Fig. 2–21). Its horizontal component is called the **body** and contains the teeth (Fig. 2–22). As described earlier for the maxilla, the *alveolar process* extends from the body and supports the teeth (Fig. 2–22). Projecting upward from the body is the **ramus**, which ends anteriorly as the **coronoid process** and posteriorly as the **condylar process** and its *condyle* (Fig. 2–22). The depression between these two structures is called the **mandibular notch**. The posteroinferior

junction between the ramus and body is referred to as the **angle** (Fig. 2–22).

A triangular-shaped eminence, the **mental protuberance**, lies on the anterior surface of the mandible (Figs. 2–9 and 2–21). The broadness of the protuberance determines the shape of the chin. The **mental foramen** is located laterally on the facial surface of the body of the mandible in the vicinity of the root of the first premolar tooth (Figs. 2–21 and 2–22). Each foramen contains blood vessels and nerves of the same name that supply the lips and chin. The **mandibular foramen** is located on the medial (lingual) surface (Fig. 2–23A) and opens into the **mandibular canal** (Fig. 2–23B). The inferior alveolar artery, vein, and nerve course through the mandibular foramen and canal to supply the mandibular teeth. Also on the lingual surface is a linear ridge known as the **my-lohyoid line** that separates two depressions (Fig. 2–23). The one superior to the ridge is the **sublingual fossa** and contains the sublingual gland. The one inferior to the ridge is the **submandibular fossa**, which contains a portion of the submandibular gland (Fig. 2–23).

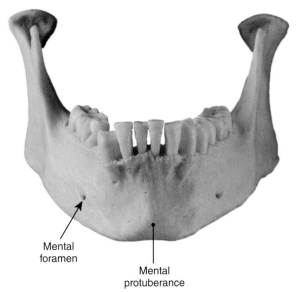

Figure 2–21 Frontal view of the mandible. The mental protuberance is a triangle-shaped elevation on the anterior surface of the mandible. The mental foramen is lateral to the protuberance. The portion of the mandible that forms the sockets of the teeth is called the *alveolar process*.

Review Question Box 2-5

1. What bones contribute to the formation of the orbital rim?
2. What bones contribute to the formation of the hard palate?
3. What surface features are found on the medial surface of the mandible?

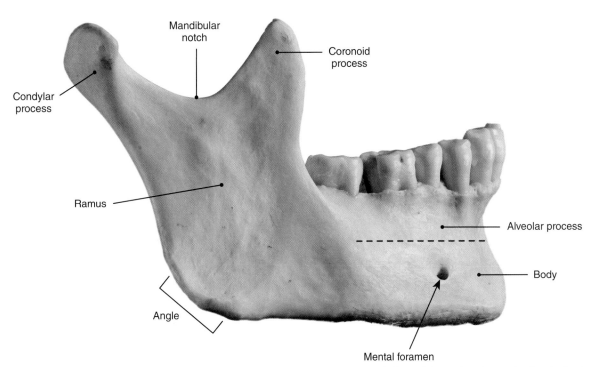

Figure 2–22 Lateral view of the mandible. The ramus of the mandible is a vertical plate of bone that is attached to its body. The posterior junction between these features is the angle. The ramus has an anterior coronoid process and posterior condylar process. The processes are separated by the mandibular notch.

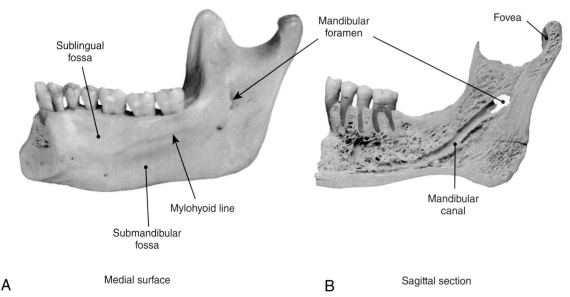

A   Medial surface   B   Sagittal section

Figure 2–23 (A) The mandibular foramen is located on the medial surface of the mandible. The mylohyoid line separates the sublingual fossa from the more inferior submandibular fossa. **(B)** Sagittal view through the mandibular canal. The inferior alveolar artery, vein, and nerve (not shown) pass through the mandibular canal to access the mandibular teeth. The fovea of the condylar process is for the attachment of muscles.

PARANASAL SINUSES

Within the *ethmoid, sphenoid, frontal,* and *maxillary* bones are epithelial-lined extensions of the nasal cavity called the **paranasal sinuses** (Fig. 2–24). The sinuses are hollow but can become filled with mucus during a sinus infection. Their functions are to lighten the weight of the skull and give resonance to our voices. Clinically speaking, the **maxillary sinus** is more important to the dental profession. The bone of the floor of the sinus is very thin and lies in close proximity to the roots of the maxillary molars (Fig. 2–24). Because the maxillary sinus and the maxillary teeth are innervated by the same nerves, a maxillary sinus infection can refer pain to the teeth. Therefore, it is necessary to determine the origin of maxillary pain before treating tooth decay. In addition, the maxillary sinus continues to enlarge throughout life, and thus the walls of the sinus become thinner. This is important to the dental clinician because the sinuses could be accidently opened during extraction of the molars (in particular, impacted third molar teeth).

Review Question Box 2-6

1. Why is the relationship of the maxillary sinus to the oral cavity important to the dental hygienist?

CERVICAL VERTEBRAE

General Features of Cervical Vertebrae

There are seven cervical vertebrae. The first two, the atlas and the axis, have their own special features and are considered individually after this general description of the other five vertebrae.

The **cervical vertebrae** are composed of an anterior mass called the **body**, which is the major load-bearing contact between adjacent vertebrae, and a **neural (vertebral) arch** that forms the **vertebral foramen** (Fig. 2–25). In the intact vertebral column, the foramina form the **vertebral canal**, which contains the spinal cord. An **intervertebral disc** of fibrocartilage separates each vertebra and acts as a shock absorber (symphysis) (Figs. 2–5 and 2–26). Projecting from the vertebral body are two processes, the **pedicles**, which form the anterolateral portion of the neural arch. The posterolateral portion is formed by the two **laminae** (singular: **lamina**). A **transverse process** extends laterally on either side of each vertebra at the point where the laminae and pedicles join. In each process, there is a **transverse foramen** (Fig. 2–25) for the passage of the **vertebral artery** and **vertebral vein** that supply the brain (Table 2–1). At the point where the two laminae join posteriorly, there is a **spinous process,** which is bifid, having two **tubercles**. Each vertebra has two **superior** and two **inferior**

articulating processes that serve as attachment sites for adjacent vertebrae (Fig. 2–26). These articulations are synovial joints. When two vertebrae are placed together, a small foramen is formed along the lateral border. This **intervertebral foramen** contains the spinal nerves emerging from the spinal cord (Fig. 2–26).

Atlas

The **atlas** is the first cervical vertebra (C1) (Fig. 2–27). The atlas has neither a body nor spinous process. Instead, there are two **lateral masses** connected by two thin arches, which are called the **anterior** and **posterior arches**. On each arch there is a **tubercle** for the attachment of muscles. The **anterior arch** is smaller and articulates with the dens of the axis (discussed in the next section). Its vertebral foramen is larger than the other vertebra to accommodate the brainstem. The superior articulating processes, which are located on the lateral masses, articulate with the occipital condyles of the

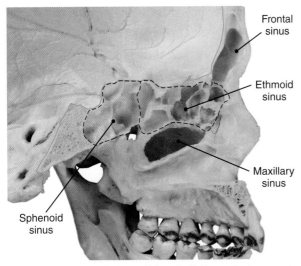

Frontal sinus

Ethmoid sinus

Maxillary sinus

Sphenoid sinus

Figure 2–24 Sagittal view of the skull through the nasal cavity. The diploë of four bones of the skull become pneumatized and are thus an extension of the respiratory system. The frontal, ethmoidal, and sphenoidal sinuses are located under the floor of the cranial cavity. The sinus of the maxillary bone is located between the orbit and oral cavity.

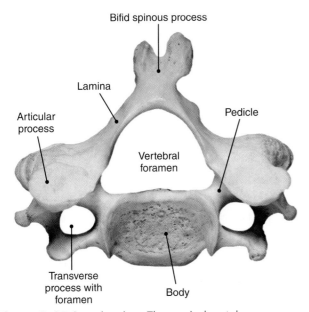

Bifid spinous process

Lamina

Articular process

Pedicle

Vertebral foramen

Transverse process with foramen

Body

Figure 2–25 Superior view. The cervical vertebrae are composed of the weight-bearing body and the neural arch that protects the spinal cord. The transverse process extends laterally from the body. The transverse foramen serves as a passageway for the vertebral artery. The pedicles form the anterolateral portion of the neural arch, and the laminae form the posterolateral component. The spinous process is located at the junction of the two laminae and is characteristically bifid.

Clinical Correlation Box 2-2

Intervertebral Disc Disorders

The intervertebral disc serves not only to join adjacent vertebrae but also to act as a shock absorber to prevent compression of the vertebral column while bending, standing, walking, and exercising. The disc is composed of two parts, the anulus fibrosus and the nucleus pulposus. The **anulus fibrosus** is the outermost layer and is formed by concentric layers of fibrocartilage. The **nucleus pulposus** is a gelatinous mass that forms the central core of the disc. During aging, the bodies of the vertebrae undergo bone loss and become more concave. The disc changes shape to maintain the joint. As a result, there can be a decrease in height during aging. The disc can undergo other degenerative changes with age and trauma. The anulus fibrosus can become weakened, allowing the nucleus pulposus to protrude outside its normal radius but not rupturing the outer layer of fibrocartilage. This condition is called a **bulging disc** and does not cause pain unless the bulge impinges on the nerves in the spinal canal. If the anulus fibrosus is weakened such that the nucleus pulposus penetrates the cartilage (rupture of the cartilage), the condition is called a **herniated disc**. The herniating mass can impinge on nerve roots, which can cause the connective tissue surrounding the nerve to become inflamed. This can result in pain and numbness in the area innervated by the nerve.

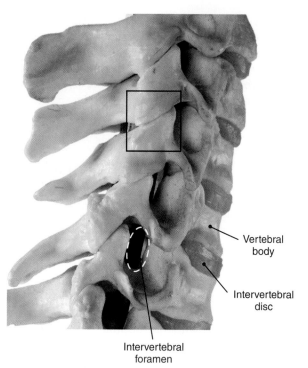

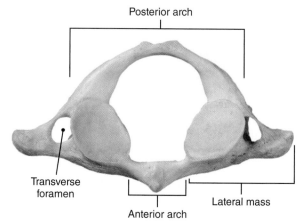

skull. A *transverse process* with a *transverse foramen* extends from the lateral mass (Fig. 2–27).

Axis

The **axis** is the second cervical vertebra (C2) and more closely resembles the other vertebrae in this region (Fig. 2–28). It is unique in having an upward projection

Figure 2–26 Lateral view. The bodies of the vertebrae are connected by the intervertebral disc. Superior and inferior articulating processes (see box) also join the adjacent vertebrae. An intervertebral foramen is formed by the union of two vertebrae. These openings serve as channels for the spinal nerves that exit the spinal cord.

Figure 2–27 Inferior view. The atlas is the first cervical vertebra (C1). The atlas articulates with the occipital condyles superiorly and the axis inferiorly. The atlas is atypical in that it lacks a body and is composed of an anterior and a posterior arch attached to a lateral mass.

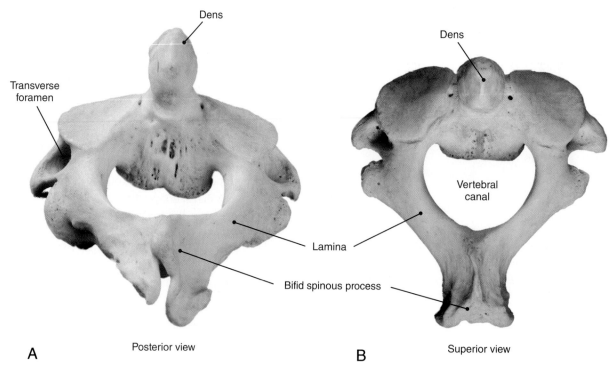

Figure 2–28 (A) Posterior and **(B)** anterior view of the axis, which is the second cervical vertebra (C2). It has the same features as a typical cervical vertebra, with the exception of the dens attached to its body.

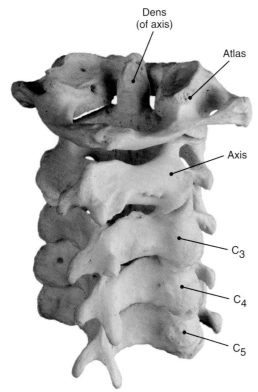

Dens
(of axis)

Atlas

Axis

C₃

C₄

C₅

Figure 2–29 Posterior view. The dens articulates with the anterior arch of the atlas, which allows for rotation of the neck.

arising from the body, the **dens**, sometimes called the **odontoid** (toothlike) **process**. This serves as a pivot for the rotation of the atlas. When the head is turned, the atlas rotates on the dens of the axis (Fig. 2–29).

Review Question Box 2-7

1. Compare the structure of the atlas to a typical cervical vertebra.
2. What structure is uniquely characteristic to the axis? What is its function?

SUMMARY

The skull and vertebrae are the portions of the skeleton that support and protect the structures of the head and neck. Bones also serve as attachment sites for muscles, which is the mechanical basis for movement. In addition, bones are a reservoir for calcium, and bone marrow produces the cells of the peripheral blood. The skull also contains the five organs of special senses: taste, smell, vision, hearing, and equilibrium. Although bones are characterized by size and shape, all bones are made of compact and spongy bone. Bones articulate at the joints. Joints are classified as fibrous, cartilaginous, or synovial. Fibrous joints include the sutures of the skull and the attachment of the roots of the teeth to the bone, a gomphosis. The cartilaginous joints are characteristic of the vertebral column, in which the intervertebral disc joins adjacent vertebrae (symphysis). The growth plate of developing long bone is also a cartilaginous joint. The synovial joint is a mobile joint; the temporomandibular joint is an example in the head.

The skull is divided into a neurocranium, which surrounds the skull, and the viscerocranium, which is composed of the bones of the facial skeleton. The cranial base is the portion of the neurocranium on which the brain rests. The sphenoid bone is the center of the cranial base to which the parietal, temporal, frontal, ethmoid, and occipital bones are attached. The base is characterized by several foramina, apertures, and fissures for the passage of nerves and blood vessels to and from the skull. The facial skeleton is composed of the nasal, zygomatic, maxillary, lacrimal, and palatine bones as well as the inferior nasal concha, vomer, and mandible.

Bones have surface markings in the form of elevations or depressions that are caused by the attachment of muscles, whereas openings are created for nerves and blood vessels.

The cervical vertebrae protect the cervical portion of the spinal cord. The typical cervical vertebra is composed of a body, which bears weight; spinous and transverse processes for the attachment of muscles; and a neural arch that forms the vertebral foramen. The arch is formed by the pedicles that attach the body to the transverse process and the laminae that join the transverse processes to the spinous process. The first cervical vertebra, the atlas, is atypical because it does not possess a body or transverse processes. The atlas is attached to the skull by the occipital condyles. The second cervical vertebra, the axis, has an additional process called the dens. The dens articulates with the atlas to allow rotation of the skull on the cervical vertebrae.

The skull is very complex and may seem overwhelming at first, but coloring and labeling diagrams of the skull and palpating the structures on yourself will make your study much easier.

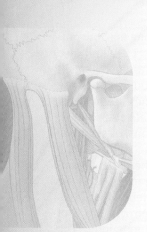

LEARNING LAB
Exercises for review, practice, and study

Laboratory Activity 2-1

Palpating Surface Skeletal Features of the Head and Neck

The surface of our body takes on the form of the underlying structures. Palpation (touching with your fingers) will help you learn anatomy as well as help you locate structures in the clinic.

Objective: In this exercise, you will palpate surface features related to the bones of the skull and the neck using yourself as a model.

Materials Needed: Plastic gloves (If working with a partner)

Step 1: Start by placing your fingers on your forehead and note that it is formed by the *frontal bone*. On the back of your head, feel for a large bump superior to the attachment of the neck. This structure is the *external occipital protuberance* of the occipital bone. Extending to the left and right of the protuberance is a linear elevation called the *superior nuchal line*. You may be able to feel another linear elevation about a fingerwidth below and parallel to this line called the *inferior nuchal line*. Inferior to this line, you can palpate soft tissue (muscles of the neck and back) that attach to these lines.

- Return to the anterior surface of the head. With a finger, palpate the nasal bones in the midline of the face inferior to the frontal bone. The nasal bones form the bridge of the nose; the nostrils are formed by cartilage. Now palpate the cheek bone, which is the *body* of the zygomatic *bone*. More medially, palpate the *maxillary bone*, which is inferior to the eye and lateral to the nose and is easily recognizable in individuals with teeth.

Step 2: The eyes are contained within the orbit. Only the outer rim is palpable.

- Start along the superior border of the rim, which is a feature of the *frontal bone*. The lateral border is formed by the *frontal bone* superiorly and the *zygomatic bone* inferiorly. Attempt to find the suture joining these two bones about midway on the lateral orbital rim. (Do not be concerned if you cannot palpate the suture.) The inferior border of the rim is formed by the zygomatic bone and the maxillary bone. Some individuals may be able to palpate the suture as a slight depression in the rim about midway on the orbital rim. The *infraorbital foramen* of the maxillary bone is located just inferior to the suture. Feel for a slight depression below the orbital rim for this foramen, which is a landmark for intraoral injection. The medial border of the orbital rim is formed by the frontal bone superiorly and the maxillary bone inferiorly.
- Palpate the roots of the maxillary teeth by searching for a series of vertical elevations and depressions between the teeth. The socket and bony supporting structure surrounding the teeth form the *alveolar process*. Realize that in edentulous individuals, the bone is resorbed (bone loss).

Step 3: Now palpate the *piriform aperture*, the bony opening of the nasal cavity.
   Start by placing a finger on the left and right inferior borders (not inside) of the nostrils, glide the fingers superolaterally along the *maxillary bone*, and continue along the inferior surface of the *nasal bone*, thus outlining the aperture.

Step 4: The mandible is a very important bone for the dental hygienist.

- Start at the chin or **mentum**. Palpate the left and right sides of your mandible simultaneously using fingers of both hands. The mentum is of varying shapes; it is generally more pointed in a female and broader in a male. Feel for a triangular projection called the *mental protuberance*.
- Palpate the inferior border of the mandible to its termination at the *angle* of the mandible. Realize this represents the body of the mandible. As you did for the maxillary bone, feel for the roots of the mandibular teeth and recognize that the supporting bone is the *alveolar process*.
- Now put your fingers on the angle and move your finger superiorly onto the *ramus* of the mandible. Although you can palpate the posterior border of the ramus, the lateral border is covered by the masseter muscle, one of the muscles of mastication (chewing muscle).

- Move your finger superiorly until you feel bone arching horizontally on the side of your face. This is the *zygomatic arch*. This is formed by the temporal process of the zygomatic bone anteriorly and the zygomatic process of the temporal bone posteriorly.
- Move your fingers along the arch toward the ears. Open and close your mouth several times. You should be able to feel the movement of the *condyle* of the mandible in the temporomandibular joint (TMJ). Observe that the fleshy portion of the ear surrounds the *external auditory meatus* of the temporal bone. The relationship is very important because clicking sounds from the TMJ are clearly audible.
- Now, place your fingers posteroinferiorly to the ear and palpate the *mastoid process* of the temporal bone, which is an attachment site for muscle.

Step 5: Let's turn our attention to the neurocranium. You have already identified the frontal bone and portions of the temporal bone. The *squamous* (flat) portion of the temporal bone is a rather broad area superior to the mastoid process anteriorly to approximately midway medial to the zygomatic arch. The borders are ill defined.

- Palpate the soft tissue above the zygomatic process. This is a portion of the temporalis muscle, which, like the masseter muscle, is a muscle of mastication. Place your finger vertically along the lateral border of the orbital rim. The *greater wing of the sphenoid bone* lies deep to your finger.
- Place your fingers on the temporalis muscle and clench your teeth several times. You should be able to feel the contraction of the muscle. Palpate superiorly on this muscle until you no longer can feel the contraction. This is the attachment site to the *parietal bone*. The parietal bones are attached to each other on the superior surface of the skull in the medial plane. Attempt to palpate the *sagittal suture* between the two bones. Some individuals may be able to trace the sagittal suture to its intersection with the *coronal suture,* which is in the frontal plane and binds the frontal bones to the parietal bones.

Step 6: Finish this exercise by first palpating the *transverse processes* of the *cervical vertebrae* on the lateral side of the neck.

- Now, using your index finder and thumb, feel the soft tissue ligament that courses lengthwise on the back of your neck. This ligament (ligamentum nuchae) covers the surface of most of the *spinous processes* of the cervical vertebrae. Glide your fingers on the median plane of the neck until you feel a prominent bulge, which represents the spinous process of the seventh cervical vertebra (called the *vertebra prominens*).
- Wash your hands after finishing this exercise.

For Discussion or Thought:

1. *Why is it important for a dental hygienist to be able to palpate skeletal structures and other surface features?*

Learning Activity 2-1

Anterior View of the Skull

Match the numbered structures with the correct terms listed below.

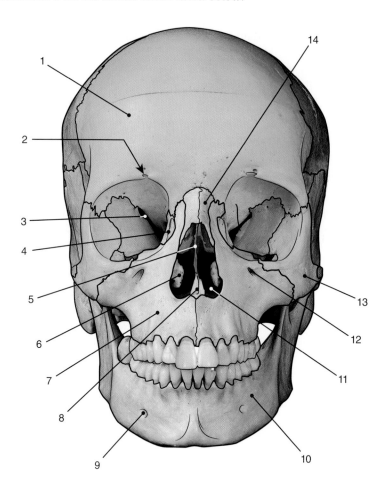

_____ Frontal bone

_____ Inferior nasal concha

_____ Infraorbital foramen

_____ Lacrimal bone

_____ Mandible

_____ Maxillary bone

_____ Mental foramen

_____ Nasal bone

_____ Perpendicular plate of ethmoid bone

_____ Piriform aperture

_____ Superior orbital fissure

_____ Supraorbital notch

_____ Vomer

_____ Zygomatic bone

Learning Activity 2-2

Lateral View of the Skull

Match the numbered structures with the correct terms listed below.

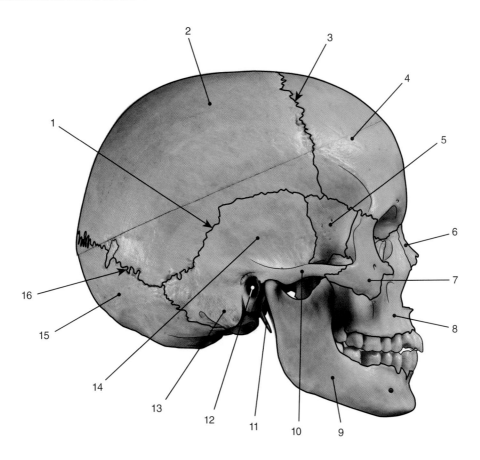

_____ Coronal suture

_____ External acoustic meatus

_____ Frontal bone

_____ Greater wing of sphenoid bone

_____ Lambdoid suture

_____ Mandible

_____ Mastoid process

_____ Maxilla

_____ Nasal bone

_____ Occipital bone

_____ Parietal bone

_____ Squamous suture

_____ Squamous portion of temporal bone

_____ Styloid process

_____ Zygomatic arch

_____ Zygomatic bone

Learning Activity 2-3

Cranial Base

Match the numbered structures with the correct terms listed below.

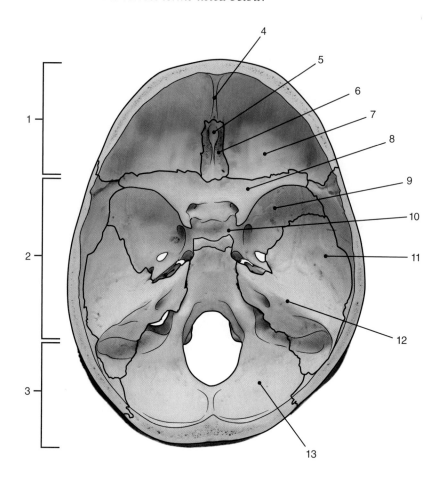

_____ Anterior cranial fossa

_____ Body of sphenoid bone

_____ Cribriform plate of ethmoid bone

_____ Greater wing of sphenoid bone

_____ Frontal crest

_____ Crista galli

_____ Lesser wing of sphenoid bone

_____ Middle cranial fossa

_____ Occipital bone

_____ Orbital plate of frontal bone

_____ Petrous ridge of temporal bone

_____ Posterior cranial fossa

_____ Squamous portion of temporal bone

Learning Activity 2-4

Inferior View of Skull

Match the numbered structures with the correct terms listed below.

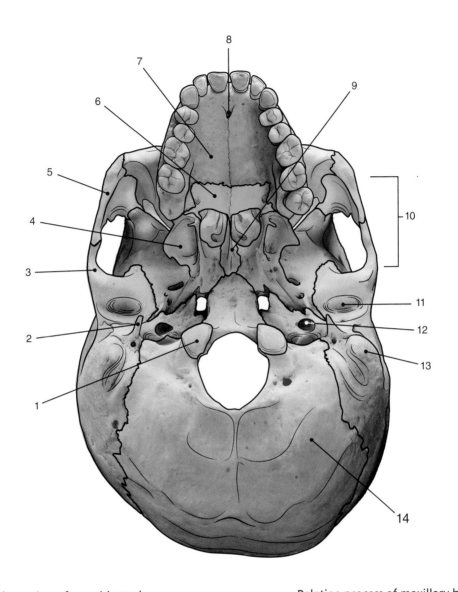

_____ External opening of carotid canal

_____ Horizontal plate of palatine bone

_____ Incisive canal

_____ Mandibular fossa

_____ Mastoid process

_____ Occipital condyle

_____ Occipital bone

_____ Palatine process of maxillary bone

_____ Pterygoid process of sphenoid bone

_____ Styloid process of temporal bone

_____ Temporal process of zygomatic bone

_____ Vomer

_____ Zygomatic arch

_____ Zygomatic process of temporal bone

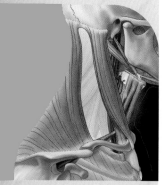

chapter

3

Regional Anatomy of the Neck

Objectives

1. Describe the compartmentalization of the neck into functional groups and the concept of dividing the neck into triangles.
2. Identify the boundaries of the anterior and posterior cervical triangles and their subsidiary triangles, and compare the major contents of each.
3. Compare the origin and insertion, innervation, and function of the muscles of the neck.

Overview

The term **neck** is defined as a constriction at the end of a bottle, a small stretch of land, or, in the case of the human body—a constriction that connects the head and trunk. Although the neck is short and narrow, it is very complex in structure and in function and is a good example of how studying regional anatomy is better than the systems approach. Let's first consider the contents of the neck.

Posteriorly, the neck is formed by the cervical vertebrae and the surrounding musculature. The vertebrae provide structural support, whereas the muscles flex, extend, and rotate the neck. In addition, the vertebrae surround and protect the spinal cord. Anteriorly, the neck contains the esophagus and trachea, which connect the entryways of the respiratory and digestive systems in the head to the functional organs in the trunk. This area of the neck also contains the vocal cords, which produce sound, and endocrine organs, which regulate the body's metabolic rate and calcium ion concentration in the blood. In addition, the salivary glands, which secrete saliva to cleanse the mouth and reduce the population of bacteria, are also located in the anterior portion of the neck. Blood vessels in the neck distribute and drain blood from the head, neck, and extremities, whereas lymphatic vessels collect lymph from the same regions. The nerves within the neck not only innervate the cervical structures but also contain nerve fibers that innervate the diaphragm and the viscera of the thorax and abdomen. The anterior cervical muscles assist in rotation of the neck, elevation and lowering of the pharynx during swallowing, and opening the mouth; as well as controlling the opening and closing of the vocal cords.

The relationship of all these structures would be difficult to understand by the systems approach. With the regional approach, the neck is divided into compartments of functional groups. Furthermore, the muscles are used to divide the neck into geometric forms—triangles—that are used to locate structures of the various organ systems.

INTRODUCTION TO THE ORGANIZATION OF THE NECK

The neck is covered on the surface by skin that rests on a layer of loose connective tissue referred to as the **superficial fascia**. The skin covering the anterior surface of the neck differs from the skin on most surfaces of the body in that it contains skeletal muscle, the **platysma muscle** (Fig. 3–1). This muscle originates from the fascia covering the pectoralis major and deltoid muscles (area of the second rib) and inserts onto the mandible and the corners of the mouth (Fig. 3–1). The platysma muscle is one of several muscles of facial expression that will be discussed in Chapter 5. Beneath the superficial fascia, there is a denser layer of connective tissue called the **deep fascia**, which covers the muscles, viscera, and neurovascular structures of the neck (Fig. 3–1). The deep fascia is further divided into three layers. The superficial layer or **investing fascia** surrounds the more superficial skeletal muscles of the neck. As a result, an outer **musculofascial collar**

is formed that functions to rotate the head and flex the neck. This layer also creates a **muscular compartment**, which contains a group of muscles that are associated with movements of the hyoid bone. A middle layer, called the **pretracheal fascia**, forms the **visceral compartment** by surrounding the visceral organs in the neck. The deep layer, or the **prevertebral fascia**, encloses the intrinsic muscles of the neck to form the **vertebral compartment**. Nerves and vessels of the **neurovascular compartment** are surrounded by the **carotid sheath**. This sheath is formed by a combination of connective tissue that originates from the blood vessels and investing and pretracheal fascia (Fig. 3–2).

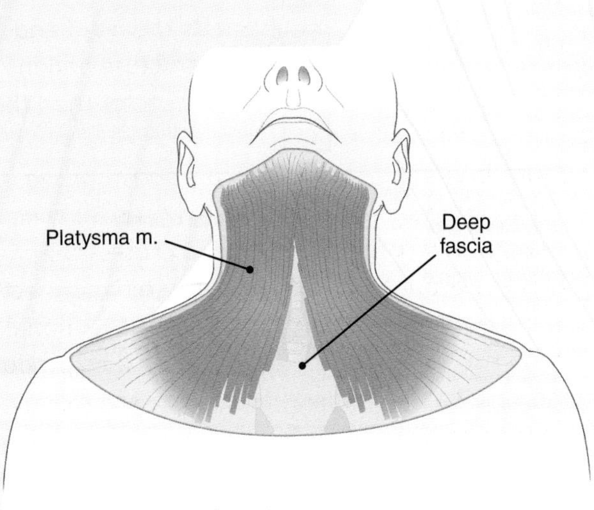

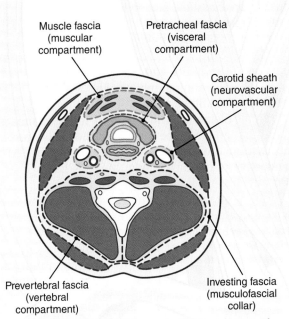

Figure 3–1 In the anterior neck, the platysma muscle is located in the superficial fascia next to the skin. The deep fascia lies underneath the platysma muscle.

Figure 3–2 Cross section of the neck. The three layers of the deep fascia compartmentalize the neck by splitting into investing fascia, muscular fascia, pretracheal fascia, prevertebral fascia, and carotid sheath, which surround structures within the neck.

To simplify the complexity of the neck from both clinical and anatomical viewpoints, the neck can be considered as a rectangular box with a top and bottom (Fig. 3–3). Three of its sides are formed by bone and muscle, whereas the fourth side is an imaginary line drawn through the median plane of the neck (Fig. 3–3). The top is formed by the investing fascia, whereas the bottom is formed by connective tissue and muscle. The rectangular neck is divided into two major triangles, namely the **anterior** and **posterior cervical triangles**, by the **sternocleidomastoid muscle**. These larger triangles are in turn divided into smaller subsidiary triangles (Fig. 3–3). Palpation of the borders of the triangles allows for the location of underlying structures such as blood vessels, nerves, glands, lymph nodes, and other muscles. Palpation of lymph nodes and salivary glands for signs of infection or cancer are essential components of a routine oral examination performed by the dental hygienist.

Review Question Box 3-1

1. What is the difference between the compartmentalization of the neck by fascia as compared to the division of the neck into triangles?

STRUCTURE OF SKELETAL MUSCLE

Muscles are classified anatomically by their appearance under the microscope as either smooth or striated. Striated muscle is subdivided into two groups: skeletal muscle and cardiac muscle. **Skeletal muscles** are those that move the joints and are grossly formed of two parts: the belly and the tendon (Fig. 3–4). The **belly** is the fleshy, middle part of the muscle that contains the contractile elements. The **tendon** is fibrous connective tissue that attaches the muscle to the skeleton, or, in the case of the muscles of facial expression, to the connective tissue of the skin. Muscles have generally two attachment sites. The **origin** of a muscle is the stationary attachment, whereas the **insertion** is the moveable attachment. As an example, the temporalis muscles, which closes the mouth (Fig. 3–4), has its origin on the bone of the skull and its insertion on the mandible (lower jaw). Note that the muscle or its tendon must cross over the joint for the contraction of the muscle to produce motion. Movements in the head and neck are not always associated with joints. For example, the muscles of facial expression affect the skin, whereas muscles attached to the hyoid bone raise and lower the bone while swallowing and speaking.

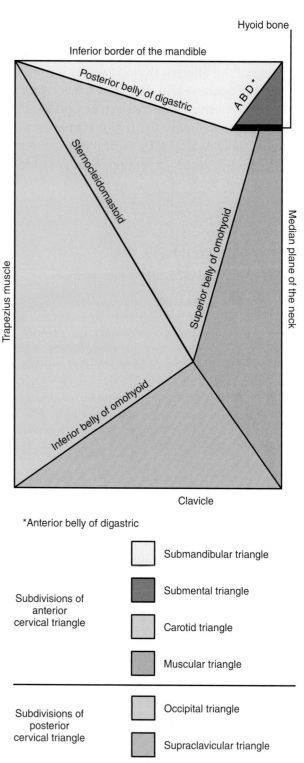

*Anterior belly of digastric

Subdivisions of anterior cervical triangle
- Submandibular triangle
- Submental triangle
- Carotid triangle
- Muscular triangle

Subdivisions of posterior cervical triangle
- Occipital triangle
- Supraclavicular triangle

Figure 3–3 In a lateral view, the neck can be compared to a rectangular box. The box is divided into two inverted right triangles by the diagonally oriented sternocleidomastoid muscle. The anterior and posterior cervical triangles are further divided into smaller triangles by cervical musculature.

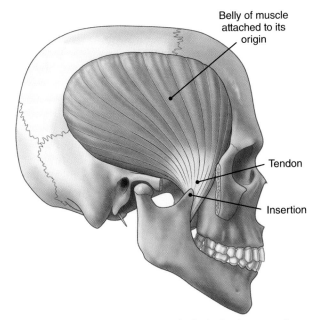

Belly of muscle attached to its origin

Tendon

Insertion

Figure 3–4 Muscles are composed of a belly that contains the contractile elements and tendons that attach muscle to bone. The origin is the immobile attachment site, whereas the insertion is the attachment to the moveable structure.

Some muscles are able to affect either attachment site. For example, muscles attached to the hyoid bone and mandible can either raise the hyoid bone during swallowing or help depress (lower) the mandible while opening the mouth.

Muscles are generally named according to (1) origin and insertion, (2) shape, or (3) function. As an example, the sternohyoid muscle originates from the sternum and attaches to the hyoid bone. The trapezius muscle of the back is named for its four-sided, diamond-shaped structure. On the other hand, the name of the levator labii superioris muscle describes its function as an elevator of the upper lip.

POSTERIOR CERVICAL TRIANGLE

The posterior boundary (side) of the triangle is the **trapezius** muscle, the anterior boundary (side) is the *sternocleidomastoid* muscle, and the inferior boundary or the base is formed by the middle third of the **clavicle** (Fig. 3–5). The trapezius muscle is a large muscle of the back. The portion that contributes to the posterior triangle originates from the external occipital protuberance of the occipital bone and inserts onto the spine of the scapula and the lateral third of the clavicle. Its major functions include movements of the scapula and support of the arm. The sternocleidomastoid muscle has two heads of

Box 3-1 Torticollis (Wryneck)

Torticollis literally means "twisted neck" and is caused by either congenital (at birth) or acquired shortening of the sternocleidomastoid muscle. The head of the individual is twisted toward the side of the lesion, whereas the chin is tilted upward toward the opposite side. Congenital torticollis can result from either malposition in the uterus or damage during childbirth. Damaged muscle can become fibrous, leading to the permanent shortening of the muscle. Acquired torticollis can be caused secondarily to previous conditions such as scars, injury to the vertebrae, inflammation of glands, and several others.

origin, the clavicular and the sternal heads, and inserts onto the mastoid process of the temporal bone. This muscle's function is to tilt and rotate the head (Table 3–1). Both muscles are innervated by the **accessory nerve (XI)**.

The *investing fascia*, which forms the roof of the triangle (Fig. 3–5), is attached posteriorly to the spines of the cervical vertebrae and splits to enclose the trapezius muscle (Fig. 3–2). After encircling the muscle, the two layers of the investing fascia fuse together and form the *roof* of the triangle. The fascia then splits to enclose the sternocleidomastoid muscle (Fig. 3–2) and fuses along the median plane of the neck. The *floor* of the triangle is formed by a carpetlike layer of fascia called the *prevertebral fascia*, which covers several muscles (Fig. 3–6), including the **anterior, middle,** and **posterior scalene muscles**, as well as the **levator scapulae** muscle (Fig. 3–7). The scalene muscles originate from the transverse process of the cervical vertebrae and attach to the first and second ribs. Contraction of these muscles flexes the neck and elevates the first and second ribs during forceful inspiration. The levator scapulae muscle also originates from the transverse processes of cervical vertebrae but inserts onto the scapula. Contraction of this muscle elevates the scapula. The scalene muscles and the levator scapulae muscle are innervated by branches of the **brachial plexus** (Table 3–1).

The posterior cervical triangle is divided into two smaller triangles by the **inferior belly of the omohyoid muscle**. The **occipital triangle**, which is the larger of the two triangles, is bordered by the trapezius muscle, the sternocleidomastoid muscle, and the inferior belly of the omohyoid muscle (Figs. 3–3 and 3–8). The smaller **supraclavicular triangle** is bordered by the inferior belly of the omohyoid muscle, the sternocleidomastoid muscle, and the clavicle (Fig. 3–8).

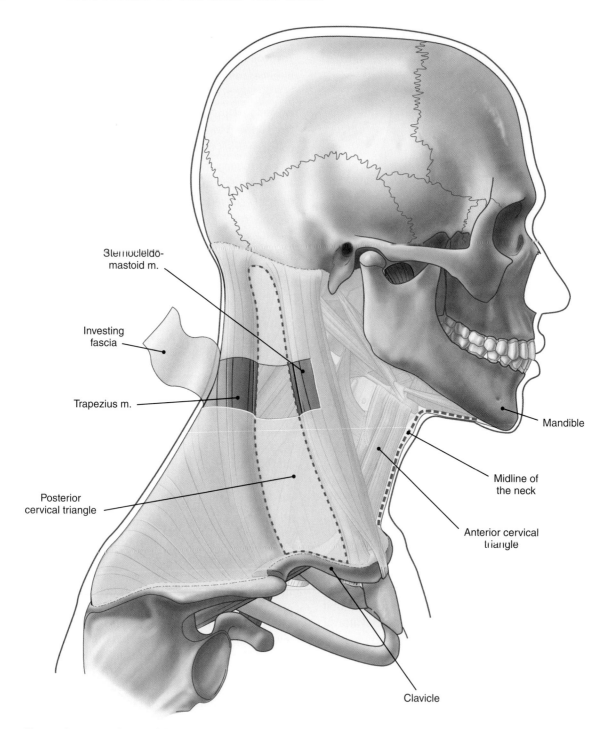

Sternocleido-
mastoid m.

Investing
fascia

Trapezius m.

Posterior
cervical triangle

Mandible

Midline of
the neck

Anterior cervical
triangle

Clavicle

Figure 3–5 Lateral view of the neck. The neck is divided into anterior and posterior cervical triangles by the sternocleidomastoid muscle. The investing fascia forms the roof of the triangles and encloses both the sternocleidomastoid and trapezius muscles.

Several structures of interest to the dental hygienist are located in, or pass through, the triangle. The *accessory nerve (XI)* passes along the roof of the occipital triangle to innervate the sternocleidomastoid and trapezius muscles (Fig. 3–6). The **subclavian artery** and **vein** are located in the supraclavicular triangle, whereas the **external jugular vein** penetrates the investing fascia to reach the subclavian vein (Fig. 3–7). Branches of the subclavian artery and tributaries of the subclavian vein also pass through the posterior

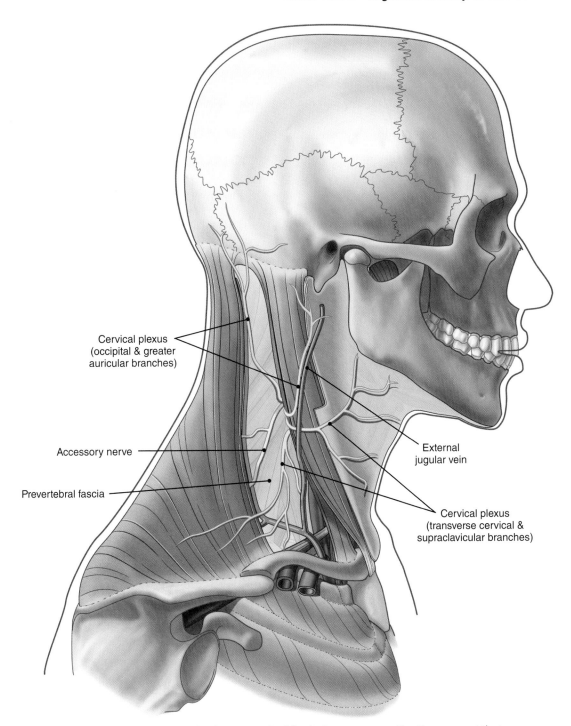

Cervical plexus
(occipital & greater
auricular branches)

Accessory nerve

Prevertebral fascia

External
jugular vein

Cervical plexus
(transverse cervical &
supraclavicular branches)

Figure 3–6 Lateral view of the neck. The prevertebral fascia forms a connective tissue carpet that creates a portion of the floor of the posterior cervical triangle. The muscles of the floor are covered by the connective tissue. The accessory nerve, cutaneous branches of the cervical plexus, and the external jugular vein pass through the triangle.

triangles but are generally not encountered by the dental hygienist because they supply muscles of the neck and scapula. The roots and trunks of the *brachial plexus (C5 to C8, T1)* emerge between the muscles of the floor of the posterior cervical triangle (Fig. 3–7)

to reach the upper extremity. In addition, cutaneous (skin) nerves from the **cervical plexus (C1 to C4)** pass through the triangle to reach the skin of the neck and shoulder (Fig. 3–6).

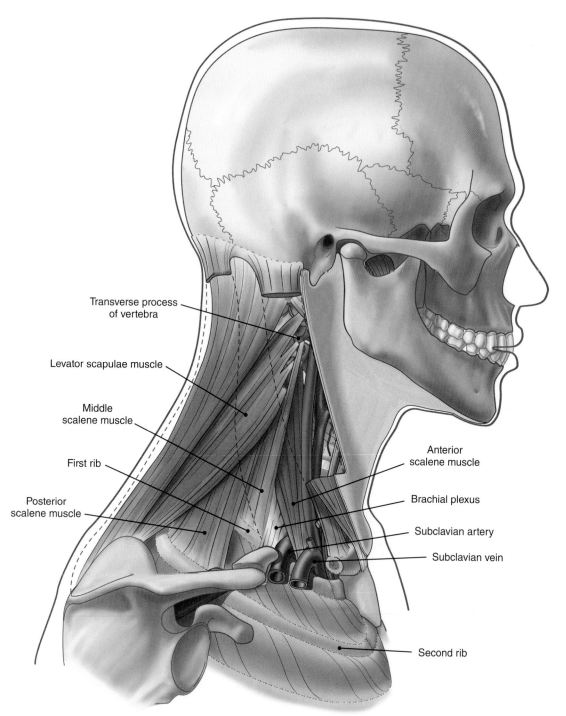

Transverse process
of vertebra

Levator scapulae muscle

Middle
scalene muscle

First rib

Posterior
scalene muscle

Anterior
scalene muscle

Brachial plexus

Subclavian artery

Subclavian vein

Second rib

Figure 3–7 In this lateral view of the neck, the trapezius and sternocleidomastoid muscles (dashed lines) have been cut to better visualize the floor of the posterior cervical triangle. The prevertebral fascia has been removed to expose the muscles of the floor of the posterior cervical triangle. The subclavian vein lies superficial to the anterior scalene muscle, whereas the subclavian artery and brachial plexus separate the anterior and middle scalene muscles.

The subclavian vessels and the brachial plexus can be used to distinguish the anterior scalene from the middle scalene muscle. The subclavian vein lies anterior or superficial to the anterior scalene muscle (Fig. 3–7). On the other hand, the subclavian artery and the brachial plexus are situated in between the anterior and middle scalene muscles (Fig. 3–7). The posterior scalene muscle is located deep and in between the middle scalene and levator scapulae muscles (Fig. 3–7).

Review Question Box 3-2

1. What is the relationship of the investing fascia and prevertebral fascia to the posterior cervical triangle?
2. What forms the boundaries of the posterior cervical triangle?
3. How does subdividing the posterior cervical triangle to smaller triangles convey structural relationships?
4. How is it possible to distinguish the muscles of the floor of the posterior cervical triangle?

ANTERIOR CERVICAL TRIANGLE

The *anterior cervical triangle* (Fig. 3–5) is inverted compared to the posterior cervical triangle in that the base is formed by a line drawn along the lower margin of the *mandible* to the mastoid process, whereas the sides are formed by the *sternocleidomastoid muscle* and an imaginary vertical line drawn from the chin to the manubrium (the *median plane* of the neck). This triangle is divided into several smaller triangles by the omohyoid and digastric muscles (Fig. 3–3). These triangles are the following:

a. Submandibular or digastric triangles (2)
b. Submental triangle (1)
c. Muscular triangles (2)
d. Carotid triangles (2)

The *omohyoid* muscle is composed of a *superior belly* and an *inferior belly*, which are connected by an *intermediate tendon* (Fig. 3–8). The inferior belly arises from the upper border of the scapula and inserts into an intermediate tendon that is attached to the clavicle by a sling of connective tissue. The superior belly ascends almost vertically to attach to the body of the hyoid bone. Both bellies depress (move downward) the hyoid bone while swallowing and speaking (Table 3–1). The **digastric** muscle is located inferior to the mandible. This muscle also has two bellies that are connected by an intermediate tendon (Figs. 3–8 and 3–9). The *posterior belly* arises from the mastoid process of the temporal bone and inserts onto its *intermediate tendon*, which is attached to the body of the hyoid bone by a connective tissue sling. The *anterior belly* sweeps anteriorly and superiorly to attach onto the mandible. Both bellies assist in either depressing the mandible or steadying the hyoid bone while swallowing and speaking (Table 3–1). The innervation of the digastric muscle is unusual in that the anterior belly is innervated by the **trigeminal nerve** (**V**) and the posterior belly is innervated by the **facial nerve** (**VII**).

Review Question Box 3-3

1. What are the boundaries of the anterior cervical triangle?
2. How are the digastric and omohyoid muscles similar in structure?

Submandibular Triangle

The inferior border of the *body of the mandible* and the *anterior* and *posterior bellies* of the *digastric muscle* form the boundaries of the **submandibular triangle** (Figs. 3–3 and 3–9). The triangle contains the **submandibular gland** and the **submandibular lymph nodes** and is crossed by the **facial artery** and **vein** as they course over the inferior border of the mandible to reach the face (Fig. 3–9). In addition to these visceral structures, the **stylohyoid muscle** is located within the triangle (Fig. 3–9). This muscle, which is innervated by the facial nerve (VII), arises from the styloid process of the temporal bone and inserts onto the hyoid bone. When contracted, the muscle elevates and retracts the hyoid bone (Table 3–1). The triangle is separated from the oral cavity by the **mylohyoid muscle** (Fig. 3–9) and other muscles of the floor of the mouth to be discussed in Chapter 8.

Review Question Box 3-4

1. Why does a proper dental examination include palpating the submandibular triangle?
2. What are the boundaries of the submandibular triangle?

Submental Triangle

The **submental triangle** is a small, unpaired area between the *anterior bellies* of the *digastric muscles* and the **hyoid bone** (Fig. 3–10). This triangle receives its name because it lies beneath the chin or **mentum**. The presence of the **submental lymph nodes** is of clinical interest to the dental hygienist. These nodes drain the incisor teeth, tip of the tongue, and anterior portion of the floor of the mouth. Enlargement of these lymph nodes can be a sign of inflammation or cancer in the oral cavity. The submental triangle is separated from the oral cavity by the *mylohyoid muscle* and other muscles of the floor of the mouth.

1. How is the submental triangle unique to the other triangles?
2. Why should palpation of the submental triangle be included in a dental examination?

Muscular Triangle

The *superior belly of the omohyoid muscle*, the anterior border *of the sternocleidomastoid muscle*, and the *anterior median plane* of the neck form the borders of the **muscular triangle** (Figs. 3–3 and 3–10). The latter receives its name because it contains the *infrahyoid* muscles. These muscles are also called the *strap* muscles because of their long, slender shape. The infrahyoid muscles act as a functional group to depress (lower) the hyoid bone while swallowing and speaking (Fig. 3–10; Table 3–1).

The muscles are divided into superficial and deep groups and are named according to their origins and their respective insertions onto the sternum, hyoid bone, and thyroid cartilage. Superficially, the *superior belly of the omohyoid muscle* is located lateral to the **sternohyoid muscle**. The sternohyoid muscle originates from the manubrium of the sternum and inserts onto the hyoid bone. The two deep muscles are the **sternothyroid** and **thyrohyoid** (Fig. 3–10). All these muscles, with the exception of the thyrohyoid, are innervated by branches of the **ansa cervicalis**, which is a nerve loop formed from spinal roots *C1 to*

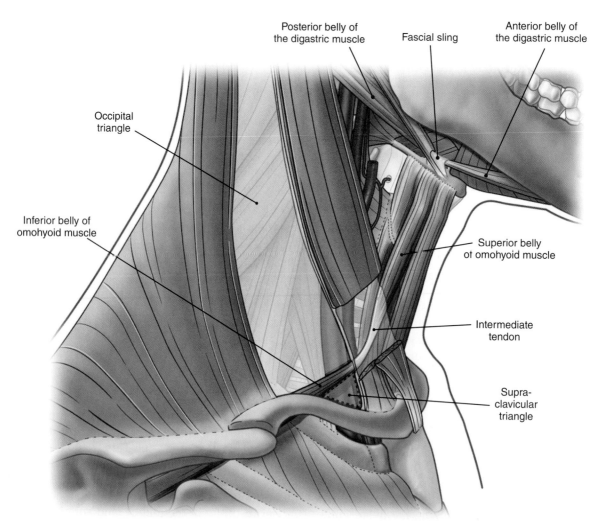

Figure 3–8 Lateral view of the neck. The inferior and superior bellies of the omohyoid muscle are separated by an intermediate tendon that is attached to the clavicle by a connective tissue sling. The inferior belly divides the posterior cervical triangle into the larger occipital triangle and the smaller supraclavicular triangle. Similarly, the anterior and posterior bellies of the diagastric muscle are connected by an intermediate tendon located in the fascial sling.

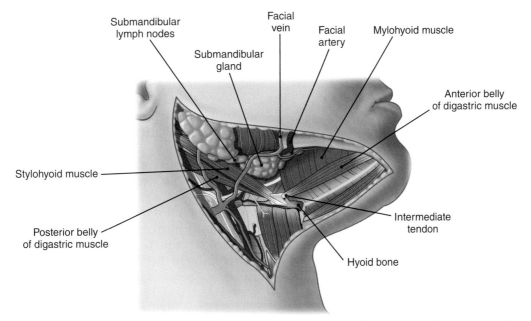

Figure 3–9 Lateral view of the neck. The submandibular triangle is bordered by the inferior border of the mandible and the anterior and posterior bellies of the digastric muscle, which are joined by an intermediate tendon that attaches to the hyoid bone by a connective tissue sling. The triangle contains the submandibular gland, the submandibular lymph nodes, the stylohyoid muscle, and the facial artery and vein. The mylohyoid muscle separates the triangle from the floor of the mouth.

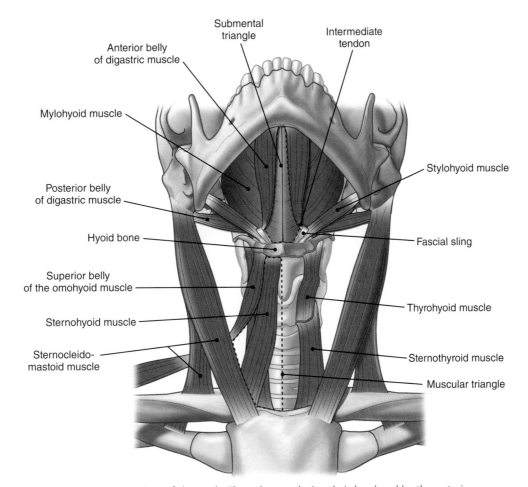

Figure 3–10 Anterior view of the neck. The submental triangle is bordered by the anterior and posterior bellies of the digastric muscle and the hyoid bone. The triangle contains lymph nodes and is separated from the floor of the mouth by the mylohyoid muscle. The muscular triangle contains the strap muscles. The superior belly of the omohyoid and the sternohyoid muscles are superficial to the deep group composed of the sternothyroid and thyrohyoid muscles.

C3 that comprise part of the cervical plexus. The thyrohyoid muscle is innervated directly by spinal nerve C1 (Table 3–1).

Review Question Box 3-6

1. Is the superior belly of the omohyoid muscle actually within the muscular triangle?
2. What is the ansa cervicalis?
3. What effect would the contraction of the infrahyoid muscles have on the hyoid bone?

Carotid Triangle

The *posterior belly of the digastric*, the *superior belly of the omohyoid*, and *the anterior border of the sternocleidomastoid* muscles form the boundaries of the carotid triangle (Figs. 3–3 and 3–11A). Within the triangle, the common carotid artery, the internal carotid artery, the internal jugular vein, and the vagus nerve are enclosed in a dense, tubular sheath of connective tissue called the *carotid sheath* (Figs. 3–2 and 3–11A). The sheath extends from the base of the skull to merge with the connective tissue of the great vessels of the heart. The **common carotid artery** bifurcates (divides) into the **internal carotid** and **external carotid arteries** (Figs. 3–11A and 3–11B). The internal carotid artery is one of two major arteries that supply

the brain, whereas the external carotid is the major distributing artery to the head and neck. Five branches of the external carotid artery arise in this triangle: (1) the superior thyroid artery, (2) the ascending pharyngeal artery, (3) the lingual artery, (4) the facial artery, and (5) the occipital artery (to be discussed in Chapter 11). In addition, there are several important nerves. The **hypoglossal nerve** courses through the triangle en route to innervate the tongue. The *ansa cervicalis*, which is formed by the motor fibers of C1 to C3 of the cervical plexus, innervates the strap muscles that are located in the muscular triangle (Fig. 3–11B). The *vagus nerve* is a complex nerve that supplies taste fibers to the epiglottis; motor fibers to the muscles of the pharynx, larynx, and palate; and autonomic and sensory fibers to the viscera of the thorax and abdomen (to be discussed in Chapter 15). The **internal jugular vein**, also located in the triangle (Fig. 3–11B), carries deoxygenated blood from the brain and from structures of the neck to the great veins of the heart (to be discussed in Chapter 11).

Review Question Box 3-7

1. What muscle separates the carotid triangle from the submandibular triangle?
2. What compartment of the neck lies in the carotid triangle?
3. What nerves are located within the carotid triangle?
4. To which structures does the term "carotid triangle" refer?

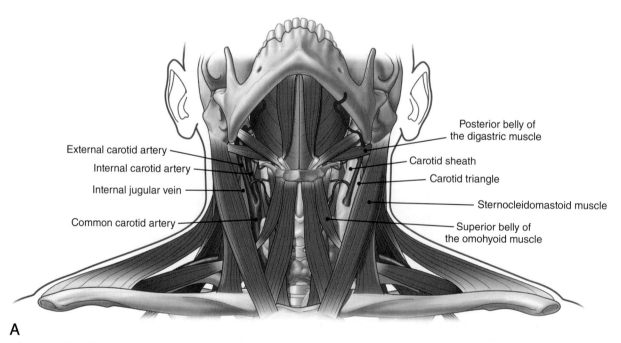

Figure 3–11 (A) Anterior view of the neck. The carotid triangle is enclosed by the sternocleidomastoid, superior belly of the omohyoid, and posterior belly of the digastric muscles. On the left side, the carotid sheath encloses major blood vessels and nerves, whereas on the right side the sheath has been removed to reveal its contents.

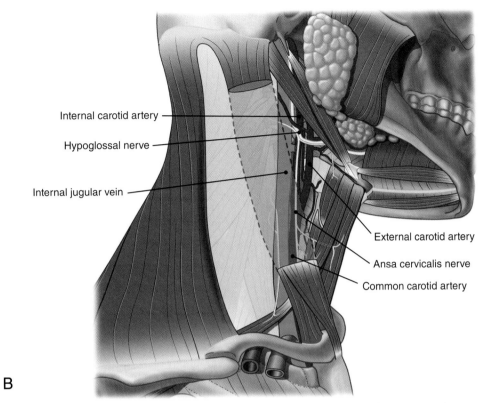

Internal carotid artery

Hypoglossal nerve

Internal jugular vein

External carotid artery

Ansa cervicalis nerve

Common carotid artery

B

Figure 3–11—cont'd (B) Lateral view of the neck. The carotid sheath has been removed to expose the internal jugular vein, the common carotid artery, and the internal carotid artery. The hypoglossal nerve and the ansa cervicalis are located superficial to the sheath. The vagus nerve is hidden by the vessels. Five branches of the external carotid artery are located within the triangle for which the triangle is named.

TABLE 3–1	Muscles of the Triangles of the Neck			
Muscle	**Origin**	**Insertion**	**Action**	**Innervation**
Sternocleidomastoid	Sternum and clavicle	Mastoid process of the temporal bone	Tilts and rotates the head	Accessory nerve
Trapezius (superior fibers)	External occipital protuberance	Spine of the scapula and lateral one-third of the clavicle	Moves the scapula and supports the arm	Accessory nerve
Anterior scalene	Transverse processes of the cervical vertebrae	First rib	Elevates the rib during forced breathing	Brachial plexus
Middle scalene	Transverse processes of the cervical vertebrae	First rib	Elevates the rib during forced breathing	Brachial plexus
Posterior scalene	Transverse processes of the cervical vertebrae	Second rib	Elevates the rib during forced breathing	Brachial plexus
Levator scapulae	Transverse processes of the cervical vertebrae	Superomedial border of the scapula	Elevates the scapula	Brachial plexus
Superior belly of the omohyoid	Upper border of the scapula	Hyoid bone	Depresses the hyoid bone while swallowing and speaking	Ansa cervicalis
Inferior belly of the omohyoid	Upper border of the scapula	Hyoid bone	Depresses the hyoid bone while swallowing and speaking	Ansa cervicalis

continued

TABLE 3–1	Muscles of the Triangles of the Neck—cont'd			
Muscle	Origin	Insertion	Action	Innervation
Anterior belly of the digastric	Mandible	Hyoid bone	Assists in depressing the mandible; raises and steadies the hyoid bone during swallowing and speaking	Trigeminal nerve
Posterior belly of the digastric	Mastoid process	Hyoid bone	Assists in depressing the mandible; raises and steadies the hyoid bone during swallowing and speaking	Facial nerve
Stylohyoid	Styloid process	Hyoid bone	Elevates and retracts the hyoid bone	Facial nerve
Sternohyoid	Manubrium	Hyoid bone	Depresses the hyoid bone while swallowing and speaking	Ansa cervicalis
Sternothyroid	Manubrium	Thyroid cartilage	Depresses the hyoid bone while swallowing and speaking	Ansa cervicalis
Thyrohyoid	Thyroid cartilage	Hyoid bone	Depresses the hyoid bone while swallowing and speaking	C1

SUMMARY

The neck is a complex structure that contains components of many organ systems. The structural relationships can be better understood by dividing the neck into fascial compartments and triangles. The neck is covered by skin and superficial fascia. The skin on the anterior surface of the neck contains the platysma muscle, a muscle of facial expression. The next layer of fascia beneath the superficial layer is called the deep fascia. This layer is complex and is subdivided into the investing fascia, the pretracheal fascia, the prevertebral fascia, and the carotid sheath. These fascial layers divide the neck into tubular compartments that separate muscles, viscera, blood vessels, and nerves. The neck is divided into anterior and posterior cervical triangles by the sternocleidomastoid muscles to localize structures. Other muscles in the neck divide these primary triangles into smaller triangles that allow structures to be pinpointed more accurately.

LEARNING LAB

Exercises for review, practice, and study

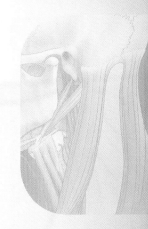

Laboratory Activity 3-1

Draw and Label the Triangles of the Neck

Learning the complexity of the neck can be simplified by learning to draw and label the boundaries of the cervical triangles of the neck and then assigning what structures can be found within the triangles.

Objective: In this exercise, you will draw and label the boundaries of the neck using Figure 3.3 as a guide. The exact dimensions are not important but are given to you to aid in drawing the diagram and allow you space to label structures. Do not be concerned about the accuracy of your measurements with a ruler. Anatomically, recognize that the triangles of the neck are the areas between but do not include the boundaries that create the space.

Materials Needed: Ruler, paper, and pencil. *Optional:* Photocopy of Figure 3.3.

Step 1: First, draw a rectangle that is 8 inches high and 5½ inches wide. Label the rectangle to represent boundaries of the lateral view of the neck.

- The upper side of the rectangle is the *inferior border* of the *mandible*.
- The left side is the *trapezius muscle*.
- The lower side is the *middle third* of the *clavicle*.
- The right side is an imaginary line drawn through the *median plane* of the neck.

Step 2: Draw a diagonal line from the upper left-hand corner to the lower right-hand corner. The rectangle has been divided into two inverted right triangles.

- Label the triangle on the left as the *posterior cervical triangle* and the triangle on the right as the *anterior cervical triangle*.
- The diagonal line represents the *sternocleidomastoid muscle*.

Step 3: Starting in the upper right-hand corner (where the mandible and median plane of the neck intersect), measure downward a distance of 1½ inches and extend a horizontal line approximately 1 inch to the left (inside the anterior cervical triangle).

- Label this line the *hyoid bone*.

Step 4: Begin in the lower right-hand corner (where the clavicle and the median plane of the neck intersect), and measure 3 inches along the diagonal line (*sternocleidomastoid muscle*) and mark the line.

- Start at the lower left-hand corner (intersection of the clavicle and the trapezius muscle), and draw a line to the 3-inch mark and continue upward to the midpoint of the line representing the *hyoid bone*.
- Label the line in the posterior triangle of the neck (left triangle) as the *inferior belly of the omohyoid muscle*, and the line in the anterior triangle of the neck (inverted right triangle) as the *superior belly of the omohyoid muscle*.

Step 5: For the next line, begin at the upper left-hand corner (intersection of the mandible with the trapezius muscle) of the posterior cervical triangle, and draw a line to the distal end of the line representing the hyoid bone.

- Label this line as the *posterior belly of the digastric muscle*.

Step 6: Finally, draw a line from the upper right-hand corner (intersection of the mandible and the median plane of the neck) of the anterior cervical triangle to the same point on the distal end of the hyoid bone.

- Label this line as the *anterior belly of the digastric bone*.

Step 7:   Note that the posterior cervical triangle has been divided into two smaller triangles, and the anterior cervical triangle has been divided into four. To complete the diagram, label these smaller triangles.

- In the posterior cervical triangle, the *occipital triangle* is outlined by the trapezius, the sternocleidomastoid, and the inferior belly of the omohyoid muscles.
- The *supraclavicular triangle* is bordered by the inferior belly of the omohyoid muscle, the sternocleidomastoid muscle, and the clavicle.
- In the anterior cervical triangle, the *submental triangle* is formed by the two anterior bellies of the digastric and the hyoid bone. Why is the median plane of the neck not included? If you answered that the submental triangle is a single triangle, you are correct.
- The *submandibular triangle* is bordered by the anterior and posterior bellies of the digastric muscle and the inferior border of the mandible.
- The *carotid triangle* is enclosed by the sternocleidomastoid, the superior belly of the omohyoid, and the posterior belly of the digastric muscles.
- The *muscular triangle* is formed by the superior belly of the omohyoid muscle, the sternocleidomastoid muscle, and the median plane of the neck.

Step 8:   Realize that the neck is a three-dimensional structure and is represented by a triangular box with four sides, a top, and a bottom. You have drawn the four sides. The cover of the box represents the *investing fascia* of the neck, which forms the *roof* of the triangle. The bottom of the box is equivalent to the *floor* of the posterior triangle of the neck, formed by the prevertebral fascia and muscle.

For Discussion or Thought:

1. *What side of the neck is represented?*

2. *How would drawing a line from the upper right-hand corner to the lower left-hand corner affect the labeling of the diagram?*

Learning Activity 3-1

Triangles and Muscles of the Neck

Match the numbered structures with the correct terms listed to the right.

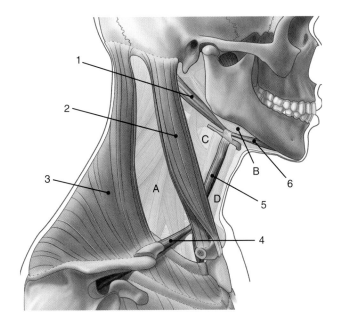

_____ Anterior belly of digastric muscle

_____ Carotid triangle

_____ Inferior belly of the omohyoid muscle

_____ Muscular triangle

_____ Posterior belly of the digastric muscle

_____ Posterior triangle (specifically occipital triangle)

_____ Sternocleidomastoid muscle

_____ Submandibular triangle

_____ Superior belly of the omohyoid muscle

_____ Trapezius muscle

Learning Activity 3-2

Posterior Cervical Triangle

Match the numbered structures with the correct terms listed to the right.

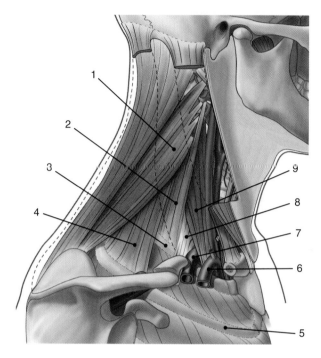

_____ Anterior scalene muscle

_____ Brachial plexus

_____ First rib

_____ Levator scapulae muscle

_____ Middle scalene muscle

_____ Posterior scalene muscle

_____ Second rib

_____ Subclavian artery

_____ Subclavian vein

Learning Activity 3-3

Submental and Muscular Triangles

Match the numbered structures with the correct terms listed below.

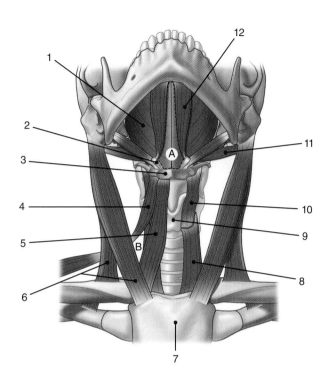

_____ Anterior belly of digastric muscle

_____ Connective tissue sling

_____ Hyoid bone

_____ Muscular triangle

_____ Mylohyoid muscle

_____ Posterior belly of the digastric muscle

_____ Sternocleidomastoid muscle

_____ Sternohyoid muscle

_____ Sternothyroid muscle

_____ Sternum

_____ Superior belly of the omohyoid muscle

_____ Submental triangle

_____ Thyrohyoid muscle

_____ Thyroid cartilage

Learning Activity 3-4

Contents of the Submandibular and Carotid Triangle

Match the numbered structures with the correct terms listed to the right.

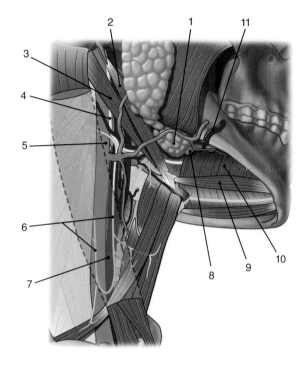

_____ Ansa cervicalis

_____ Anterior belly of the digastric muscle

_____ Common carotid artery

_____ Facial artery

_____ Hypoglossal nerve

_____ Internal jugular vein

_____ Lymph node

_____ Mylohyoid muscle

_____ Posterior belly of the digastric muscle

_____ Stylohyoid muscle

_____ Submandibular gland

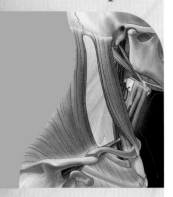

4

Pharynx, Larynx, and Soft Palate

Objectives

1. Identify and compare the boundaries of the three subdivisions of the pharynx.
2. Identify the muscles of the soft palate and pharynx and know their functions and innervations.
3. Identify and compare the structural features of the oro-, naso-, and laryngeal pharynx and larynx.

Overview

How does air from the nose reach the lungs, and how does food from the mouth reach the stomach? Many would say that the air must pass through the "windpipe" or trachea to enter into the lungs and that food must pass through the esophagus to reach the stomach. However, air and food must first pass through another passageway: the pharynx. The pharynx is a semimuscular tube that connects the nasal cavity to the trachea and the mouth to the esophagus.

INTRODUCTION TO THE PHARYNX, LARYNX, AND SOFT PALATE

The **pharynx** is a shared passageway of the respiratory and the digestive systems. It is divided into three parts: (1) the *nasopharynx*, (2) the *oropharynx*, and (3) the *laryngeal pharynx* (Fig. 4–1). Inspired air from the nasal cavity passes into the nasopharynx via two openings in the posterior wall of the nasal cavity. Similarly, ingested food and fluid enter the oropharynx through an opening between the pharynx and the oral cavity. Food and fluids

from the mouth and air from the nose cross paths in the pharynx to enter into the trachea and the esophagus. Air entering the nasopharynx from the nasal cavities courses in an anteroinferior direction to enter the respiratory passages; conversely, food and fluids from the oral cavity course in a posteroinferior direction to enter the esophagus (Fig. 4–1). Because of this unusual arrangement, the pharynx has been adapted to protect food from entering the airways. The soft palate, which extends from the posterior surface of the hard palate, acts as flap that can be elevated to prevent food and fluid from refluxing into

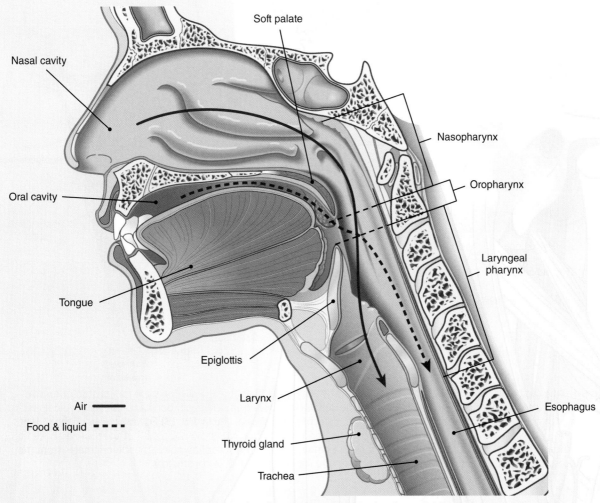

Figure 4–1 A sagittal section through the head and neck demonstrates the three divisions of the pharynx. The oropharynx lies posterior to the mouth between the dashed lines. The oropharynx is separated from the nasopharynx superiorly by the soft palate and the laryngeal pharynx and inferiorly by the epiglottis. The pathways for food (red arrow) and air (blue arrow) cross in the pharynx.

the nasal cavity. Elevation of the epiglottis of the larynx protects the opening of the airways and prevents ingested material from entering the lungs.

The larynx and the soft palate are not considered a part of the pharynx, but are included in this chapter because of their anatomical and functional relationships.

MUSCLES OF THE PHARYNGEAL WALL

Although the *pharynx* is described as a tubular muscular organ, only the posterolateral portion of the pharynx is enclosed by muscle (Figs. 4–2A and 4–2B). The muscular wall is composed of three circularly arranged constrictor muscles and three pairs of longitudinally oriented muscles. The constrictor muscles constrict or narrow the pharynx, thus forcing the bolus of food toward the esophagus.

The longitudinal muscles raise and widen the superior end of the pharynx while swallowing.

Constrictor Muscles

The constrictor muscles overlap as if stacking three funnels on top of each other (Figs. 4–2A and 4–2B). The **superior pharyngeal constrictor muscle** arises from the **pterygomandibular raphe** (Fig. 4–3) and its attachment to the **pterygoid hamulus** of the medial pterygoid plate of the sphenoid bone (Fig. 4–3) and the body of the **mandible** (Fig. 4–2A). The superior constrictor shares the same line of attachment as the **buccinator muscle** (muscle of facial expression), which is the pterygomandibular raphe (Fig. 4–3). The **middle pharyngeal constrictor muscle** arises from the lower end of the **stylohyoid ligament** and the **hyoid bone** (Fig. 4–2A).

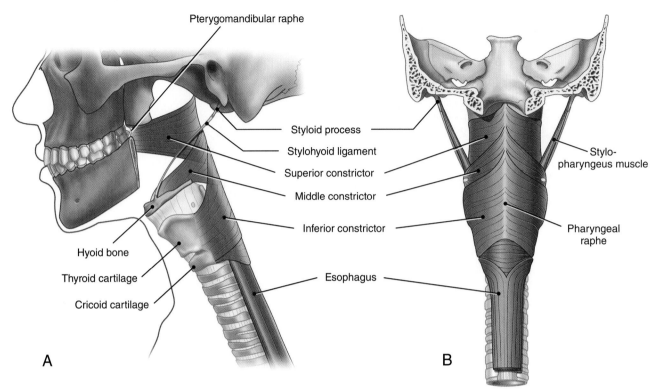

Figure 4–2 (A) Lateral view of the overlapping muscles of the external pharyngeal wall. The superior constrictor muscle originates from the pterygomandibular raphe, the middle constrictor arises from the hyoid bone and the stylohyoid ligament, and the inferior constrictor originates from the thyroid and cricoid cartilages of the larynx. **(B)** Posterior view of the muscles of the external pharyngeal wall. The superior, middle, and inferior constrictor muscles overlap so that the muscle above fits inside the muscle below. These muscles insert onto the pharyngeal raphe. The stylopharyngeus muscle originates from the styloid process and inserts in the pharyngeal wall between the superior and middle constrictors.

The **inferior pharyngeal constrictor muscle** arises from the **thyroid** and **cricoid cartilages** (Fig. 4–2A). All three muscles insert on a connective tissue partition, the **pharyngeal raphe**, which courses along the posterior median plane of the pharynx (Fig. 4–2B). The sequential constriction (**peristalsis**) of these muscles pushes the bolus of food from the oral cavity toward the stomach (Table 4–1).

Longitudinal Muscles

The three longitudinal muscles that contribute to the pharyngeal wall are the stylopharyngeus, palatopharyngeus, and the salpingopharyngeus muscles. The actions of all three muscles are to elevate and to widen the superior portion of the pharynx during swallowing. Of the three muscles, only the stylopharyngeus can be viewed from the exterior surface. The **stylopharyngeus muscle** arises from the **styloid process** of the temporal bone and inserts onto the lateral wall of the pharynx between the superior and middle constrictor muscles and thyroid cartilage (Fig. 4–2B). The salpingopharyngeus muscle arises from the cartilages of the auditory tube and will be discussed with the nasopharynx. The palatopharyngeus muscle is a shared muscle of the soft palate and the oropharynx and will be discussed in a later section.

All of the muscles of the pharynx are innervated by the **vagus nerve** (**X**), except for the stylopharyngeus muscle, which is innervated by the **glossopharyngeal nerve** (**IX**) (Table 4–1).

Review Question Box 4-1

1. What is the significance of the overlapping of the constrictor muscles? (*Hint: Think about the passage of food and fluids through the pharynx.*)

INTERNAL STRUCTURE OF THE PHARYNX

As already mentioned, the pharynx is a shared passageway of the respiratory and digestive systems. It is divided into three subdivisions: (1) nasopharynx, (2) oropharynx, and (3) laryngeal pharynx. The nasopharynx and oropharynx are separated by the **soft palate**, whereas the oropharynx and laryngeal pharynx are separated by the **epiglottis** (Fig. 4–4). Each subdivision has unique internal features.

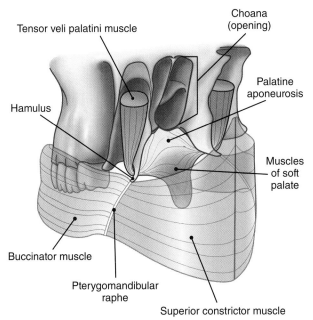

Figure 4–3 The pharynx has been cut through a horizontal plane of the nasopharynx just superior to the attachment of the buccinator to the mandible (not shown). The superior constrictor of the pharynx and the buccinator muscle of the face share a common attached site called the *pterygomandibular raphe*. The choanae are the posterior openings of the nasal cavity into the nasopharynx. The tensor veli palatini muscle and other muscles of the soft palate attach to the palatine aponeurosis, which extends from the posterior border of the hard palate.

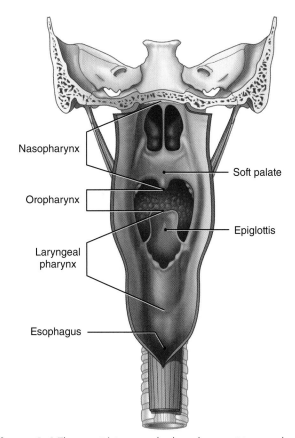

Figure 4–4 The constrictor muscles have been cut to reveal the internal structure of the pharynx. The nasal cavities are connected posterior to the nasopharynx via the choana. This portion of the pharynx is separated from the owl-shaped oropharynx by the soft palate. The laryngeal pharynx lies posteriorly to the larynx and is separated from the oropharynx by the epiglottis. The laryngeal pharynx is the entranceway into the esophagus.

Nasopharynx

Although the **nasopharynx** is a tubular structure, only the posterior wall is formed by muscle. The nasopharynx is located posterior to the nasal cavities (Figs. 4–1 and 4–4). The anterior wall is characterized by two openings, or **choanae**, that connect the nasal cavity and the nasopharynx (Figs. 4–3 and 4–9). The **pharyngeal tonsils** are located along the superior wall of the nasopharynx posterior to the choana (Fig. 4–5A). The tonsils sample the

inhaled air for antigens (foreign substances). When inflamed, these structures are called the *adenoids*; however, these tonsils generally degenerate with age.

The openings of the **auditory** (eustachian) **tubes** are located on the lateral wall of the nasopharynx.

TABLE 4–1	Muscles of the Pharynx			
Muscle	**Origin**	**Insertion**	**Action**	**Innervation**
Superior pharyngeal constrictor	Pterygoid hamulus, pterygo-mandibular ligament, and the posterior end of the mylohyoid line	Pharyngeal raphe	Constricts the pharynx	Vagus nerve
Middle pharyngeal constrictor	Stylohyoid ligament and lesser horn of the hyoid bone	Pharyngeal raphe	Constricts the pharynx	Vagus nerve
Inferior pharyngeal constrictor	Thyroid and cricoid cartilages	Pharyngeal raphe	Constricts the pharynx	Vagus nerve
Stylopharyngeus	Styloid process	Lateral pharyngeal wall	Elevates the pharynx during swallowing	Glossopharyngeal nerve
Salpingopharyngeus	Auditory tube	Lateral pharyngeal wall	Elevates the pharynx during swallowing	Vagus nerve

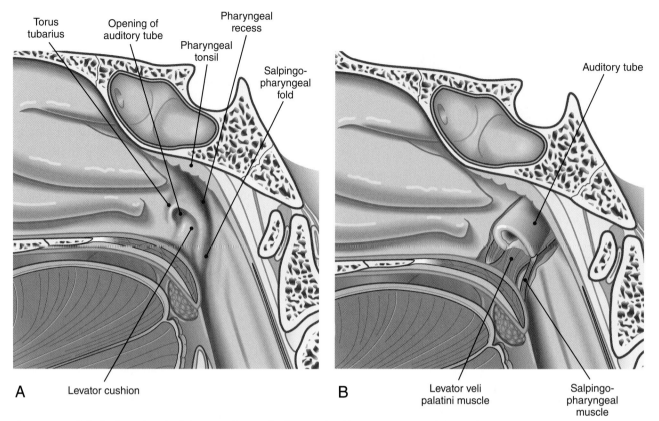

Figure 4–5 (A) The lateral wall of the nasopharynx is characterized by the opening of the auditory tube that is shielded by the torus tubarius. The pharyngeal tonsils are located superior to the torus. The salpingopharyngeal fold arises from the posterior surface of the torus and the levator cushion extends medially from the opening of the auditory tube. The pharyngeal recess lies posterior to this fold. **(B)** The mucosa of the lateral wall has been removed to reveal the cartilage of the auditory tube, the origin of the salpingopharyngeus muscle, and the insertion of the levator veli palatini muscle on the soft palate.

The opening is partially shielded by a horseshoe-shaped fold of mucosa called the **torus tubarius** (Fig. 4–5A). Posterior to this structure, the nasopharynx expands laterally to form the **pharyngeal recess** (Fig. 4–5A). Extending inferiorly from the torus tubarius is a fold of mucosa, the **salpingopharyngeal fold** (Fig. 4–5A) that overlies the **salpingopharyngeal muscle**, one of the longitudinal muscles of the pharynx. This slender muscle arises from the cartilages of the auditory tube (*salpingo* refers to the auditory tube) and inserts onto the lateral pharyngeal wall (Fig. 4–5B; Table 4–1). The levator cushion is a fold of mucosa that extends medially from the auditory tube (Fig. 4–5A). The mucosa covers the levator veli palatini muscle of the palate, which will be discussed in a later section (Fig. 4–5B).

Review Question Box 4-2

1. What is the difference between the torus tubarius and the auditory tube?
2. What structures produce the folds in the nasopharynx?

Oropharynx and Soft Palate
Oropharynx

The **oropharynx** is located posterior to the oral cavity and is separated from the nasopharynx by the *soft palate* (Fig. 4–4). From an anterior view, there are two vertical folds of oral mucosa that are separated by the **palatine tonsils**. The folds resemble a column or pillar and many clinicians refer to them as the **anterior** and **posterior tonsillar pillars** (Fig. 4–6A), but are referred to anatomically as the palatoglossal and palatopharyngeal folds (Fig. 4–6B). The **palatoglossal folds** extend from the free border of the soft palate and attach to the lateral surface of the tongue, whereas the **palatopharyngeal folds** blend with the lateral wall of the oropharynx (Figs. 4–6B, 4–7A, and 4–8). Anatomists refer to the anterior tonsillar pillars as the *palatoglossal folds* (Fig. 4–7A) because the mucosa covers the **palatoglossus muscles** of the soft palate (Fig. 4–7B). Likewise, the posterior tonsillar pillars are called the *palatopharyngeal folds* (Fig. 4–7A) because the mucosa covers the **palatopharyngeus muscle** (Fig. 4–7B). The *palatine tonsils* lie in a depression

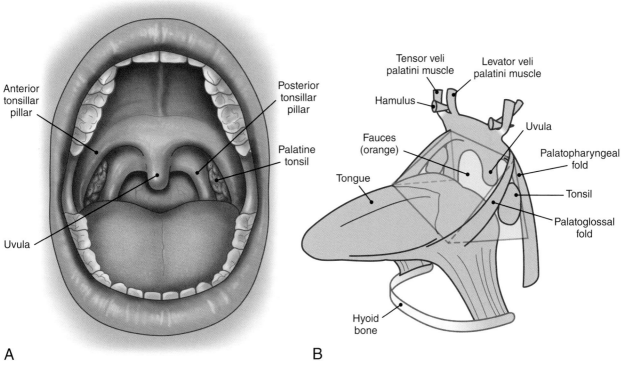

Figure 4–6 (A) The anterior view of the open mouth illustrates how the anterior and posterior tonsillar pillars enclose the palatine tonsils. The uvula is the conspicuous downward projection of the free border of the soft palate. **(B)** The fauces or throat is the pyramidal space between the anterior tonsillar pillars (glossopharyngeal folds) and the posterior tonsillar pillar (palatopharyngeal folds) and the tongue. The planar opening between the anterior tonsillar pillars (glossopharyngeal folds) is known as the *isthmus of the fauces.*

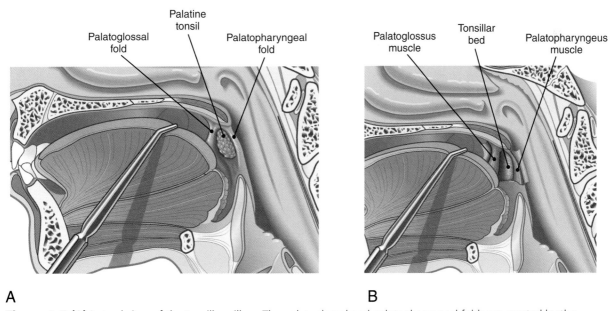

Figure 4–7 (A) Lateral view of the tonsillar pillars. The palatoglossal and palatopharyngeal folds are created by the mucosa covering underlying muscles of the same name. The palatine tonsils lie in between the two folds. **(B)** The mucosa has been removed to reveal the palatopharyngeus muscle and the palatoglossus muscle. The palatoglossus muscle inserts into the tongue, whereas the palatopharyngeus muscle inserts onto the lateral pharyngeal wall. The palatine tonsil has been removed to show the tonsillar bed.

between the palatoglossal and palatopharyngeal folds called the **tonsillar bed** (Fig. 4–7B). The merging of the two palatoglossal folds forms an archway called the *palatoglossal arch*, which separates the oral cavity and the oral pharynx. The palatopharyngeal folds form a similar arch called the *palatopharyngeal arch*, which separates the oropharynx from the nasopharynx. The pyramidal space bordered by the palatoglossal and palatopharyngeal folds (arches), the palatine tonsils, and the dorsal surface of the tongue is called the **fauces** or *throat* (Figs. 4–6B and 4–8). The entranceway into the throat is formed by the palatoglossal arch and is called the **isthmus of the fauces** (Fig. 4–6B). When the palatine tonsils become inflamed, the fauces is narrowed and the throat becomes sore.

In addition to the features of the lateral wall, other structures are found along the anterior wall of the oropharynx. The tongue is divided into two parts by a V-shaped line called the *sulcus terminalis* (Fig. 4–8). The posterior one-third or the **root** of the tongue is located in

the oropharynx. The root's surface is covered by the **lingual tonsils** (Fig. 4–8). As with the palatine tonsils, the lingual tonsils sample the oral cavity for antigens. The tongue is attached to the epiglottis by three folds of the mucosa. A single **median** and two **lateral glossoepiglottic folds** extend from the base of the tongue and attach to mucosa of the *epiglottis* of the larynx (Fig. 4–8). The folds create spaces or depressions located in between the folds. These spaces are collectively called the **epiglottic vallec- ulae** and represent areas where food or other ingested for- eign objects (such as small objects swallowed by children) can be trapped in the throat. It is also possible that debris from dental procedures, such excess dental materials, can be swallowed and trapped in these spaces and cause the patient to choke and gag. (Reflexes associated with the oral cavity will be discussed in Chapter 19.)

Box 4-1 Swallowing

Swallowing is a very complex sequence of contractions and relaxations of muscles that not only include the muscles of the tongue and pharynx, but other muscles that are attached to the hyoid bone. There is still some question on the exact sequence of muscle contractions. However, swallowing has been divided into three stages.

Stage 1: In the first stage, the contraction of muscles is voluntary. The food is rolled into a bolus, compressed against the palate, and pushed from the mouth into the oropharynx. These movements mainly involve the muscles of the tongue and soft palate.

Stage 2: The muscle contractions in stage 2 are involuntary and rapid. The soft palate is tensed and elevated to compress the soft palate against the posterior wall of the pharynx. The elevation of the soft palate seals off the nasopharynx from the oropharynx and laryngopharynx. The longitudinal muscles of the pharynx and suprahyoid muscles contract to widen and shorten the pharynx to receive the bolus of food.

Stage 3: The contraction of the circular muscles of the pharynx is involuntary. The sequential contraction of all three constrictor muscles forces the bolus of food inferiorly into the esophagus.

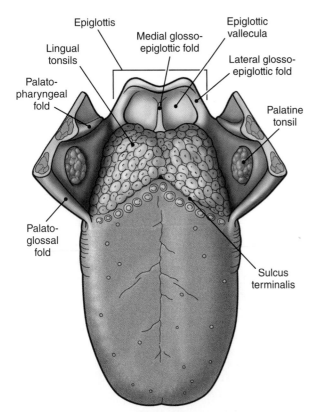

Figure 4–8 The roof of the fauces has been cut to expose the root or posterior one-third of the tongue, which is the floor of the fauces. The isthmus (entranceway) of the fauces is bounded by the two palatoglossal folds that form the palatoglossal arch. The root of the tongue is located in the oropharynx and is covered by the lingual tonsils. It is separated from the anterior two-third or body of the tongue by the V-shaped sulcus termi- nalis. The root of the tongue is attached to the epiglottis by the two lateral glossoepiglottic folds and median epiglottic fold. The depressions between the lateral and median folds are the epiglottic valleculae.

Labels in figure:
Epiglottis
Lingual tonsils
Medial glosso- epiglottic fold
Epiglottic vallecula
Lateral glosso- epiglottic fold
Palato- pharyngeal fold
Palatine tonsil
Palato- glossal fold
Sulcus terminalis

Review Question Box 4-3

1. Compare the tonsillar pillars to the palatoglossal and palatopharyngeal folds.
2. What is the difference between folds and arches?
3. What is the fauces and its boundaries?
4. Why are tonsils present at the entranceways into the pharynx?

Soft Palate

The *soft palate* is the soft tissue portion of the palate that separates the oropharynx and the nasopharynx (Fig. 4–4). Its purpose is to prevent food and fluid from moving upward into the nasal cavities. Although the soft palate and pharynx are different structures, their muscles intermingle and share common attachment sites. Five pairs of muscles form the soft palate: (1) palatoglossus, (2) palatopharyngeus, (3) uvular, (4) levator veli palatini, and (5) tensor veli palatine muscles. The contraction of these muscle tense, elevate, and shape the soft palate to seal the lumen (opening or passageway inside a tubular organ) of the nasopharynx (Table 4–2).

Palatoglossus Muscle

The *palatoglossus muscle* originates from the palatine aponeurosis and inserts onto the lateral part of the tongue (Fig. 4–7B). The **palatine aponeurosis** is a dense layer of connective tissue that extends from the posterior end of the hard palate for the attachment of muscles (Fig. 4–3). Contraction of the palatoglossus muscle (1) pulls the sides of the tongue upwards and backwards, (2) pulls down on the lateral edges of the soft palate, and (3) narrows the space between the right and left palatoglossal folds (narrows the fauces) (Table 4–1).

Palatopharyngeus Muscle

The *palatopharyngeus muscle* originates from the posterior portion of the hard palate and the palatine aponeurosis, passes behind the palatine tonsil, and inserts onto the lateral wall of the pharynx (Figs. 4–7B and 4–9). It functions to (1) narrow the fauces and (2) elevate and widen the pharynx behind the tongue

in preparation for accepting food from the oral cavity (Table 4–2).

Uvular Muscle

The **uvula** is a small tongue-shaped structure that hangs inferiorly into the pharynx from the posterior free border of the soft palate (Fig. 4–6). Reflection of the mucosa reveals that the uvula is composed of two bands of muscle, collectively called the **uvular muscle** (Fig. 4–9), which originates from the posterior nasal spine of the hard palate and courses posteriorly to attach to the mucosa of the uvula. When this muscle contracts, it shortens and broadens the uvula. As a result, the uvula changes shape to adapt to the posterior pharyngeal wall to seal the nasopharynx from the oropharynx while swallowing (Table 4–2).

Levator Veli Palatini Muscle

The **levator veli palatini muscle** (Fig. 4–9) originates from the petrous portion of the temporal bone. The fibers run downward and medially to insert onto the palatine aponeurosis (Fig. 4–5B) Contraction of the muscle pulls on the aponeurosis, which allows it to elevate the soft palate during swallowing (Table 4–2).

Tensor Veli Palatini Muscle

The **tensor veli palatini muscle** originates from the scaphoid fossa (base of the medial pterygoid plate of the sphenoid bone) and the cartilage of the auditory tube. The fibers run inferiorly and anteriorly and pass laterally around the pterygoid hamulus of the medial pterygoid plate, then medially onto the palatine aponeurosis (Fig. 4–9). The action of this muscle is to tense the soft palate and open the auditory tube when swallowing and yawning. The motor innervation to muscles of the palate

TABLE 4–2	Muscles of the Soft Palate			
Muscle	**Origin**	**Insertion**	**Action**	**Innervation**
Uvular	Posterior nasal spine	Mucosa of the uvula	Shortens and broadens the uvula	Vagus nerve
Palatoglossus	Palatine aponeurosis	Lateral part of the tongue	(1) Pulls the sides of the tongue upwards and backwards; (2) pulls down on the lateral edges of the soft palate; and (3) narrows the space between the right and left palatoglossal folds	Vagus nerve
Palatopharyngeus	Hard palate and palatine aponeurosis	Lateral pharyngeal wall	(1) Narrows the fauces; and (2) elevates and dilates the pharynx behind the tongue	Vagus nerve
Levator veli palatini	Petrous portion of the temporal bone	Palatine aponeurosis	Elevates the soft palate during swallowing	Vagus nerve
Tensor veli palatini	Scaphoid fossa and cartilage of the auditory tube	Palatine aponeurosis	(1) Tenses the soft palate; and (2) opens auditory tube when yawning and swallowing	Trigeminal nerve

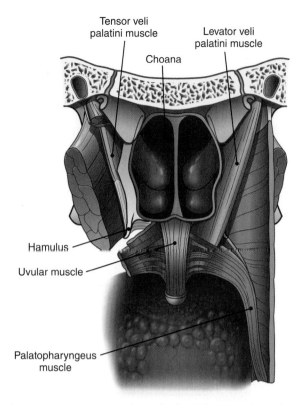

Tensor veli palatini muscle

Levator veli palatini muscle

Choana

Hamulus

Uvular muscle

Palatopharyngeus muscle

Figure 4–9 A posterior view of a frontal section through the pharynx demonstrates the choana of the nasal cavity and the muscles of the soft palate. The uvular muscle is the longitudinal band of muscle of the uvula. The levator veli palatini muscle arises from the petrous portion of the temporal bone and angles diagonally to insert onto the palatine aponeurosis deep within the soft palate. The tensor veli palatini muscle arises from the base of the medial pterygoid plate and the auditory tube and courses inferiorly in a vertical direction. The muscle then turns under the hamulus of the sphenoid bone to insert onto the palatine aponeurosis.

is the *vagus nerve* (I), with the exception of the tensor veli palatini muscle, which is innervated by the **trigeminal nerve** (**V**) (Table 4–2).

Review Question Box 4-4

1. What structure is partially located in the nasopharynx and the oropharynx?
2. How do the palatal muscles adapt the soft palate for swallowing?
3. How does the motor innervation of the tensor veli palatini differ from the other muscles of the palate?

Laryngeal Pharynx and Larynx

The **laryngeal pharynx** is located posterior to the larynx or voice box (Fig. 4-4). Its surface features

consist of the epiglottis, the aryepiglottic folds, and the piriform recess. Because the boundary between the laryngeal pharynx and the larynx are shared, these two related regions will be discussed together. The skeleton of the **larynx** is formed by cartilage and is covered by mucosa (epithelium and connective tissue). The *thyroid* (shield-shaped*) cartilage* is the largest of the cartilages and is formed by two laminae of cartilage that are fused anteriorly in the median plane of the neck (Fig. 4–10A). Superiorly, the cartilage is characterized by a V-shaped indentation called the *thyroid notch*. At the closed end of the "V," the thyroid cartilage protrudes as the **laryngeal protuberance** (Adam's apple) (Fig. 4–10A). The *epiglottic cartilage* is attached inferiorly to the cricoid cartilage by a sheet of connective tissue and extends superiorly to protect the opening of the larynx (Fig. 4–10B). The *cricoid cartilage* is located inferior to the thyroid cartilage and is the only cartilage of the larynx to form a completely enclosed ring (Figs. 4–10A and 4–10B). There are two **arytenoid cartilages**, which look like two birds perched on top of the posterosuperior surface of the cricoid cartilage (Fig. 4–10B). The vocal cords and the muscles that control them are attached to the arytenoid cartilage. These small cartilages are connected to the epiglottis by a sheet of connective tissue covered by mucosa. The fold of mucosa that covers the free edge of the connective sheet is called the **aryepiglottic fold** (Fig. 4–11). The thyroid and the cricoid cartilages are attached by the **median cricothyroid ligament** (Fig. 4–10A), which is the site for emergency airway procedures.

The *superior aperture* of the larynx is bounded laterally by the *aryepiglottic folds* that extend from the arytenoid cartilage to the epiglottis (Fig. 4–11). The **piriform recess** is a lateral expansion of the laryngeal pharynx inferior to the aryepiglottic fold (Fig. 4–11). Internally, the opening of the larynx narrows into a

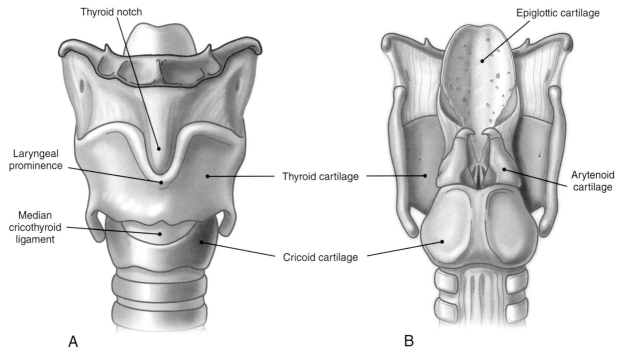

Figure 4–10 **(A)** Anterior view of the laryngeal skeleton. The thyroid, cricoid, and epiglottic cartilages form the basic structure of the larynx. The laminae of the thyroid cartilage fuse to form the laryngeal prominence and the thyroid notch. The thyroid and cricoid cartilages are joined by the median cricothyroid ligament. **(B)** The posterior view of the laryngeal skeleton. The thyroid cartilage is incomplete, whereas the cricoid cartilage is a complete ring. The arytenoid cartilages appear as two birds perched on the cricoid cartilage.

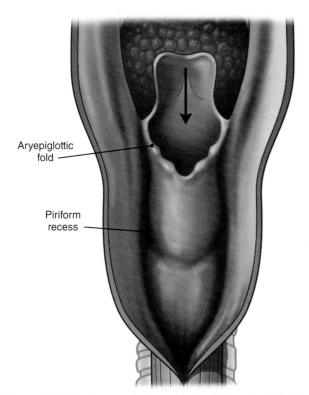

Figure 4–11 The laryngeal pharynx is located posterior to the larynx. The superior laryngeal aperture (arrow) is bounded by the aryepiglottic folds. The piriform recess is located lateral to the larynx.

Box 4-3 Emergency Airway Procedure

When an individual stops breathing, one of the first steps in treatment is to clear the airway. The tongue should be pulled forward to ensure that the tongue is not swallowed. The oral cavity and throat should be cleared of any foreign material. If the individual is choking and gasping for air, an object may be lodged deeper in the pharynx. Abdominal thrust procedures, such as the Heimlich maneuver, can be performed to dislodge the object. Once all procedures are exhausted and the episode is a medical emergency (an action that could lead to death), the airway can be opened by incising the skin and the median cricothyroid ligament between the thyroid cartilage and the cricoid cartilage. A tube can then be placed in the opening to establish controlled breathing. The point of access into the airway is close to the surface and there are no major vessels or organs that can be damaged. A *tracheotomy* is the procedure to allow ventilation of the airway, and is performed in the operating room to control bleeding and damage to surrounding structures.

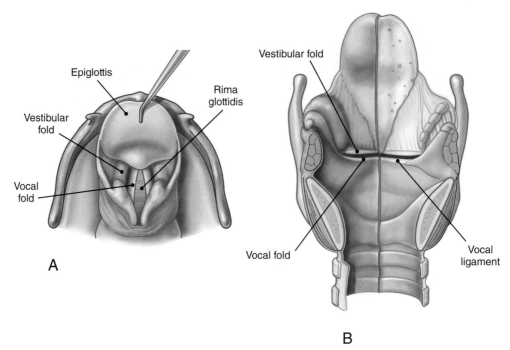

Figure 4–12 (A) Superior view of the larynx. The rima glottidis is the narrow slit between the vocal folds. **(B)** The posterior wall has been opened to expose the interior of the larynx. The vestibular fold is superior to the vocal fold. On the left side, the mucosa has been stripped away to reveal the vocal cords underneath the vocal folds.

narrow slit, the **rima glottidis**, which is bounded by a pair of horizontal folds from the lateral wall (Fig. 4–12A). The superior folds are called the **vestibular folds** or "false vocal" cords, whereas the mucosae of inferior folds, called the **vocal folds**, cover the connective tissue that forms the true vocal cords (Fig. 4–12B). The vocal folds and the rima glottidis are collectively called the **glottis**. The muscles of the larynx act upon the vestibular and vocal folds to open and close the rima glottidis, whereas other laryngeal muscles control the tension on the vocal folds, which vibrate and produce sound. The muscles of the vestibular folds seal the airway and increase abdominal pressure (the so-called *Valsalva maneuver*) to perform weight lifting, excretory functions such as urination and defecation, and "pushing" during childbirth.

Review Question Box 4-5

1. Is the larynx in the laryngealpharynx? Why?
2. What structure is attached to the laryngealpharynx inferiorly?
3. What is the difference between the superior laryngeal aperture and the rima glottidis?
4. What is the significance of the anterior space between the thyroid and cricoid cartilages?

SUMMARY

The pharynx is a shared passageway of the respiratory and digestive systems. The pharynx is divided into three parts. Superiorly, the nasopharynx connects to the nasal cavity by the choanae and to the middle ear by the opening of the auditory tube. The soft palate separates the nasopharynx from the oropharynx that lies posterior to, and is connected to, the oral cavity by the isthmus of the fauces. The oropharynx is separated inferiorly from the laryngopharynx by the epiglottis.

The soft palate is a flap that prevents the reflux of food and fluids into the nasal cavity. Contraction of the palatal muscles tenses, elevates, and shapes the soft palate to fit the contours of the posterior wall, effectively sealing off the nasopharynx.

The fauces is the portion of the oropharynx that is bordered anteriorly by the palatoglossal arch and posteriorly by the palatopharyngeal folds. The palatine tonsil is located between the two arches. The root of the tongue and the lingual tonsils are other major structures of the oropharynx.

The laryngeal pharynx is located posterior to the larynx and connects to the esophagus inferiorly. The larynx is not part of the pharynx. The laryngeal cartilages prevent the collapse of the airway. The vocal folds contain the true vocal cords, which produce sound. The vestibular folds or "false vocal cords" contain muscles that, when contracted, seal the airway.

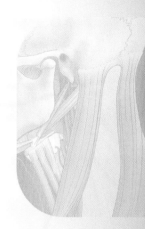

LEARNING LAB
Exercises for review, practice, and study

Laboratory Activity 4-1

Identifying Structures of the Oropharynx and Larynx

Objective: Many structures of the pharynx cannot be viewed without special instrumentation. In this exercise, you will examine the oropharynx and palpate the laryngeal cartilages and their landmarks using your own body as a model. Be careful when placing fingers, tongue depressors, or other instruments in your mouth to position the tongue. The oral cavity is generally insensitive to reflexes; however, the uvula and fauces are very sensitive and you can initiate the gag reflex if you probe too deeply. You will study the reason for the change in sensitivity in a later chapter.

Materials Needed: A mirror (if using yourself as a model), gloves (if working with a partner), and lighting such as a small flashlight. *Optional:* Tongue depressor.

Step 1:   Begin this exercise by looking into your oral cavity with a mirror and proper lighting. Realize that the oropharynx is located posterior (behind) to the oral cavity and the tongue will block your view. The portion of the tongue that is exposed is the anterior two-thirds or body of the tongue and is located in the oral cavity. To obtain a clearer view, it is necessary to lower the tongue in the floor of the mouth.

- Identify the *uvula* in the midline of the fauces (throat). Note the posterior wall of the nasopharynx distal to the uvula.
- Now observe the lateral wall of the fauces, which is bordered by the anterior and posterior tonsillar pillars. The *palatine tonsils* are located in between the tonsillar pillars if they have not been surgically removed.
- The *anterior tonsillar pillar* is the clinical term for the *palatoglossal fold*, which covers the *palatoglossus muscle*. The two folds come together at the uvula and form the *palatoglossal arch*. The palatoglossal arch is the entranceway into the fauces.
- Likewise, the *posterior tonsillar pillar* is the clinical term for the *palatopharyngeal fold*, which covers the *palatopharyngeus muscle*. The palatoglossal folds come together at the uvula to form the *palatopharyngeal arch*. Note that these muscles contribute to the free border of the palate (the portion not attached to the hard palate).
- Realize that the fauces is the area between the *palatoglossal* and *palatopharyngeal folds*.
- In a frontal plane through the palatoglossal arch, look for the vallate papilla on the surface of the tongue. The papilla may be conspicuous in some individuals. It marks the division of the body and root of the tongue. The *root* or posterior one-third of the tongue is located in the oropharynx.

Step 2:   Direct your attention to the neck and continue the exercise by palpating the laryngeal cartilages.

- Begin by locating the *laryngeal prominence* (Adam's apple). The prominence is formed by the two lamina of the thyroid cartilage. With your fingers and thumb, start at the laryngeal prominence and palpate the extent of the cartilage. Just superior to the prominence, palpate the *thyroid notch*, a V-shaped notch on the free border of the thyroid cartilage.
- Next, move your finger inferior along the anterior surface of the thyroid cartilage. You should feel a soft area between the thyroid cartilage and the more inferior *cricoid cartilage*. Although the extent cannot be palpated, the cricoid cartilage is the only cartilage that forms a complete ring around the larynx.
- Return to the soft space between the thyroid and cricoid cartilages. Note that the skin is thin in this area and rests on membrane that connects the thyroid and cricoid cartilages. This is the site of incision for the emergency airway procedure called a *cricothyrotomy* in which a ventilating tube is placed into the airway.

For Discussion or Thought:

1. *Why is the root of the tongue not considered to be located in the oral cavity?*

2. *What is the fauces?*

3. *Why is the soft tissue space a good site for the placement of a ventilating tube in the airway when the upper air passages between the oropharynx and the larynx are obstructed?*

Learning Activity 4-1

Fauces

Match the numbered structures with the correct terms listed to the right.

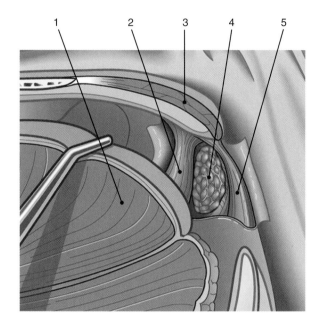

_____ Palatine tonsil

_____ Palatoglossus muscle

_____ Palatopharyngeus muscle

_____ Tongue

_____ Uvular muscle

Learning Activity 4-2

Muscles of the Soft Palate

Match the numbered structures with the correct terms listed to the right.

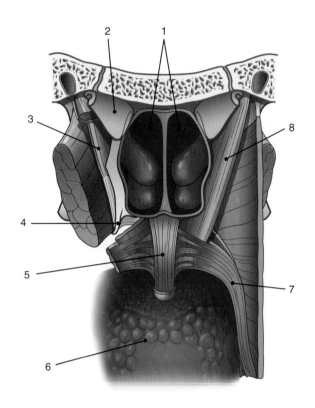

_____ Auditory tube

_____ Choanae

_____ Hamular process of pterygoid bone

_____ Levator veli palatini muscle

_____ Palatopharyngeus muscle

_____ Tensor veli palatini muscle

_____ Tongue

_____ Uvular muscle

Learning Activity 4-3

Muscles of the Pharynx

Match the numbered structures with the correct terms listed to the right.

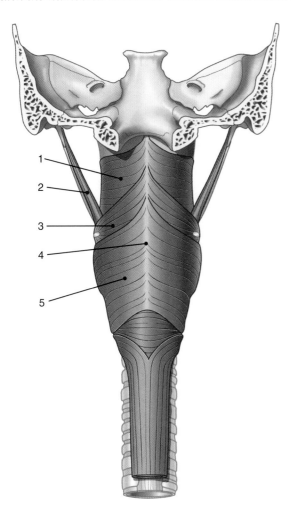

_____ Inferior constrictor muscle

_____ Middle constrictor muscle

_____ Pharyngeal raphe

_____ Stylopharyngeus muscle

_____ Superior constrictor muscle

Learning Activity 4-4

Structures of the Pharynx—Posterior View

Match the numbered structures with the correct terms listed to the right.

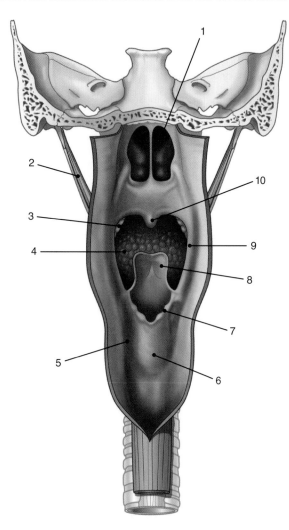

_____ Aryepiglottic fold

_____ Bulge of the cricoid cartilage

_____ Choana

_____ Epiglottis

_____ Lingual tonsil

_____ Palatine tonsil

_____ Palatopharyngeal fold

_____ Piriform recess

_____ Stylopharyngeus muscle

_____ Uvula

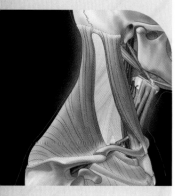

5

Muscles of Facial Expression

Objectives

1. Identify the landmarks of the superficial face.
2. Identify the muscles of facial expression, and know the actions and innervation of these muscles.

Overview

Our facial appearance plays an important role in our society. We make judgments on others by the way they look. There is no doubt that we are attracted to those we feel have pleasing features. We also judge people according to their facial expressions. We consider people who always smile as being happy and congenial. Sadness is often expressed by the wrinkling of the forehead and downward movement of the corners of the mouth. People in deep thought or who are very serious may have a stern face, without expression. Before athletic events, coaches tell their players to put on their "game face," which implies being serious and focusing. Card players put on their "poker face" to keep their opponents guessing about the cards they are playing.

Realize that when treating patients, their mouths are open and filled with instruments, and they are unable to verbally respond. Observing your patient's facial expressions will give you visual clues on the individual's comfort or discomfort during treatment.

The face can tell much more. Similar facial features suggest family relationships. Unusual placement of the eyes, the width of the mouth, and the size and dimpling of the chin are determined during embryonic development. By the end of this chapter, the expression "you're not just a pretty face" should have a whole new meaning.

INTRODUCTION TO THE MUSCLES OF FACIAL EXPRESSION

The integument of the face has been adapted by the addition of skeletal muscle in the integument's underlying connective tissue that performs functions unique to the face. This muscle layer (1) assists in the protection of the eyes by closure of the eyelids, (2) enhances chewing by confining food to the mouth by closure of the lips and the tightening of the cheeks, and (3) enhances breathing and olfaction by the flaring of the nostrils.

The muscles of facial expression are thin bundles of skeletal muscle embedded in the skin of the face, neck, scalp, and the skin surrounding the ears. Most of the muscles originate from bone and insert into the dermis of the skin. In addition to the three functions mentioned earlier, the contraction of these muscles allows our face to express the emotions of joy, sadness, surprise, and so on as in smiling, frowning, or grimacing.

The muscles of facial expression are innervated by the **facial nerve (VII)**. **Facial palsies**, which are the paralysis of facial muscles by injury or disease to the facial nerve, cause distorted facial features. This is of clinical interest to the dental hygienist because improper closure of the mouth may cause drooling from the mouth and the potential of biting on the cheek wall.

Review Question Box 5-1

1. What functions of the muscles of facial expression are important to the dental hygienist? Why are they important?
2. What is unique about the location of the muscles of facial expression?
3. How is the innervation of the facial muscles different from the muscles of the trunk?

FEATURES OF THE SUPERFICIAL FACE

Observation is a critical ingredient to any clinical evaluation. An understanding of the normal facial features can help a dental hygienist detect changes that are caused by emotions, nerve injury, aging, or facial development.

The surface of the forehead displays horizontal wrinkles in the skin that are called **forehead furrows** (Fig. 5–1). These furrows become more prominent with age. A patient's inability to wrinkle his or her forehead is an indication of damage to the facial nerve. The **supraciliary ridge** is the bony prominence above

Clinical Correlation Box 5-1

Facial Paralysis

Injury to the *facial nerve* can cause either temporary or permanent *paralysis* of the structures innervated by the nerve dependent upon the cause and site of the injury. The facial nerve has its origin in the midbrain, which could be susceptible to **stroke** and **tumors**. The nerve enters the external acoustic meatus and courses through the middle ear to reach the face. *Infections* within the middle ear can spread to the facial nerve, causing it to swell while passing through the canal. Increased pressure on the nerve can cause temporary paralysis of the facial muscles and other symptoms. The facial nerve exits the skull through the stylomastoid foramen, where it can be damaged by transverse *fractures* of the skull. The nerve then courses through the parotid gland to innervate the facial muscles. **Mumps** and tumors of the parotid gland can cause damage to branches of the facial nerve. Branches of the facial nerve can also be damaged by an aberrant needle while attempting an *inferior alveolar nerve block* (local anesthesia). Approximately 75% of facial muscle paralysis is a result of **Bell's palsy**, which is characterized paralysis or weakness of muscles on one side of the face. This results in drooping of the muscles and inability to close the eye on the affected side of the face. Secretion of saliva (dry mouth), taste to the anterior two-thirds of the tongue, and pain and temperature sensations of the skin around the ear can also be affected. Although the etiology of Bell's palsy is unknown, inflammation of the facial nerve has been linked to the *herpes zoster virus*, which affects cranial nerves. The onset of Bell's palsy is sudden; all symptoms manifest within the first 2 days. The condition gradually improves and symptoms are generally resolved within 2 months.

(superior to) the eyebrows (Fig. 5–1). In males, the supraciliary ridge is more pronounced and the forehead has a tendency to be sloped, whereas in females, the ridge is smaller and the forehead is more vertical.

The eyeballs are protected anteriorly by the **palpebrae** (singular: **palpebra**) or eyelids. The **palpebral fissure** is the space between the margins of the eyelids when they are open. The fissure is bounded medially and laterally by the **palpebral commissures** (corners) where the upper (superior) and lower (inferior) eyelids meet (Fig. 5–1).

The nose is divided into two parts. The **bridge of the nose**, formed by the fusion of the nasal bones, is the

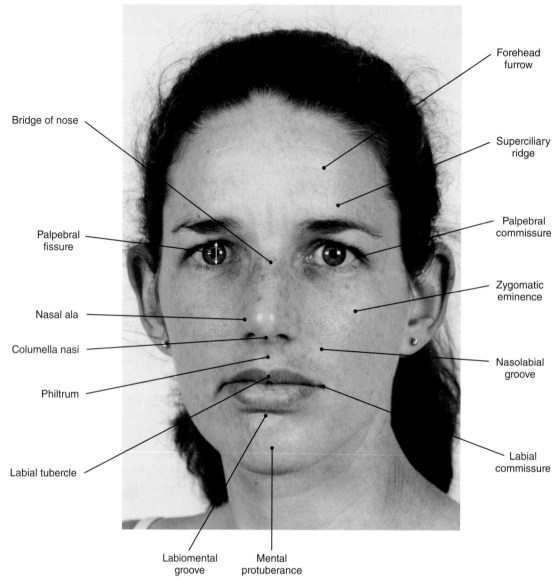

Figure 5–1 Surface features of the face can be used to evaluate a person's emotions, age, and developmental anomalies.

narrow part of the nose leading downward between the eyes toward the lower, flared part surrounding the nostrils (openings into the nasal cavities) (Fig. 5–1). The **nasal ala** is the wing of the nose, which is the flaring cartilaginous expansion that forms the outer surface of each nostril (Fig. 5–1). In between the nostrils is the **columella nasi** that represents the fleshy distal margin of the nasal septum (Fig. 5–1).

The furrow that separates the upper lip and nose from the cheek is called the **nasolabial groove** (Fig. 5–1). The groove may become more pronounced by aging and is generally related to excess skin or fat. During facial paralysis, the groove is greatly reduced or absent; thus, comparing the depth of the groove on the left versus the right side of the face can indicate damages to branches of the facial nerve, which is a cranial nerve.

In the middle of the face, the **zygomatic eminence** is the bony prominence of the cheek wall just inferior to the rim of the orbit. The upper and lower lips are joined at the **labial commissures** (Fig. 5–1). The size of the mouth is determined by the fusion of the mandible and maxillary processes during embryonic development. Just inferior to the columella, the upper lip is characterized by a vertical groove called the **philtrum** (Fig. 5–1). Because the philtrum represents a fusion site for two embryonic structures that form the upper lip, it is a site for cleft lips. The upper lip often presents a central rounded projection called the **labial tubercle** (Fig. 5–1).

The **labiomental groove** is a horizontal furrow between the lower lip and the chin. The portion of the chin that juts forward is the **mental protuberance** and

Clinical Correlation Box 5-2

Development of the Face

The structural features of the face are determined during the 4th to 6th week of embryonic development. Four paired processes—the *medial nasal process*, the *lateral nasal process*, the *maxillary process*, and the *mandibular process*—develop anterior to the brain bulge. These processes must grow and fuse anteriorly to form the various features of the face. The fusion of the medial nasal processes forms the midline structures of the face, the *bridge* and *dorsum* of

the nose, and the *philtrum* of the upper lip. The fusion of the medial nasal process and the maxillary process forms the upper lip and underlying structures, whereas the fusion of the mandibular processes form the lower lip and structure of the jaw. The *alae* (wings) of the nose are formed by the lateral nasal process, and the maxillary process forms the *zygomatic eminence* (cheekbone). Fusion of the maxillary and mandibular process also determines the size of the opening of the mouth.

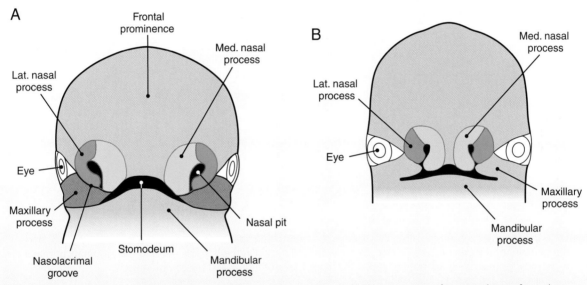

Four paired structures—the medial nasal, lateral nasal, maxillary, and mandibular processes—fuse together to form the face. The stomodeum is the primitive mouth and the frontal prominence becomes the forehead. **(A)** The eyes and nostrils are far apart. **(B)** With further development, the eyes and nostrils migrate medially. The nostrils fuse to form the nose and the eyes become aligned into their anterior location.

is related to the shape of the chin or **mentum** (Fig. 5–1). This portion of the jaw is more rounded in females than in males.

MUSCLES OF FACIAL EXPRESSION

Because of the complex names, the study of the muscles of facial expression may seem to be a daunting task. However, understanding that the muscles are generally named according to their location, origin, function, and size will make the task easier. As an example, the zygomaticus major muscle arises from the zygomatic arch, and is called *major* because it is larger than a smaller muscle of the same origin, the zygomaticus minor. The levator anguli oris muscle is inserted onto, and elevates, the corners of the mouth.

The muscles are presented according to regions of the face beginning with the mouth because of the importance to the dental hygienist and ends with the scalp and ears, which are of lesser importance. Although the functions of individual muscles are given, it is important to realize that multiple muscles contract synergistically (act together) to produce an expression such as a smile.

Muscles of the Mouth

The **orbicularis oris muscle** surrounds the opening of the mouth and is the main intrinsic muscle of the lips (Fig. 5–2). Compared to the normal mouth (Fig. 5–3A), the action of the muscle is to close, compress, and pucker the lips (Fig 5–3B). At its periphery, the orbicularis oris

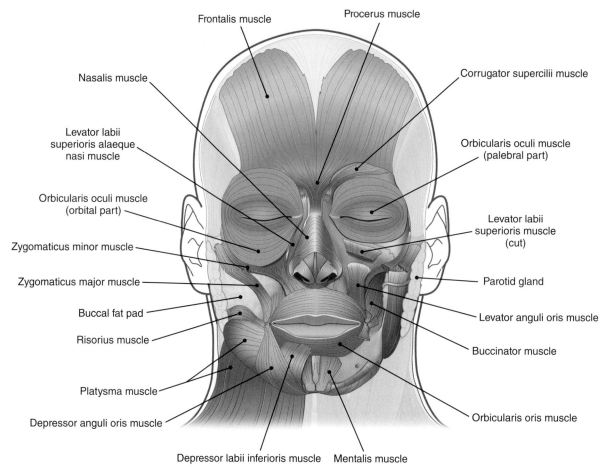

Figure 5–2 The facial muscles can alter the shape of the mouth and lips, close the eyelids, elevate the eyelids, and alter the tautness of the skin of the forehead, cheek wall, and neck. On the left side, fat and the zygomaticus major and minor muscles have been removed to reveal the deeper levator anguli and buccinator muscles.

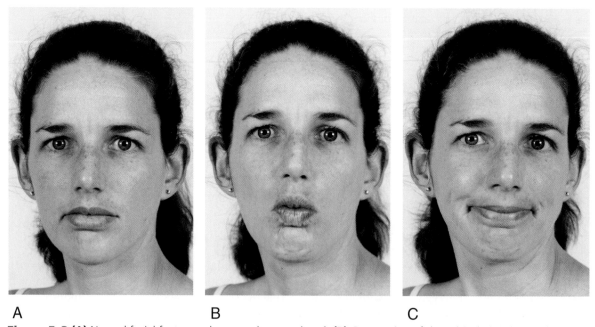

A   B   C

Figure 5–3 (A) Normal facial features when muscles are relaxed. **(B)** Contraction of the orbicularis oris muscles purses the lips. **(C)** The risorius muscle causes the labial commissures to extend laterally, producing a grimace.

muscle is joined by other muscles that affect the shape of the mouth. The **risorius muscle** arises from the connective tissue (fascia) over the parotid gland and inserts onto the corner of the mouth (Fig. 5–2). This muscle pulls the corners of the mouth laterally (Fig. 5–3C). Superior to the insertion of the risorius is the **zygomaticus major muscle**, which originates from the zygomatic bone. Its fibers run downward and forward to its insertion onto the angle of the mouth (Fig. 5–2). Its function is to elevate the corners of the mouth as in smiling (Fig. 5–4A). The zygomaticus minor, the levator labii superioris, and levator labii superioris alaeque nasi muscles merge with the orbicularis oris muscle superior and medial to the insertion of the zygomaticus major muscle. The **zygomaticus minor muscle** arises from the zygomatic bone and is smaller than the zygomaticus major (Fig. 5–2). Medially, the **levator labii superioris muscle** arises from the lower rim of the orbit (Fig. 5–2), whereas the **levator labii superioris alaeque nasi muscle**, which is closest to the median plane, arises from the frontal process of the maxilla (Fig. 5–2). This muscle inserts onto the ala of the nose, as well as the upper lip. The function of these three muscles is to raise the upper lip (Fig. 5–4B). In addition, the levator labii superioris alaeque nasi muscle raises the ala of the nose to allow more air to enter the nose. The remaining muscle of the upper lip lies deep to these three muscles and is called the **levator anguli oris** (Fig. 5–2). This muscle arises from the canine fossa of the maxilla and, as the name implies, raises the corners of the mouth (Fig. 5–4C).

Three muscles join the orbicularis oris along the lower lip. The **depressor anguli oris muscle** inserts onto the corner of the mouth from a broad origin along the lower border of the mandible (Fig. 5–2). This triangle-shaped muscle pulls the corners of the mouth downward indicating sadness (Fig. 5–5A). The **depressor labii inferioris muscle** is inserted medial to the insertion of the depressor anguli oris and also has its origin from the lower border of the mandible (Fig. 5–2). This muscle is partially overlapped by the depressor anguli muscle. The function of the depressor labii inferioris is to depress or pull down the lower lip. The **platysma muscle** is actually a muscle of the neck (Figs. 5–2 and 5–5B). It originates from the fascia covering the pectoralis major and deltoid muscles and inserts onto the inferior border of the mandible and the skin near the corners of the mouth. Therefore, the contraction of the platysma causes wrinkling of the skin of the neck, depresses the corners of the mouth, and assists in the depression of the mandible (Fig. 5–5B).

The **mentalis muscle** originates on the anterior surface of the mandible just below the lateral incisors (Fig. 5–2). The fibers run inferiorly toward the midline to insert onto the skin of the chin. Contraction of the mentalis raises and pushes up the lower lip, causing wrinkling of the skin of the chin (Fig. 5–5C). The **buccinator muscle**, although considered a muscle of facial expression, assists in the process of mastication (Fig. 5–2). This muscle originates from the **pterygomandibular raphe** (see Fig. 4–3), a band of connective tissue fibers that runs from the pterygoid hamulus down to the

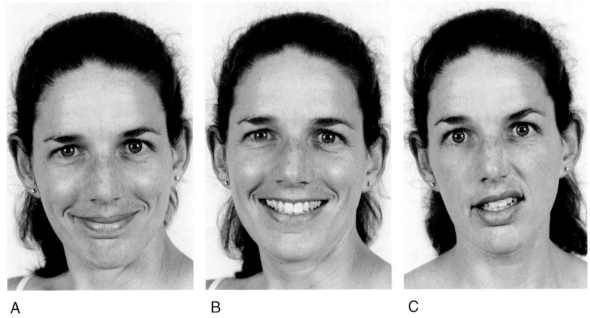

A   B   C

Figure 5–4 (A) The zygomaticus major muscle elevates the corners of the mouth to produce a smile. **(B)** Contracting the elevators of the lip along with the zygomaticus major produces a smile that exposes the teeth. **(C)** Contracting the zygomaticus major and levator anguli muscles elevates the labial commissure on the left side.

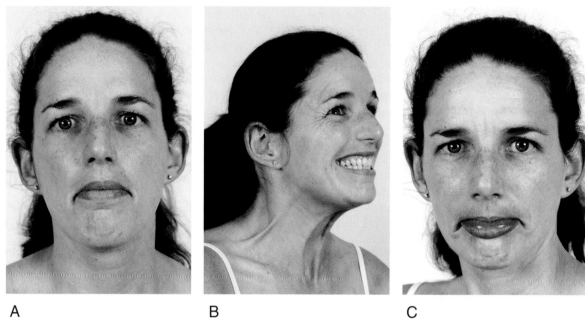

A   B   C

Figure 5–5 (A) The depressor anguli oris causes the corners of mouth to turn downward. **(B)** Although the platysma causes wrinkling of the skin, the neck has been stretched to outline the borders of the muscle. **(C)** The mentalis muscle causes protrusion of the lower lip and wrinkling of the skin of the chin.

medial surface of the mandible and inserts deeply into the corner of mouth. This is the major muscle of the cheek and causes tautness (tightness) in the cheek wall during chewing. This muscle prevents food from building up in the buccal vestibule by pressing the cheek against the teeth during the chewing cycle.

Muscles of the Eyes

The **orbicularis oculi muscle** totally encircles the eye. The muscle has two parts: the portion surrounding the eye is called the *orbital* portion and the portion found in the eyelids is called the *palpebral* portion (Fig. 5–2). The function of this muscle is to close the eyelid (Fig. 5–6A). The **corrugator supercilii muscle** runs from the bridge of the nose upward and laterally along the superciliary ridge (Fig. 5–2). The muscle pulls the eyebrow medially and downward during frowning and as a result causes vertical wrinkles in the skin of the forehead (Fig. 5–6C). The **procerus muscle** fibers run vertically from the nose to insert onto the medial aspect of the eyebrow (Fig. 5–6C). This muscle also causes the eyebrow to move medially and downward, producing horizontal wrinkles on the bridge of the nose (Fig. 5–6C).

Muscles of the Scalp

The major muscle of the scalp is the **occipitofrontalis** or **epicranius muscle**. This muscle is composed of two muscles. The **occipitalis muscle**, which is posterior in location, is attached to the superior nuchal line of the occipital bone (Fig. 5–7). The **frontalis muscle**, which is located anteriorly, covers the forehead and blends with other facial muscles to insert onto the skin deep to the eyebrow (Fig. 5–7). A broad, tough connective sheath or **aponeurosis** connects the two muscle groups over most of the superior surface of the cranium. The most noticeable function of the epicranius is apparent by viewing the horizontal wrinkles of the forehead by contracting the frontalis muscle (Fig. 5–6B).

Muscles of the Nose and Ears

The muscles of the nose and ears are generally not a concern to the dental hygienist. The **nasalis muscle** functions to open and close the nostrils (Fig. 5–7). The anterior auricular, superior auricular, and posterior auricular muscles are named according to their position around the ears (Fig. 5–7). Although some individuals can wiggle their ears, these muscles are generally poorly developed in humans.

Review Question Box 5-2

1. Contraction of what muscles indicates sadness?
2. Contraction of what muscles indicates happiness?
3. What muscle(s) do you use when squinting to bright light?
4. What muscle(s) is (are) used to keep food in the oral cavity while chewing?

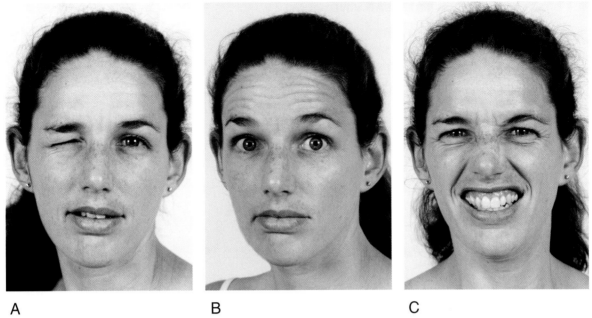

Figure 5–6 (A) The right eyelid has been closed by the orbicularis oculi muscle. **(B)** Contraction of the frontalis muscle produces the horizontal furrows and elevation of the eyebrows. **(C)** Contraction of the corrugator supercilii muscles causes the eyebrows to move in a medial direction and produces vertical folds of the skin between the brows. Contraction of the procerus muscle accompanied by the nasalis muscle, causes horizontal furrows along the root of the nose and the expansion of the nares.

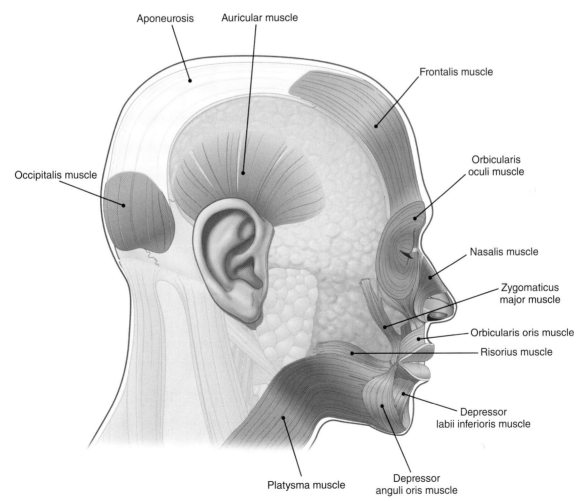

Figure 5–7 The muscles of the ear are best seen on a lateral view of the head. The epicranius muscle is composed of the frontalis and occipitalis muscles separated by a connective tissue aponeurosis. Other facial muscles are indicated.

SUMMARY

The bony features of the face are genetic and are determined during human development. Improper fusion of the embryonic processes that form the face results in facial anomalies such as cleft lips. The muscles of facial expression are unusual in that they are found in the superficial fascia of the skin and they are affected by emotions. The muscles are innervated by the facial nerve and injury to the nerve can cause loss of muscle function. Observing a patient's face can offer clues to developmental problems and damage to the facial nerve, as well as serve as visual cues for detecting a patient's anxiety regarding dental procedures.

LEARNING LAB

Exercises for review, practice, and study

Laboratory Activity 5-1

Observing Facial Features

Objective: Facial features vary among individuals and can serve as signs of mode changes and nerve disorders. In this exercise, you will compare surface features of several individuals. First, start by identifying the features on yourself and then comparing the surface features to classmates, friends, family, or even pictures in a magazine or other media. Remember, there is no perfect face and variations between the left and right sides are normal.

Materials Needed: A mirror, and pictures of faces from photographs, magazines, or other media.

Step 1: Using a mirror, start your study by assessing the entire face. Look at the slope of your forehead, the size and shape of your nose, the placement of your eyes and ears, and the width of your mouth. Look at the general shape of your chin and determine if there is dimpling. How do these features compare to others?

Step 2: Continue your study of observing facial features by returning to the forehead. This region is called the *upper face* and is relevant for the testing of the facial nerve.

- Identify the *horizontal furrows* and realize that the furrows are shallow in younger individuals and become deeper with age. Note that the foreheads of women are generally more vertical than males. Locate the *superciliary ridge*, which is deep to the eyebrows. This ridge bulges more in males than females.

Step 3: Turn your attention to the lower face (inferior to the eyebrows). Compare the distance between your eyes with several individuals. The position of the eyes relative to the nose is variable and is determined during embryonic development.

Step 4: Now look at your mouth and identify the *labial commissures* or corners of the mouth. Compare the width of your mouth to other individuals.

Step 5: Draw an imaginary line perpendicular to labial commissures of the mouth toward the eyes. The average mouth is approximately the same as the interpupillary distance.

- Mouths of larger widths are called **macrostomia** and narrower mouths are called **microstomia**. These terms do not refer to anything abnormal as long as the face is symmetrical.
- Realize that individuals who have small mouths will not be able to open their mouths as wide, which could require alternate strategies when providing dental care.

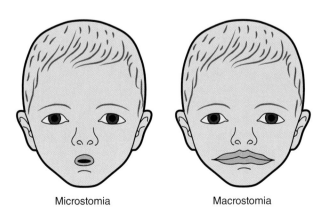

Microstomia   Macrostomia

The size of the mouth is determined by the fusion of the mandibular and maxillary processes. **(A)** *Microstomia* or small mouth. **(B)** *Macrostomia* or large mouth.

Step 6:   Now examine the nasolabial area.

- Identify the *ala* or wing of the nose, which is the soft tissue and cartilage that surrounds the nostril.
- Identify the *columella nasi*, which is the vertical column of soft tissue that separates the two nostrils. This represents the anteriormost portion of the nasal septum.
- Just inferior to the columella, identify a vertical depression of the upper lip called the *philtrum*. In the median plane, look for a small inferiorly directed projection of the lip called the *labial tubercle*.
- Look for vertical scars in the depression and raised edges of the philtrum. It is possible that the scars indicate corrective surgery for cleft lips. Realize that both improper placement of teeth and malocclusion usually accompany cleft lips, but can be corrected by orthodontic procedures.
- Identify the *nasolabial groove* extending from the ala of the nose toward the mouth and the *labiomental groove* between the lower lip and chin. The nasolabial groove can be of varying depths, depending on the age and amount of fat in the individual's face. The absence of a nasolabial groove on one side of the face could indicate damage to the *facial nerve*.

Step 7:   Determine the shape of the chin. Is it rounded or "squared"? The chin of a female is generally round as opposed to a male and is proportional to the width of the mental protuberance.

- Look for dimples. Dimpling results from the degree of fusion between the bones that form the jaw (mandible) during embryonic development.

Step 8:   Conclude this exercise by examining the position of the ears. Are they approximately horizontal from each other? In some development disorders, one ear will appear to be much lower than the other and the cheek wall may be poorly developed on one side (asymmetrical).

For Discussion or Thought:

Remember that there is a normal range of variation in facial features. The purpose of the exercise is to recognize normal variations.

1. *What makes a face abnormal?*

Clinical Correlation Box 5-3

Cleft Lips

Dental hygienists are most likely to encounter two types of clefts lips: median cleft lip and lateral cleft lip. *Median cleft lip* results from the improper fusion between the two medial nasal processes and is characterized by the absence of a philtrum. Improper fusion of the medial nasal and the maxillary processes can cause either *unilateral* or *bilateral cleft lip*. The clefts appear along the lateral edges of the philtrum. Dimpling of the chin, *median cleft chin*, is variable and results from the incomplete fusion of the two mandibular processes in the median plane.

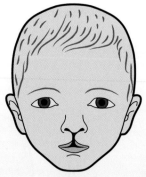
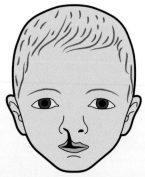

Median cleft lip   Lateral cleft lip

(A) A *median cleft lip* results from the improper fusion of the two medial nasal processes. **(B)** A *lateral cleft lip* results from the improper fusion of the medial nasal process to the maxillary process.

Learning Activity 5-1

Muscles of Facial Expression

Match the numbered structures with the correct terms listed to the right.

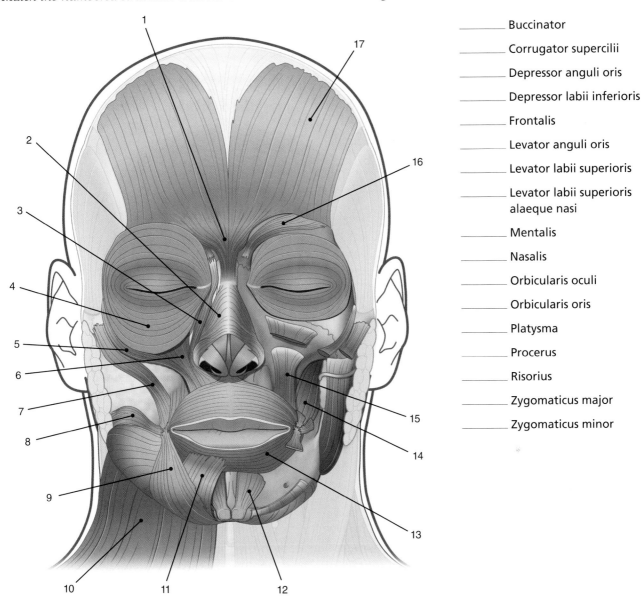

_____ Buccinator

_____ Corrugator supercilii

_____ Depressor anguli oris

_____ Depressor labii inferioris

_____ Frontalis

_____ Levator anguli oris

_____ Levator labii superioris

_____ Levator labii superioris alaeque nasi

_____ Mentalis

_____ Nasalis

_____ Orbicularis oculi

_____ Orbicularis oris

_____ Platysma

_____ Procerus

_____ Risorius

_____ Zygomaticus major

_____ Zygomaticus minor

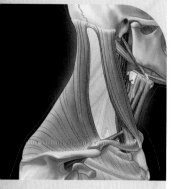

chapter

6

Nasal Cavity and Paranasal Sinuses

Objectives

1. Distinguish between the conducting and respiratory divisions of the respiratory system and their functions.
2. Identify the bones of the external nose and the structures of the medial and lateral walls of the nasal cavity.
3. Identify the paranasal sinuses and explain their functions and clinical significance.
4. Discuss the drainage of the paranasal sinuses into the nasal cavities.

Overview

Noses come in a variety of shapes and sizes. However, the nose's internal structure is designed to channel air along two functionally different pathways. As you inhale, air is directed to the olfactory region located on the roof of the nasal cavity. The mucous membranes in this area contain olfactory (smell) receptors. The sense of smell helps distinguish pleasant odors, such as flowers, from unpleasant odors of chemicals and biological wastes. Additionally, the aroma from freshly prepared foods or sweets (such as chocolate) can stimulate the release of saliva with the anticipation of eating something tasty. On the other hand, the lateral walls of the nasal cavity are designed to swirl the air over the mucous membranes to regulate the temperature and humidity of the air, as well as trap dust and pollutants to prevent them from entering the lungs.

Our sinuses (paranasal) can be a source of discomfort for many. Sinuses can become infected and produce copious amounts of mucus. Of course, we feel this as stuffiness, and the sinuses are common sources of headaches. The paranasal sinuses are extensions of the nasal cavity. The pneumatization (filling with air cells) of the bones containing the sinuses lightens the cranium (head) and contributes to the resonance of our voices. Of the four sinuses, the maxillary sinus is clinically important to the dental hygienist. Nerves that supply the sinus also innervate the maxillary teeth. Therefore, individuals with a maxillary sinus infection frequently complain of toothaches, and the dental hygienist must learn to distinguish among the symptoms to properly treat the patient.

INTRODUCTION

The **nose** is the entranceway into the air passageways of the **respiratory system**. The respiratory system is divided into a **conducting division** that begins at the nose, and includes the nasopharynx, larynx, trachea, bronchi, and bronchioles. These passageways warm and humidify the inspired air, as well as filter and trap pollutants before entering the more sensitive structures of the **respiratory division** within the lungs where gas exchange actually takes place.

The nose is a combination of bones and cartilages that form the *external nose* and the **nasal cavities**. The nose not only conditions and cleanses the air, but also contains receptors for the sense of smell. Furthermore, the nasal cavities receive drainage from the **paranasal sinuses** (mucus) and drainage from the **nasolacrimal duct** (tears). The nose contains many blood vessels and is innervated by sensory fibers of the **trigeminal (V)** and **olfactory (I) nerves**.

The *paranasal sinuses* are extensions of the nasal cavity that invaded the diploë (the spongy bone of the flat bones of the skull) of the maxillary, sphenoid, frontal, and ethmoid bones. Their functions are to reduce the weight of the skull and to provide resonance to our voice. However, they are more clinically relevant because of sinus infections. Infections of the maxillary sinus are often confused with pain associated with problems (such as caries) of the maxillary molars.

NOSE AND NASAL CAVITIES

External Nose

The external nose is covered by skin and is divided into two parts: the dorsum and the ala. The **dorsum** is the anterior crest of the nose, whereas the **alae** (singular: **ala**) or wings are its lateral expansions (Fig. 6–1). The dorsum begins as the root of the nose (Fig. 6–2), at the junction of the two nasal bones and the frontal bone, and extends from the face to the tip of the nose. The **bridge of the nose** is the superior portion of the dorsum that is formed by the **nasal bones** (Figs. 6–1 and 6–2). The **nostrils** are the openings into the nasal cavities and are separated by a vertical column of tissue called the **columella nasi** (Fig. 6–1). The external nose is attached to the **piriform aperture**, a pear-shaped opening into the cranium. The aperture is bordered by the *nasal bones* and portions of the *maxillary bones* (Fig. 6–2).

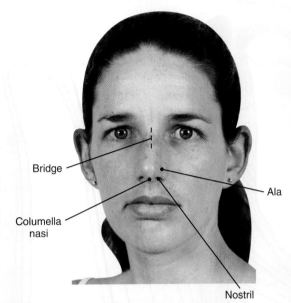

Figure 6–1 The bridge is formed by the nasal bones, whereas the ala is formed by cartilage. The fleshy columella nasi separates the nostrils.

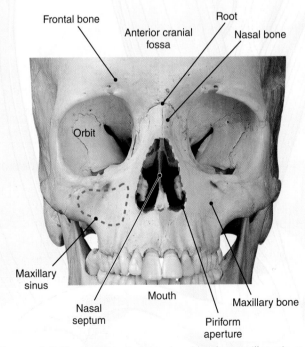

Figure 6–2 The nasal cavity is bordered by the maxillary sinus (outlined in blue), orbits, anterior cranial fossa, and oral cavity. The nasal cavities are triangular in shape and are separated by the nasal septum. The piriform aperture is highlighted in blue.

Nasal Cavity

The interior of the nose resembles a triangular space sub-divided into two right triangular *nasal cavities* separated by the **nasal septum**. The nasal cavities are located inferior to the **anterior cranial cavity**, superior to the **oral cavity**, and medial to the **orbit** and **maxillary sinus** (Fig. 6–2). The apex or roof of the nasal cavity is formed mainly by the **cribriform plate** of the ethmoid bone flanked anteriorly by the nasal and frontal bones and posteriorly by the body of the sphenoid bone (Fig. 6–3). Olfactory nerve fibers (fila olfactoria) traverse the openings in the cribriform plate to enter into the cranial cavity (Fig. 6–3). The **hard palate**, which is composed by the palatine bones and the maxilla, forms the base of the cavities and separates them from the oral cavity (Fig. 6–3). The lateral wall is characterized by a series of three scroll-like bones known as the superior, middle, and inferior nasal conchae (Fig. 6–3). The **superior** and **middle nasal conchae** are processes of the **ethmoid bone**, whereas the

inferior nasal concha is a separate and independent bone (Fig. 6–3). The posterolateral wall is formed by the *perpendicular plate of the palatine bone* and the *medial pterygoid plate of the sphenoid bone* (Fig. 6–3). Anteriorly, the cavity is enclosed mainly by the nasal bones, the maxillary bones (Fig. 6–3), and nasal cartilages.

Posteriorly, the nasal cavities open into the nasopharynx through two openings called the **choanae** (singular: **choana**) (see Fig. 2–18). The *perpendicular plate of ethmoid bone*, the **vomer**, and the **septal cartilage**, form the medial wall or *nasal septum* that separates the two nasal cavities (Fig. 6–4).

The *inferior nasal conchae* are the largest of the nasal conchae and are more anteriorly located. The *middle nasal conchae* are intermediate in size, and the *superior nasal conchae* are the smallest and are situated more posteriorly in the nasal cavity. The conchae are covered with a highly vascular mucous membrane that contains glands and cilia (Fig. 6–5). The *glands* secrete a fluid and mucus to trap dirt and pollutants, whereas the *cilia* move

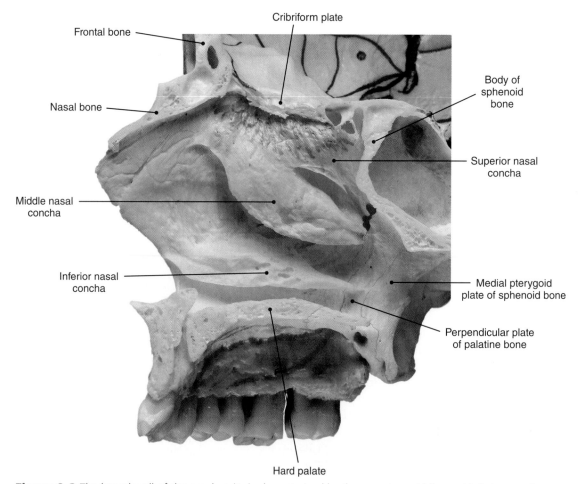

Figure 6–3 The lateral wall of the nasal cavity is characterized by the superior, middle, and inferior nasal conchae. The roof is formed by the frontal bone, the cribriform plate of the ethmoid bone, and the body of the sphenoid bone. Fila olfactoria on the surface of the superior nasal concha enter the anterior cranial cavity through the cribriform plate. The hard palate separates the nasal cavity from the oral cavity below.

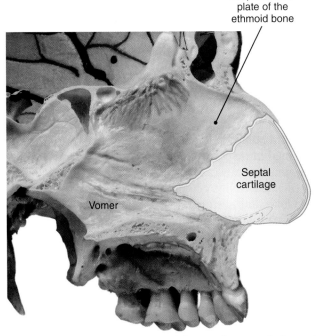

Figure 6–4 The skeletal portion of the nasal septum is formed principally by the ethmoid bone, vomer, and septal cartilage.

will study in the next section, each meatus also contains the openings (**ostium**, plural: ostia) of the paranasal sinuses and the nasolacrimal duct.

Review Question Box 6-1

1. Why are passageways into the lungs called the *conducting division of the respiratory system*?
2. What is the difference between the piriform aperture and the choanae?
3. In comparing the nasal conchae, what is unique about the inferior nasal conchae?
4. What effect would shearing forces have on the structures that pass through the cribriform plate of the ethmoid bone?

PARANASAL SINUSES

The paranasal sinuses are air-filled cells (sacs) located in the *frontal* (Fig. 6–6A), *maxillary* (Figs. 6–6A and 6–6B), *ethmoid* (Fig. 6–7), and *sphenoid bones* (Fig. 6–8). The sacs are lined by the same type of mucous membranes found in the nasal cavity. The *frontal sinus* empties into the anterior aspect of the middle nasal meatus (Fig. 6–9). The ethmoidal sinus is a complex of small air cells that are divided into anterior,

the mucus toward the oropharynx to be swallowed. Inferior to each nasal concha is a space or a **meatus** (Fig. 6–5). Air passes from anterior to posterior through the meatuses, where the air is cleansed and humidified by the mucous membranes of the nasal conchae. As you

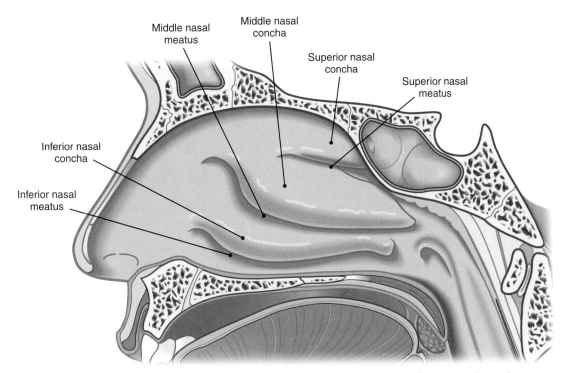

Figure 6–5 The meatuses are depressions in the lateral wall of the nasal cavity inferior to each concha that serve as air passageways through the nasal cavity.

A common place for nosebleeds (**epistaxis**) is **Kiesselbach's area** along the anterior region of the nasal septum where four of the major blood vessels that supply the septum anastomose (interconnect) with each other. These arteries include the superior labial artery (branch of the facial artery), the sphenopalatine artery (a branch of the maxillary artery), the greater palatine artery (a branch of the maxillary artery), and the anterior ethmoidal artery (a branch of the ophthalmic artery). The blood vessels will be discussed in Chapter 11. The most common causes of nosebleeds are trauma to the anterior portion of the nose, placing foreign objects such as a finger into the nose, inflammation, and drying of the mucosa. When profuse bleeding occurs, the nose must be packed with gauze to place pressure on the vessels to prevent further bleeding.

into the middle meatus, is the largest and has the most clinical significance to the dental clinician. The maxillary sinus is situated inferior to the orbit and superior to the oral cavity (Fig. 6–6A). The roots of the maxillary molars and premolars are separated from the maxillary sinus by a thin layer of bone (Fig. 6–6B). Extractions of these teeth can cause exposure of the maxillary sinus. Patients should also be warned not to blow their nose for 24 hours after extraction of maxillary premolars or molars so as not to rupture the thin lining of bone between the alveolus (tooth socket) and the floor of the sinus. Exposure of the maxillary sinus to the oral cavity could cause infection. Additionally, the maxillary sinuses receive their nerve supply from the same branches of the maxillary nerve that supplies the teeth. It is not uncommon for a patient with a head cold or sinus infection to interpret the pain as a toothache from a pulpal infection. The *posterior ethmoidal sinus* drains into the superior nasal meatus, whereas the *sphenoid sinus* drains into the **sphenoethmoidal recess** (Fig. 6–9), which is a space posterior to the superior nasal concha and anterior to the body of the sphenoid bone. The *nasolacrimal duct* carries tears from the eyes and drains into the anterior aspect of the inferior nasal meatus (Fig. 6–9).

middle, and posterior ethmoidal sinuses, although the boundary between groups of sinuses is indistinct (see Figs. 6–5 and 6–8). The *anterior* and *middle ethmoidal sinuses* also drain into the middle nasal meatus (Fig. 6–9). The *maxillary sinus*, which drains

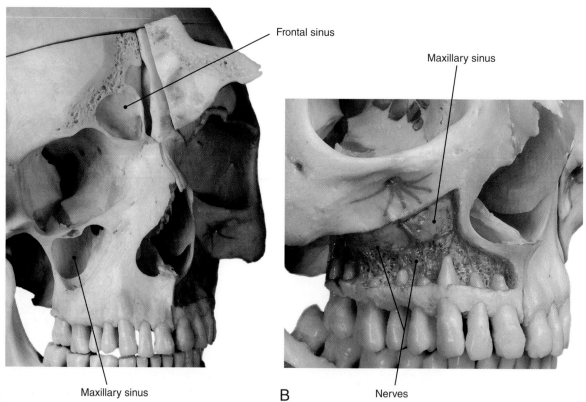

Figure 6–6 (A) The frontal bone has been opened to expose the frontal sinus. The maxillary sinus is superior to the maxillary teeth. **(B)** The nerves that innervate the maxillary teeth are separated from the maxillary sinus by a thin plate of bone.

Review Question Box 6-2

1. What structures drain into the middle nasal meatus?
2. Why does crying result in a "runny nose"?
3. What questions could you ask your patients that would help you to distinguish pain originating in the maxillary sinus from pain from the pulp of a molar tooth?

Ethmoid sinus air cells

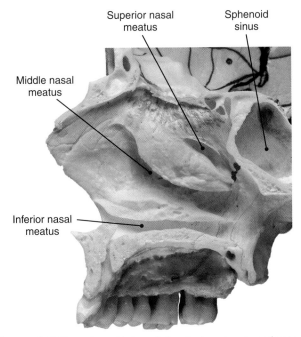

Figure 6–7 The air cells of the ethmoid sinus can be seen with illumination of the orbit.

Superior nasal meatus

Sphenoid sinus

Middle nasal meatus

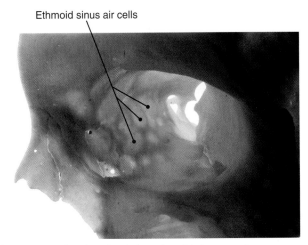

Inferior nasal meatus

Figure 6–8 The sphenoid sinus is located posterosuperior to the nasal cavity. The nasal meatuses lie inferior to the corresponding concha.

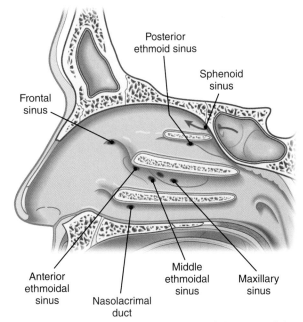

Posterior ethmoid sinus

Sphenoid sinus

Frontal sinus

Anterior ethmoidal sinus

Nasolacrimal duct

Middle ethmoidal sinus

Maxillary sinus

Figure 6–9 The openings of the paranasal sinuses and the nasolacrimal duct into the meatuses are indicated. The sphenoid sinus empties into the sphenoethmoid recess located above the superior nasal concha.

Box 6-2 Development of the Paranasal Sinuses

Only the *maxillary* and the *ethmoidal sinuses* are present at birth and are rudimentary in size. Around 2 years of age, anterior ethmoidal air cells begin to invade the diploë of the frontal bone to form the frontal sinus, whereas posterior ethmoidal air cells penetrate the sphenoid bone to form the sphenoid sinus. The expansion of air cells into the diploë is called **pneumatization** and results in the formation of the *frontal* and *sphenoid sinuses*. Enlargement of the sinusoids continues throughout life. In regard to the maxillary sinus, the bone of the floor that separates the sinus from the maxillary molars can become very thin, and as a result can be torn with the extraction of molars, particularly impacted third molars.

SUMMARY

The nose is the entranceway into the respiratory system. The nasal cavities clean and humidify the air (condition the air) before entering the delicate tissues of the lungs. The nasal cavity also contains the nerve receptors for the sense of smell. The nasal cavities are separated by the nasal septum formed by the vomer, the perpendicular plate of the ethmoid bone, the septal cartilage, and the columella nasi. The bones of the

Box 6-3 Sinus Drainage

The paranasal sinuses are extensions of the nasal cavity and part of their normal function is to produce nasal fluid and mucus to trap and remove air pollutants. The mucus traps the pollutants and the fluid produces a film under the mucus that allows the cilia to beat and move the mucus of the sinuses into the nasal passages. In the upright position, the frontal sinuses can drain by gravity into the middle nasal meatus. The opening of the maxillary sinus is located along its superomedial wall. To enhance drainage of the maxillary sinus on a particular side—that is, the left side—it is necessary to tilt the head to the right in a horizontal plane. This would also aid the drainage of the ethmoidal sinuses. To enhance drainage of the sphenoidal sinus by gravity, the head must be tilted forward in the prone position. The drainage from the sinuses moves posteriorly to the nasopharynx and is eventually swallowed. Overproduction of nasal fluids and mucus because of sinus infections, odors, and other irritants can irritate the throat and cause a sore throat.

lateral wall are modified to form three shell-shaped structures called conchae. Inferior to each concha is a depression called a nasal meatus. Air passes through the meatuses and swirls along the mucous membranes, which are rich in blood vessels and glands. The vessels warm and humidify the air, whereas the glands secrete mucus to trap dust and pollutants.

The paranasal sinuses are extensions of the nasal cavities. The diploë of the frontal, sphenoid, ethmoid, and maxillary bones become pneumatized with air sacs. The sinuses drain into the meatuses and recesses associated with the nasal conchae. The maxillary sinus is clinically important to the dental hygienist because the sensory nerves for pain that supply the maxillary teeth also supply the maxillary sinus. Infections of the maxillary sinus can be referred as pain to the maxillary teeth, particularly the molar teeth. It is necessary for the dental hygienist to determine the source of the pain.

Clinical Case 6.1

One of your patients is a 27-year-old male triathlete who has been bicycle training in the local park. He complains of pain in the left maxillary molar and premolar teeth. The pain has been present for 3 weeks, so he decided to come in for a dental examination because he has experienced pain while chewing on the left side. In reviewing his medical history, you discovered that he has seasonal allergies that are accompanied by mild headaches and sinus infections (sinusitis). Other than taking aspirin for muscle pain associated with his training, he does not take any medications and is in good health. His oral hygiene is good; though he has some generalized gingivitis, he does not have any periodontal pockets. You note that he has a small carious lesion of the right second mandibular molar tooth. Bitewing radiographs show no periodontal bone loss and no other caries. The only abnormality revealed by maxillary right posterior periapical radiographs is thickening of the mucous membrane lining (from inflammation) in the left maxillary sinus.

1. What is the probable source of his pain?
2. What is the anatomical basis for this diagnosis?

Learning Activity 6-1

Lateral Wall of the Nasal Cavity

Match the numbered structures with the correct terms listed to the right.

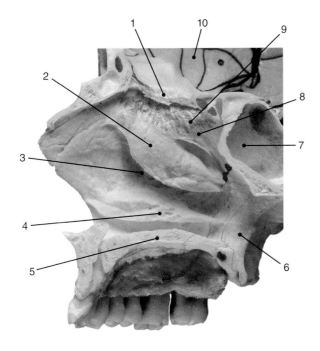

_____ Anterior cranial fossa

_____ Cribriform plate of the ethmoid bone

_____ Fila olfactoria

_____ Hard palate

_____ Inferior nasal concha

_____ Medial pterygoid process

_____ Middle nasal concha

_____ Middle nasal meatus

_____ Sphenoid sinus

_____ Superior nasal concha

Learning Activity 6-2

Nasal Septum

Match the numbered structures with the correct terms listed to the right.

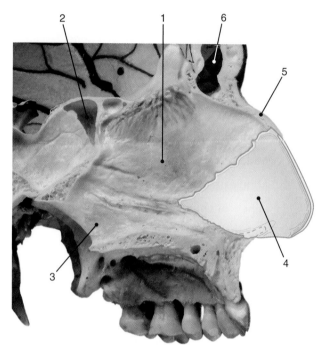

_____ Frontal sinus

_____ Nasal bone

_____ Nasal cartilage

_____ Perpendicular plate of the ethmoid bone

_____ Sphenoid sinus

_____ Vomer

Learning Activity 6-3

Openings in the Lateral Nasal Wall

Match the numbered structures with the correct terms listed to the right.

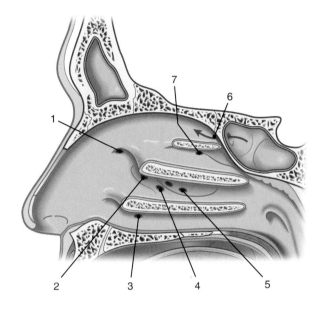

_____ Anterior ethmoid sinus

_____ Frontal sinus

_____ Maxillary sinus

_____ Middle ethmoid sinus

_____ Nasolacrimal duct

_____ Posterior ethmoid sinus

_____ Sphenoid sinus

7

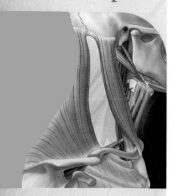

Muscles of Mastication and the Temporomandibular Joint

Objectives

1. Identify the boundaries of the temporal and infratemporal fossae.
2. Distinguish between primary muscles of mastication versus secondary muscles of mastication and know the origins and insertions, innervations, and actions of these muscles.
3. Identify the components of the temporomandibular joint and describe the movements of the joint.

Overview

Everyday, we open and close our mouths to eat, to speak, and for other routine activities. Opening and closing the mouth is similar to walking. We consciously start the movement and continue the activity without much thought. So let's consider what happens when we eat. First, we open our mouths—or another way of saying this is that we lower the jaw (mandible). Depending on the firmness of the food, we close our jaw with considerable force. Then we begin a chewing cycle, in which we alternately open and close the jaw until the food is properly ground for swallowing.

What muscles do we use to open and close our mouths? What muscles do we use to keep food in our mouths while chewing? There are four muscles whose primary function is to open and close the mouth. This group is called the *muscles of mastication*. In addition, there are several muscles whose secondary function is to assist in lowering the jaw and to maintain food in the mouth. This group of muscles is called the *accessory muscles of mastication*. The movement of the jaw occurs at the articulation between the head (condyle) of the mandible and a depression (mandibular fossa) of the temporal bone, known as the *temporo-mandibular joint*.

INTRODUCTION

The *primary muscles of mastication* are responsible for the opening and closing of the mandible during mastication (chewing). These muscles control the movements associated with the **temporomandibular joint** (**TMJ**). In addition, there are several **accessory muscles of mastication** that assist in chewing, but also have other nonrelated functions. The four primary muscles of mastication are the **temporalis**, **medial pterygoid**, **lateral pterygoid**, and **masseter muscles**.

The proper function of these muscles, the structural integrity of the TMJ, and the motor and sensory innervation of these structures are of major importance to the dental hygienist. The hygienist should understand that motor fibers of the muscular branches of the **mandibular division** or **nerve (V3)** of the trigeminal nerve innervate the muscles of mastication, whereas the **auriculotemporal nerve** of V3 supplies sensory fibers to the TMJ. With the exception of the masseter muscle, these muscles are located in either the temporal fossa or the infratemporal fossa, whereas the TMJ is located exclusively in the infratemporal fossa of the skull.

TEMPORAL AND INFRATEMPORAL FOSSAE

Temporal Fossa

The **temporal fossa** is a space that is located superior to the zygomatic arch (Fig. 7–1) and contains the temporalis muscle. Its medial boundary is the bony origin of the temporalis muscle, which is formed by portions of the **temporal**, **frontal**, and **parietal bones**, as well as the **greater wing of the sphenoid bone** (Fig. 7–1). The lateral boundary is the temporalis fascia, which covers the temporalis muscle, and will be discussed later in the chapter.

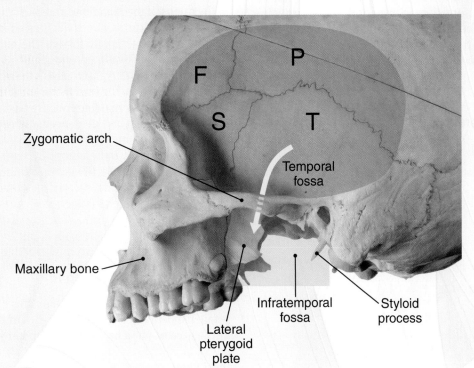

Figure 7–1 The temporal fossa (orange shade) lies superior to the zygomatic arch. The space is bound medially by the frontal bone (F), the parietal bone (P), the greater wing of the sphenoid bone (S), and the temporal bone (T). The infratemporal fossa is a rectangular space (blue shade) inferior to the zygomatic arch. The superior border is a horizontal plane drawn through the inferior border of the zygomatic arch. The anterior border is the posterior surface of the maxillary bone, whereas the posterior border is represented by the styloid process. The medial border is formed by the lateral pterygoid plate, whereas the lateral border is the medial surface of the mandible. The temporal and infratemporal fossae are connected by a narrow passageway medial to the zygomatic arch (yellow arrow) through which the tendon of the temporalis muscle passes to insert on the mandible. The mandible has been removed for a better view of the space.

Infratemporal Fossa

The **infratemporal fossa** is a large, rectangular space (Fig. 7–1) that has incomplete bony boundaries. It contains the medial and lateral pterygoid muscles, and the tendinous portion of the temporalis muscle. As will be studied in later chapters, several nerves and blood vessels of clinical importance to the dental hygienist are also located in this space. The relationships of structures located in the fossa are important clinical consideration for intraoral injections (Chapter 18). The superior boundary, or roof, of this fossa is represented by a horizontal plane drawn from the zygomatic process to the infratemporal crest of the greater wing of the sphenoid bone (Fig. 7–1). The anterior boundary is formed by the posterior, or infratemporal, surface of the maxilla, whereas a frontal plane through the styloid process of the temporal bone is the posterior boundary (Fig. 7–1). The lateral pterygoid plate of the sphenoid bone forms the medial boundary, whereas the medial surface of the ramus of the mandible forms the lateral boundary. A horizontal plane through the inferior surface of the mandible indicates the inferior limit, or floor, of the fossa. The temporal and infratemporal fossae are continuous through a narrow space medial to the zygomatic arch (Fig. 7–2), through which the tendon of the temporalis muscle passes to insert on the mandible.

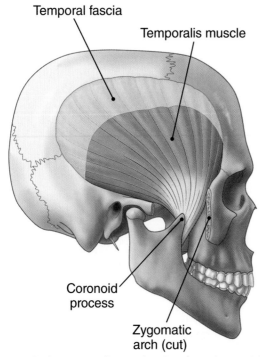

Figure 7–2 The temporalis muscle arises from the cranial bones of the medial border of the temporal fossa and the temporalis fascia. Its tendon passes deep to the zygomatic arch to insert onto the coronoid process of the mandible in the infratemporal fossa.

Temporal fascia

Temporalis muscle

Coronoid process

Zygomatic arch (cut)

Muscles of Mastication

Temporalis Muscle

The *temporalis muscle* arises from the cranial bones that form the medial boundary of the temporal fossa (sphenoid, frontal, parietal, and temporal bones) and the **temporal fascia** on the superficial surface of the muscle (Figs. 7–1 and 7–2). The muscle resembles the shape of a fan. It is broad at its origin and tapers inferiorly as it passes medial to the **zygomatic arch** to insert onto the **coronoid process** and the anterior border of the **ramus** of the mandible (Fig. 7–2). Most of the fibers run vertically; however, the posterior fibers course in a more horizontal direction to pass over the ear. The principal action of this muscle is to elevate the jaw, as in closing the mouth. In addition, contraction of the posterior fibers causes the mandible to be pulled backward. The backward movement of the mandible is called **retrusion** (Table 7–1).

Masseter

The *masseter muscle* lies on the superficial (lateral) surface of the ramus of the mandible, and thus is the only primary muscle of mastication that is not located in either the temporal or the infratemporal fossae. The masseter muscle is partially covered by the parotid gland (Fig. 7–3). In fact, the *duct of the parotid gland* passes superficially over this muscle to penetrate the buccinator muscle as it courses to the oral cavity. The masseter muscle has two heads of origin: the superficial and deep heads, which arise from the inferior border of the *zygomatic arch*. The *superficial head* is larger and arises more anteriorly than the deep head. The superficial muscle fibers run obliquely downward, whereas the *deep fibers* run vertically downward (Fig. 7–6) to insert onto the lateral (superficial) surface of the ramus of the mandible. The primary action of this muscle is to elevate the jaw during mastication, but as with the temporalis muscle, it also retrudes the mandible (Table 7–1).

Lateral Pterygoid Muscle

The *lateral pterygoid muscle* also has two heads. The smaller *superior head* arises from the **infratemporal crest** of the greater wing of the sphenoid bone (Fig. 7–4). The larger *inferior head* (Figs. 7–4 and 7–5) originates from the lateral surface of the **lateral pterygoid plate** (see Fig. 2–18). The two heads run horizontally to insert onto the **mandibular condyle**, the **articular capsule** of the TMJ, and the **articular disc** of the TMJ (Figs. 7–4 and 7–5). The lateral pterygoid has two major actions: **protrusion** (forward movement) and depression of the mandible (Table 7–1).

Medial Pterygoid Muscle

The fibers of the *medial pterygoid muscle* parallel those of the superficial head of the masseter except they are located

TABLE 7-1	Primary Muscles of Mastication			
Muscle	**Origin**	**Insertion**	**Action**	**Innervation**
Temporalis	Cranial bones of the medial border of the temporal fossa and the deep fascia of the temporalis muscle	Coronoid process and the anterior border of the ramus of the mandible	Elevates and retrudes the mandible	Mandibular nerve
Masseter	Medial and inferior border of the zygomatic arch	Lateral surface of the ramus of the mandible	Superficial fibers elevate and provide limited protrusion, deep fibers retrude the mandible	Mandibular nerve
Lateral pterygoid	Superior head arises from the infratemporal surface of the greater wing of the sphenoid bone Inferior head originates from the lateral surface of the lateral pterygoid plate	Auricular capsule of the TMJ and articular disc of the joint Mandibular condyle	Protrudes and depresses the mandible; side-to-side movement while chewing	Mandibular nerve
Medial pterygoid	Superficial head: maxillary tuberosity Deep head: medial surface of the lateral pterygoid plate	Medial surface of the ramus of the mandible	Elevates and protrudes the jaw; side-to-side movement while chewing	Mandibular nerve

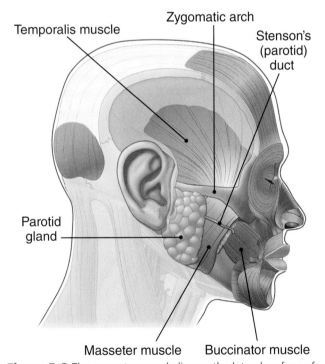

Figure 7–3 The masseter muscle lies on the lateral surface of the mandible anterior to the parotid gland. The parotid duct crosses over the surface of the muscle and penetrates the buccinator muscle to reach the oral cavity. The superficial head originates from the zygomatic process and courses obliquely downward to insert onto the angle of the mandible. The deep fibers are more vertically oriented.

on the medial surface of the ramus of the mandible. This muscle also has two origins. The smaller *superficial head* arises from the **maxillary tuberosity** just behind the third molar (Fig. 7–4). The larger *deep head* originates from the medial surface of the **lateral pterygoid plate** and **pterygoid fossa** (Fig. 7–5). The muscle inserts onto the medial surface of the *mandibular ramus* and the **pterygoid tuberosity** (Fig. 7–5). The function of this muscle is protrusion and elevation of the mandible (Table 7–1).

Review Question Box 7-1

1. What is the only muscle of mastication that opens the mouth?
2. Which muscle of mastication is not located in either the temporal or infratemporal fossae? Where is its location?
3. Define the terms *protrusion*, *retrusion*, *elevation*, and *depression* in regard to movements of the mandible.
4. What muscles form a sling around the ramus of the mandible?

ACCESSORY MUSCLES OF MASTICATION

The *accessory muscles of mastication* comprise a group of miscellaneous muscles whose secondary function is to assist the chewing process, but also have other

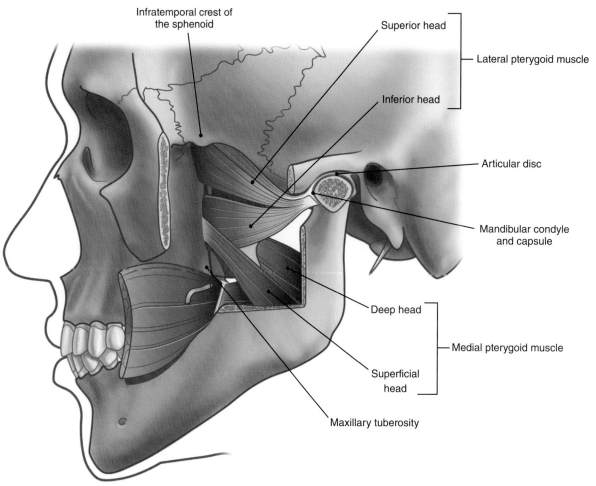

Figure 7–4 The superior head of the lateral pterygoid muscle originates from the infratemporal crest of the sphenoid bone, whereas the inferior head originates from the lateral pterygoid plate covered by the inferior head of the lateral pterygoid muscle. The superior head inserts onto the articular disc, and the inferior head inserts onto the articular capsule and mandibular condyle.

Box 7-1 Masticator Space

The muscles of mastication, along with their associated blood vessels and nerves, are enclosed by a connective tissue sheath (fascia) that isolates these structures into a compartment called the **masticator space**. Infections in this area can cause tonic (continual) contraction of muscles of mastication that can cause **trismus**, which is the inability to open the mouth. One of the more common etiologies of trismus is the inflammation of the soft tissue around impacted third molars. Radiation therapy, trauma, and surgery can also cause tonic contraction of the muscles of mastication. The **fascia** is attached superiorly to the superior temporal line of the temporal bone and covers the lateral superficial surface of the temporalis muscles. The fascia then attaches to the zygomatic arch and continues onto the surface of the masseter muscle. The sheath attaches to the inferior margin of the body of the mandible and then turns inward to cover the medial surface of the medial pterygoid muscle and attaches superiorly to the medial pterygoid plate.

functions related to swallowing. Unlike the primary muscles of mastication, not all of the accessory muscles are innervated by the mandibular nerve. The following are generally considered the accessory muscles of mastication.

Buccinator Muscle

The **buccinator muscle** (Fig. 7–6), which lies deep to the masseter muscle, is technically a muscle of facial expression (Chapter 5) and is innervated by the **facial**

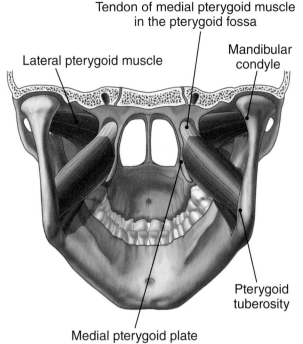

Figure 7–5 The deep head of the medial pterygoid muscle originates from the medial surface of the lateral pterygoid plate and the pterygoid fossa, which is bordered medially by the medial pterygoid plate. The muscle inserts onto the medial surface of the mandibular ramus below the mandibular foramen and onto the pterygoid tuberosity. The lateral pterygoid muscle partially covers the lateral pterygoid plate and inserts onto the mandibular condyle.

nerve (**VII**). While chewing, the buccinator keeps the cheek wall taut (tight), thus keeping the food in the oral cavity (Table 7–2).

Digastric Muscle

The **anterior** and **posterior bellies of the digastric muscle** are muscles of the neck (Chapter 3). The muscles, which are derived from two different embryonic structures, are fused at their attachment to the hyoid bone (Fig. 7–6). The anterior belly is innervated by the

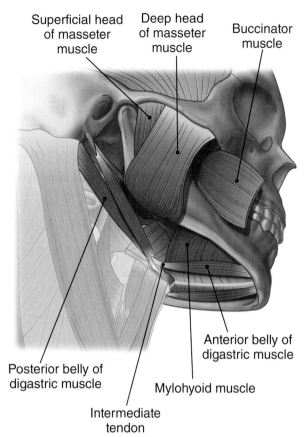

Figure 7–6 The deep and superficial heads of the masseter muscle originate from the zygomatic arch and attach to the ramus of the mandible, which is covered by the muscle. The buccinator muscle of the face and the anterior and posterior bellies of the digastric muscle are accessory muscles of mastication. The digastric muscles are joined by an intermediate tendon.

mandibular nerve (V3), whereas the posterior belly is innervated by the *facial nerve (VII)*. The posterior belly originates from the mastoid process of the temporal bone, and its tendon inserts by a sling of connective tissue attached to the hyoid bone. The anterior belly originates from the mandible and inserts on the same tendon. The common tendon is called the *intermediate tendon of the digastric muscles* (Fig. 7–6). When the

TABLE 7–2	Accessory Muscles of Mastication			
Muscle	**Origin**	**Insertion**	**Action**	**Innervation**
Buccinator	Pterygomandibular raphe	Corner of the mouth	Tightens the cheek wall while chewing	Facial nerve
Anterior belly of the digastric	Intermediate tendon on the hyoid bone	Mandible	Depresses the mandible	Mandibular nerve
Posterior belly of the digastric	Mastoid process	Intermediate tendon to the hyoid bone	Depresses the mandible	Facial nerve
Mylohyoid	Mylohyoid line of the mandible	Hyoid bone	Depresses the mandible	Mandibular nerve
Geniohyoid	Mental spine of the mandible	Hyoid bone	Depresses the mandible	C1

mandible is closed, these muscles will elevate the hyoid bone while swallowing. If the hyoid bone is held in place by the downward pull of the infrahyoid muscles, the two bellies of the digastric muscle aid in the opening of the mandible (Table 7–2).

Mylohyoid and Geniohyoid Muscles

The **mylohyoid** and **geniohyoid muscles** are muscles of the floor of the mouth (Chapter 8). These muscles are attached to the mandible and the hyoid bone (Fig. 7–7). When the mouth is closed in a fixed position, contraction of the mylohyoid muscle elevates the floor of the mouth, whereas the geniohyoid muscle raises the hyoid bone. When the hyoid bone is held in place by the infrahyoid muscles, the mylohyoid and geniohyoid muscles assist in the depression of the mandible. The mylohyoid muscle is innervated by a branch of the mandibular nerve (V3), whereas the geniohyoid is innervated by spinal nerve C1 (Table 7–2).

Review Question Box 7-2

1. Why are the accessory muscles of mastication not grouped as muscles of mastication?
2. Why is the buccinator muscle functionally different from the other accessory muscles of mastication?

TEMPOROMANDIBULAR JOINT

The *temporomandibular joint* (*TMJ*) is a freely moveable synovial joint between the **mandibular fossa** (also called the **glenoid cavity** by dental clinicians) of the *temporal bone* and the head of the *condyle* of the mandible. The joint is enclosed by a tough connective tissue capsule supported on its lateral surface by the **lateral temporomandibular ligament** (Fig. 7–8A). Internally, the capsule is lined by a synovial membrane. The membrane secretes synovial fluid, which lubricates the joint to reduce friction and wear on the articular surfaces.

Articular Surfaces

The articular surface of temporal bone is formed by the concave *mandibular fossa* (*glenoid cavity*) that is bordered anteriorly by the sloping **articular eminence** of the zygomatic process of the temporal bone (Figs. 7–9A and 7–9B). The lateral surface of the eminence is called the **articular tubercle** (Fig. 7–9B) and is an attachment site for the capsule (Fig. 7–8A). The fossa is separated from the **external acoustic meatus** by the tympanic portion of the temporal bone (Fig. 7–9A). The head of the *mandibular condyle,* which has an oblong shape, inserts obliquely into the fossa. If a line is drawn diagonally through each fossa, the lines would intersect at the foramen magnum (Fig. 7–10). Because of this arrangement, the mandible cannot be fully depressed (opened) in one motion, such as opening a door. Depressing the jaw requires two movements. The first is a hinge movement that partially opens the jaw, which is followed by a gliding movement that slides the mandibular condyle forward over the articular eminence, which allows the mandible to fully open.

Articular Capsule

As other synovial joints, the TMJ is enclosed by an *articular capsule.* The capsule is attached superiorly to the perimeter of the mandibular fossa and surrounds the articular eminence to the neck of the mandibular condyle and portions of the tendon of the lateral pterygoid muscle (Fig. 7–8A). The articular capsule is supported on its lateral surface by a thickening of the capsule known as the *lateral temporomandibular ligament.* The ligament extends superiorly from the *articular tubercle* to the mandibular condyle onto the neck of the mandibular condyle (Fig. 7–8A). It limits the posterior displacement and lateral movement of the joint. Other minor ligaments, the **stylomandibular** (Figs. 7–8A and 7–8B) and **sphenomandibular** (Fig. 7–8B) **ligaments**, help to stabilize the joint.

Joint Cavity and Articular Disc

To provide a mechanism for the movements required of the TMJ, the joint has been modified by the insertion of a disc that divides the joint into upper and lower joint spaces (Fig. 7–11). This *articular disc* has a biconcave shape with a thin intermediate zone and

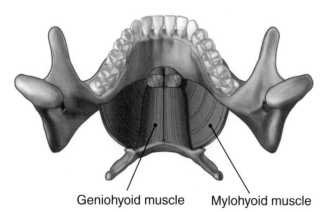

Geniohyoid muscle   Mylohyoid muscle

Figure 7–7 The mylohyoid and geniohyoid muscles are located in the floor of the mouth. These muscles assist in opening the mouth.

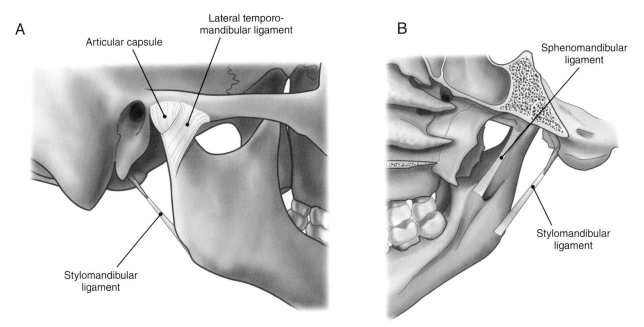

Figure 7–8 (A) The TMJ is enclosed by the articular capsule, which is reinforced by the lateral temporomandibular ligament. The ligament attaches onto the articular tubercle, and its fibers slant in a posteroinferior direction. The stylomandibular ligament is visible from the lateral **(A)** and medial **(B)** views of the mandible. **(B)** The sphenomandibular ligament is located on the medial surface of the mandible.

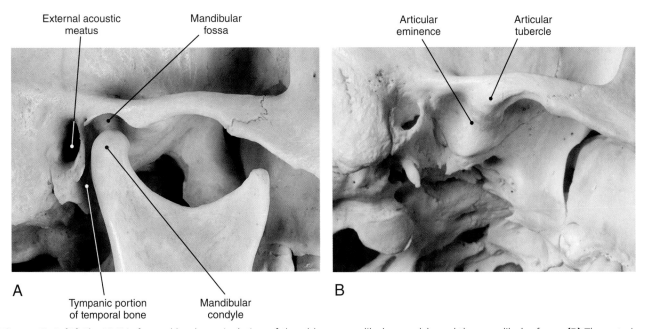

Figure 7–9 (A) The TMJ is formed by the articulation of the oblong mandibular condyle and the mandibular fossa. **(B)** The anterior sloping portion of the fossa is the articular eminence. The articular tubercle is the downward projection of bone from the zygomatic process. The TMJ is separated from the external acoustic meatus by the tympanic portion of the temporal bone.

thicker anterior and posterior zones. The area behind the articular disc is called the **retrodiscal pad** and contains the blood vessels and sensory nerves of the mandibular nerve (V3) that supply the joint. The articular disc is attached peripherally to the articular capsule and anteriorly to the *lateral pterygoid muscle*

(Fig. 7–11). The medial and lateral borders of the disc are also attached to the mandibular condyle. The disc moves forward and backward with the movement of the condyle initiated by the primary muscles of mastication, but the range of motion is limited by its attachment to the capsule.

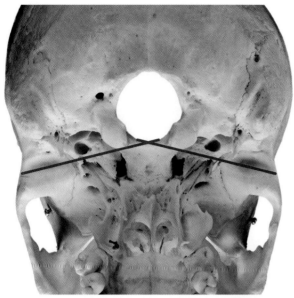

Figure 7–10 The oblique orientation of the mandibular fossae is indicated by the lines that intersect at the foramen magnum. The articulation of the condyles within the fossae prevents the opening of the mouth with a single hingelike motion.

Movements of the TMJ

As mentioned earlier, the orientation of the mandibular condyle in the fossa prevents the complete opening (depression) of the lower jaw (mandible). Thus, two movements are required to fully depress the mandible (open the mouth). As the jaw first opens, the condyle rotates (**rotational movement**) on the disc in the lower joint space (Fig. 7–12A). The movement is similar to a door opening and closing on a hinge, hence the alternate name of **hinge movement**. This movement is accomplished by gravity and contraction of several accessory muscles of mastication. To fully open the jaw, the *lateral pterygoid muscle* contracts, which causes the condyle and disc to slide (**gliding** or **translation movement**) anteriorly over the articular eminence in the upper joint space (Fig. 7–12B). The anterior movement of the mandible is called *protrusion.*

The thickness of the posterior portion of the articular disc stabilizes the joint when chewing on one side. For example, while chewing meat on the left side, the joint on the right side is slightly stretched open. This can cause wobbling and injury to the joint on the inactive (nonchewing) side. Contraction of the lateral pterygoid muscle pulls the capsule anteriorly to allow the thickened portion of the disc to support that joint. After the chewing motion has stopped, the relaxation of the lateral pterygoid slowly allows the disc to move smoothly posteriorly to its original position.

Three muscles—the temporalis, medial pterygoid, and masseter muscles—close the protruded jaw. When these muscles contract, the mandibular condyle *retrudes* (moves posteriorly) and is elevated to close the jaw.

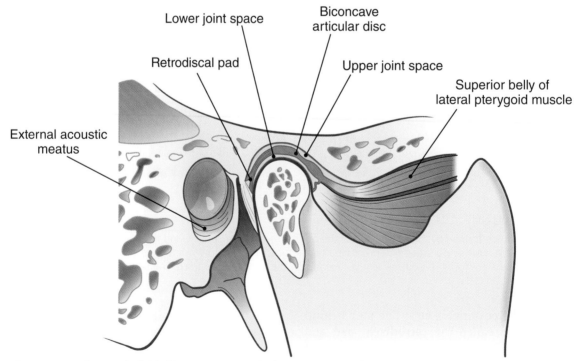

Figure 7–11 The TMJ is divided into an upper and a lower joint space by the biconcave articular disc. The thickened area posterior to the disc is the retrodiscal pad. The anterior portion of the disc is attached to the superior belly of the lateral pterygoid muscle.

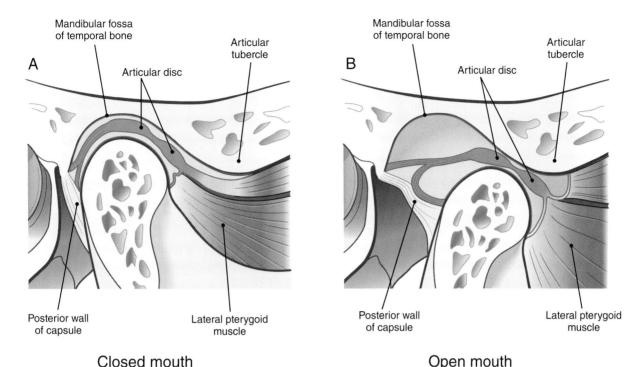

Closed mouth   Open mouth

Figure 7–12 (A) The sagittal section of the TMJ shows the position of the articular disc in a closed mouth. **(B)** The sagittal section of the open mouth illustrates the position of the mandibular condyle and articular disc on the articular eminence. The forward movement of the condyle is prevented by the thick posterior portion of the disc.

Review Question Box 7-3

1. What structural feature of the TMJ limits the depression of the mandible? How is this joint adapted to overcome this limitation?
2. What movements take place in the joint spaces of the TMJ?
3. How does the lateral pterygoid muscle depress the mandible?
4. What is the difference between the articular tubercle and the articular eminence?

Clinical Correlation Box 7-1

Dislocation of the TMJ

Anterior dislocation of the jaw can be caused by opening the mouth too wide. The initial opening of the jaw is produced by the hinge movement in the lower joint space. To continue opening the mouth, the condyle of the mandible glides onto the posterior sloping surface of the articular eminence. If the mouth is opened too widely, the condyle will become lodged on the anterior surface of the eminence. To reduce (place in the correction position) the dislocation, the mandible must be pulled inferiorly and then pushed posteriorly to slide over the articular eminence.

Clinical Correlation Box 7-2

TMJ Disorders

TMJ disorders refer to multiple conditions that place undue stress on the joint. These conditions can cause acute or chronic inflammation of the TMJ that can result in pain from the jaw and nearby areas such as the ear and neck, as well as limiting jaw movement. Stress can be caused by over opening the jaw beyond its normal range or overuse of the TMJ by repetitive movements such as grinding of the teeth (**bruxism**) and excessive chewing of gum. Other causes of TMJ disorders are trauma to the jaw, erosion of the disc, arthritis, malocclusion of the jaw, and fatigue of the muscles that stabilize the joint. Patients may complain of pain in the neck and shoulder, headaches, pain and ringing (**tinnitus**) in the ears, painful clicking when opening and closing the jaw, stiffness of the muscles of mastication, and reduced ability to move the mandible.

SUMMARY

Opening and closing the mouth requires the depression (opening) and elevation (closing) of the mandible. These movements require muscles acting on the temporomandibular joint. The TMJ is formed by the articulation of the mandibular condyle with the mandibular fossa (glenoid cavity) of the temporal bone. The TMJ is a synovial joint that is surrounded by an articular capsule, which is reinforced by the lateral temporomandibular ligament. The complete depression of the jaw is hindered because of the diagonal orientation of the mandibular condyle in the mandibular fossa. To perform the required movements, an articular disc modifies the synovial space into an upper and lower joint space. The initial downward movement is a rotation (hinge) of the mandibular condyle in the lower joint space. For full depression, the articular disc and condyle move forward onto the articular eminence. To close the mouth, the condyle and disc are retruded (moved posteriorly into the mandibular fossa).

There are four primary muscles of mastication that are innervated by motor fibers of the mandibular division (V3) of the trigeminal nerve. The temporalis, medial pterygoid, and masseter muscles elevate and retrude the jaw. The lateral pterygoid muscle depresses the jaw and protrudes the mandible by pulling the mandibular condyle and articular disc onto the articular eminence. Several accessory muscles assist in opening the mouth. Their innervations are variable. The anterior belly of the digastric muscle of the neck and the mylohyoid muscle of the floor of the mouth are innervated by the mandibular nerve (V3), whereas the posterior belly of the digastric muscle of the neck is innervated by the facial nerve (VII), and the geniohyoid muscle of the floor of the mouth is innervated by a spinal nerve (C1). While chewing, the buccinator muscle of the face—which is innervated by the facial nerve (VII)—tightens the cheek wall to keep food in the oral cavity. Sensory information from the TMJ is carried by afferent fibers of the mandibular nerve (V3)

LEARNING LAB
Exercises for review, practice, and study

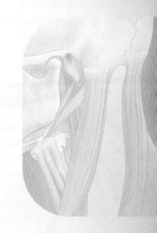

Laboratory Activity 7-1

Palpating the TMJ and Related Muscles

Objective: The structure and movements of the TMJ are important to the dental profession. Although the TMJ and its associated muscles cannot be dissected, several of its features can be determined by palpation. In this exercise, you will palpate surface features related to the *TMJ* using yourself as a model or a partner.

Materials Needed: If you do this exercise with a partner, wear gloves.

Step 1: Begin your study by identifying the masseter and temporalis muscles.

- Place your fingers on the ramus of the mandible. With your mouth closed, gently bite down on your teeth. You should be able to feel the contraction of the *masseter muscle*, which is a powerful chewing muscle of mastication.
- Now place your fingers on the skin of the temporal region superior to the zygomatic arch and gently bite down on your teeth. You should feel the contraction of the fan-shaped *temporalis muscle*, which is also a powerful chewing muscle.

Step 2: Let's now locate the TMJ.

- Using both hands, place your fingers on the inferior border of both zygomatic arches and slide your fingers toward the ear while slightly opening and closing the jaw (mandible).
- You should feel the movement of the *mandibular condyle* within the joint.

Step 3: Demonstrate the two movements associated with the TMJ.

- Slightly depress (open) and elevate (close) the mandible. Notice that the condyle is moving in a hingelike motion. This *hinge (rotational) movement* is taking place in the *lower joint space*.
- Now open your mouth wider, but do not hyperextend the jaw. Do you feel a different motion to the mandibular condyle? The answer should be yes. The condyle and the articular disc are moving forward onto the mandibular eminence, allowing the mouth to be opened wider. This is the *gliding movement* that takes place in the *upper joint space*.
- Realize as the mandible is depressed that it is being protruded (moving forward) at the same time. What muscle opens and *protrudes* the jaw? If your answer is the *lateral pterygoid muscle*, you are correct. Do other muscles of mastication assist in the protrusion of the mandible? If so, can you name the muscles? Once again, the answer is yes, and even though the *masseter* and *medial pterygoid muscles* close the mouth they can also protrude the jaw. Realize that, when closing the mouth, the mandible is *elevated* and *retruded* (moves backward). The *medial pterygoid muscle* elevates the mandible, whereas the *temporalis* and the *masseter muscles* elevate and retrude the mandible.

Step 4: Next, study the side-to-side motion of the mandible that occurs during the chewing cycle.

- Once again, place the fingers of both hands on the TMJ. Slowly move the jaw from side to side. While moving the mandible to the right, note that the mandibular condyle moves to the right. What prevents the lateral dislocation of the mandibular condyle? If your answer is the *lateral temporomandibular ligament*, you are correct. Recall that this ligament is a lateral thickening of the articular capsule.
- Now rotate the jaw to the left, and note that the left mandibular condyle moves to the left.

For Discussion or Thought:

1. *Why would it be difficult to palpate the medial and lateral pterygoid muscles?*

2. *Did you hear any clicking sounds while depressing and elevating the mandible? Clicking sounds are more prevalent in women and represent the movement of the articular disc along the articular eminence. If pain accompanies the clicking sounds, this could indicate a TMJ disorder.*

Learning Activity 7-1

Primary Muscles of Mastication

Match the numbered structures with the correct terms listed to the right.

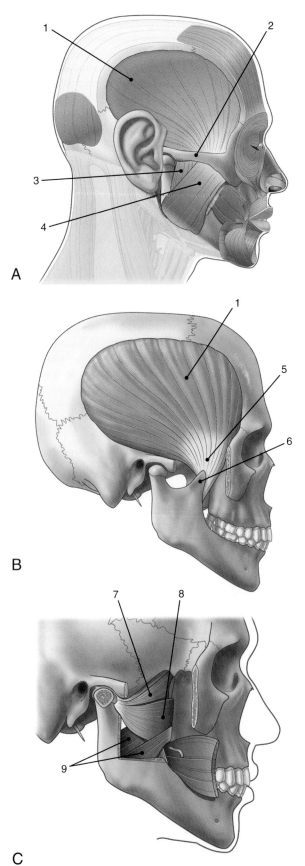

_____ Coronoid process

_____ Deep head of the masseter muscle

_____ Inferior head of the lateral pterygoid muscle

_____ Medial pterygoid muscle

_____ Superficial head of the masseter muscle

_____ Superior head of the lateral pterygoid muscle

_____ Temporalis muscle

_____ Tendon of the temporalis muscle

_____ Zygomatic arch

Learning Activity 7-2

Bones of the Temporomandibular Joint—Sagittal View

Match the numbered structures with the correct terms listed to the right.

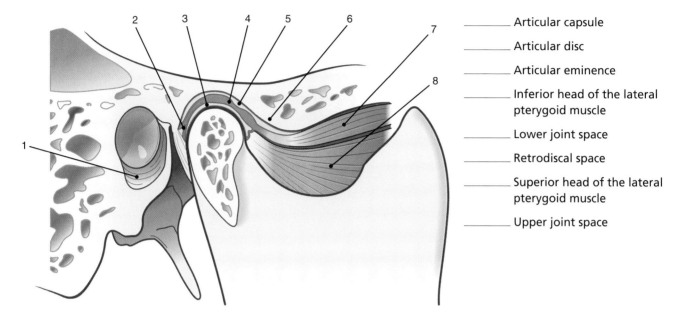

_____ Articular capsule

_____ Articular disc

_____ Articular eminence

_____ Inferior head of the lateral
pterygoid muscle

_____ Lower joint space

_____ Retrodiscal space

_____ Superior head of the lateral
pterygoid muscle

_____ Upper joint space

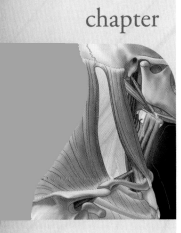

8

Oral Cavity

Objectives

1. Distinguish between the following terms: *mouth*, *oral cavity*, and *vestibule*.
2. Identify the major landmarks of the mouth.
3. Identify the muscles that form the floor of the mouth, and know their actions and innervation.
4. Identify the components of the teeth; compare the number of teeth in a child and an adult; distinguish among the tooth surfaces and describe their relationships to the surrounding tissues.
5. Identify the extrinsic and intrinsic muscles of the tongue and discuss their function and innervation.

Overview

The word *mouth* refers to an entranceway or exit point, such as the opening of a jar or the entrance into a waterway (for example, mouth of the Mississippi River). In the human body, the mouth is the entranceway into the digestive system. The walls surrounding the mouth have been adapted to enhance this function. The most obvious adaptations, which are the foundation of the dental hygiene profession, are the teeth and jaws. The anterior teeth are used for tearing, whereas the posterior teeth grind or pulverize the food. The closing and opening of the jaw, along with the contraction of the buccinator muscle, help maintain food within the mouth, whereas chewing provides the force for tearing and grinding. The tongue is used to roll the food into a bolus in preparation for swallowing. Additionally, the tongue is equipped with taste buds that help us determine whether food is safe to eat. The walls of the mouth contain small glands that produce about 5% of the saliva that is used to moisten the food, cleanse the mouth, and initiate the digestion of carbohydrates.

In this chapter, the major surface landmarks of the oral cavity and the underlying gross anatomical structures that are critical for proper intraoral examinations are discussed.

INTRODUCTION

The mouth is divided into the **oral vestibule** (Figs. 8–1A and 8–1B), the space between the teeth and the cheek and lips, and the **oral cavity** (Fig. 8–1A), which is the space in between the teeth that extends posteriorly to the entrance of the throat (anterior tonsillar pillars).

ORAL VESTIBULE

The vestibule is subdivided into two parts depending upon the relationship of the teeth to the wall of the cheek or the lip. The **buccal vestibule** is the space between the teeth and the cheek wall, whereas the **labial vestibule** is the space between the teeth and the lips (Fig. 8–1B). The superior and inferior limits of the vestibule form V-shaped depressions known as either the **vestibular**

fornix or the **mucobuccal fold** (Fig. 8–2). This surface feature represents the line of flexure where the **mucosa** (epithelium and underlying connective tissue) of the lip and cheek pass onto the surface of the alveolar bone of the mandible and maxilla (Fig. 8–2).

There are several landmarks of interest to the dental hygienist within the vestibule. The lower lip is attached to the alveolar mucosa of the mandible and the upper lip is attached to the maxilla by a fold of mucosa called the **labial frenulum** (Fig. 8–2). With proper lighting, numerous small glands are visible through the lining mucosa of the lips. These **labial glands** (Fig. 8–3) comprise one of a group of minor salivary glands that contribute 5% of the saliva to the oral cavity.

Another prominent landmark of the vestibule is the **parotid papilla**, which is located on the cheek (buccal) wall opposite the second maxillary molar (Fig. 8–4).

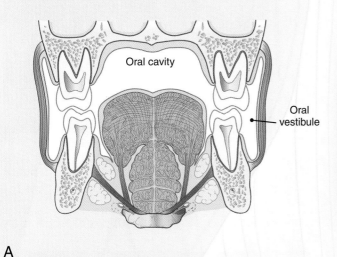

Oral cavity

Oral vestibule

A

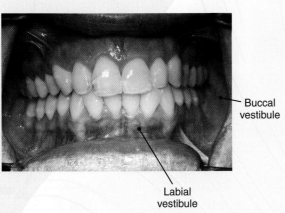

Buccal vestibule

Labial vestibule

B

Figure 8–1 (A) The mouth is divided by the teeth into the oral vestibule and the oral cavity (proper). The vestibule lies lateral to the teeth, whereas the oral cavity is surrounded by the teeth. **(B)** The buccal vestibule is the space between the teeth and the cheek wall, whereas the labial vestibule lies between the teeth and the lips.

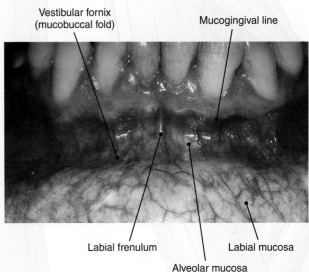

Vestibular fornix (mucobuccal fold)

Mucogingival line

Labial frenulum

Labial mucosa

Alveolar mucosa

Figure 8–2 The vestibular fornix, also called the *mucobuccal fold*, represents the reflection of the alveolar mucosa onto the wall of the cheeks and lips. The lips are attached to the alveolar mucosa by the labial frenulum. The attachment of the inferior lip to the mandibular alveolar mucosa is indicated.

Box 8-1 Minor Salivary Glands

The glands of the lip, hard and soft palates, cheek walls, and the tongue are called either **minor** or **intrinsic** because of their diminutive size and their location inside the wall of mouth. Irritation of the ducts of the labial glands—such as rubbing of orthodontic appliances on the lip—can cause blockage of the ducts of these glands, which results in the swelling of the gland. A swollen gland is known as a **mucocele**.

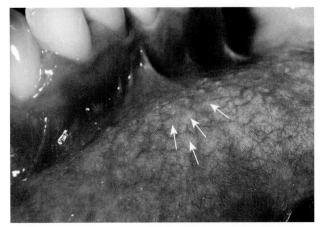

Labial glands (white arrows)

Figure 8–3 The labial intrinsic salivary glands are visible through the mucosa of the lip.

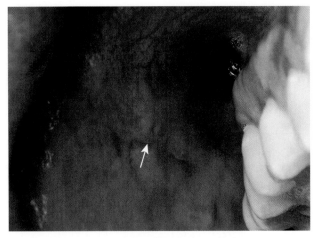

Parotid papilla (white arrow)

Figure 8–4 The duct of the parotid gland empties into the buccal vestibule by an opening on the parotid papilla (arrow) located on the cheek wall opposite the second maxillary molar.

The papilla is an elevation of the mucosal lining of the cheek on which the duct of the parotid gland opens into the vestibule. Other important features of the buccal mucosa include Fordyce spots and the linea alba. **Fordyce spots** (referred to clinically as **Fordyce granules**) are sebaceous glands that open into the oral cavity (Fig. 8–5). This is unusual in that sebaceous glands generally empty into the hair follicles of the skin. The **linea alba** is a white horizontal line of keratinized epithelium on the cheek wall that is caused by the grinding of the teeth (Fig. 8–6). The lining mucosa of the cheek wall is normally a nonkeratinized epithelium. It is important for the dental hygienist to realize that unexplained keratinization of the epithelium of the cheek wall usually indicates a pathological change deep to the surface epithelium.

Review Question Box 8-1

1. What is the difference between the vestibule and the vestibular fornix?
2. What are Fordyce spots (granules)?
3. What is the difference between a frenulum and a papilla?

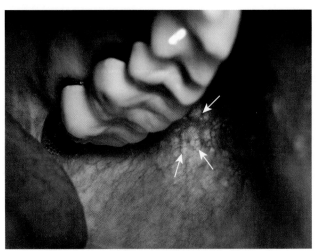

Fordyce granulations (white arrows)

Figure 8–5 Fordyce granulations are sebaceous glands (arrows) located in the buccal mucosa.

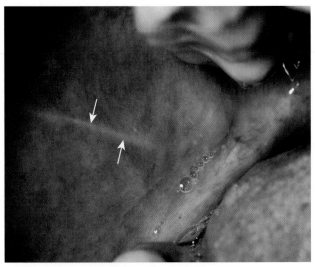

Linea alba (white arrows)

Figure 8–6 The linea alba (arrows) is a line of keratinized epithelium along the buccal mucosa caused by abrasions along the occlusal line of the maxillary and mandibular teeth.

TEETH AND SURROUNDING TISSUE

Gingiva

The teeth separate the vestibule from the oral cavity. The teeth are surrounded by a layer of mucosa called the **gingiva** (gums). The gingiva is further subdivided according to its location. The **attached gingiva** is the portion of the gingiva that is attached directly to either the bone or the tooth surface (Fig. 8–7). The nonattached, moveable margin of the gingiva is called the **free gingiva** (Fig. 8–7), whereas the sulcus (space between the teeth and gums) is lined by the **sulcular gingiva**. In between adjacent teeth is the tent-shaped **interdental papilla** (Fig. 8–7). The light pink-colored gingiva is separated from the darker red **alveolar mucosa** of the mandible and maxilla by the **mucogingival line**. The **col** is the portion of the gingiva that is located in between the contact points between adjacent teeth. Although it is not easily visible, the col has a concave surface. The col becomes flattened by bone loss due to periodontal disease.

Review Question Box 8-2

1. What is the difference between attached gingiva and free gingiva?
2. What is the difference between the interdental gingiva and the col?

Teeth

The details of tooth structure and nomenclature are discussed in dental anatomy textbooks. This section will summarize the general features of teeth, as opposed to discussing the specific features of each tooth.

There is a total of 20 **deciduous** (primary) teeth in children: 10 teeth on the mandibular and 10 on the maxillary arches. The arches are divided into four quadrants: left and right upper maxillary quadrants and left and right lower mandibular quadrants. Each quadrant contains 1 central incisor, 1 lateral incisor, 1 canine, and 1st and 2nd molar teeth. In the adult, there are 32 permanent teeth. After the shedding of the deciduous teeth, the incisors and canines are replaced by their adult counterparts; however, the deciduous molars are replaced by the permanent 1st and 2nd premolars. The 1st, 2nd, and 3rd molars develop independently from the deciduous teeth as outgrowths of the distal portions of the mandibular and maxillary arches (Figs. 8–8A and 8–8B).

The tooth is composed of a crown and a root (roots), which surround the connective tissue of the **pulp**. The **anatomical crown** of the tooth is composed of **enamel** and **dentin**, whereas the **root** is composed of *dentin* (Fig. 8–9). Enamel is a mineralized, noncellular tissue that protects the underlying dentin and pulp, in addition to providing a grinding surface for mastication. The surface of the root is covered by cementum, but is

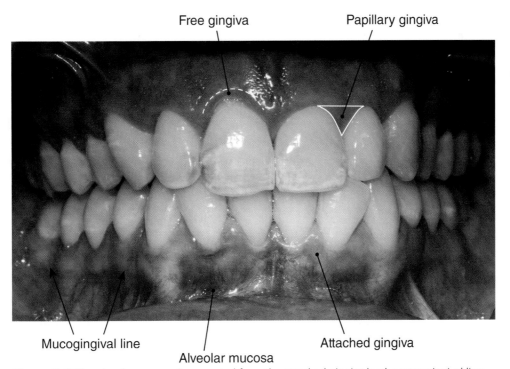

Free gingiva   Papillary gingiva

Mucogingival line   Attached gingiva

Alveolar mucosa

Figure 8–7 The alveolar mucosa is separated from the attached gingiva by the mucogingival line (arrows). The papillary gingiva is the triangle-shaped area between adjacent teeth. The free gingiva is the nonattached margin of the gingiva, which is separated from the tooth by a sulcus.

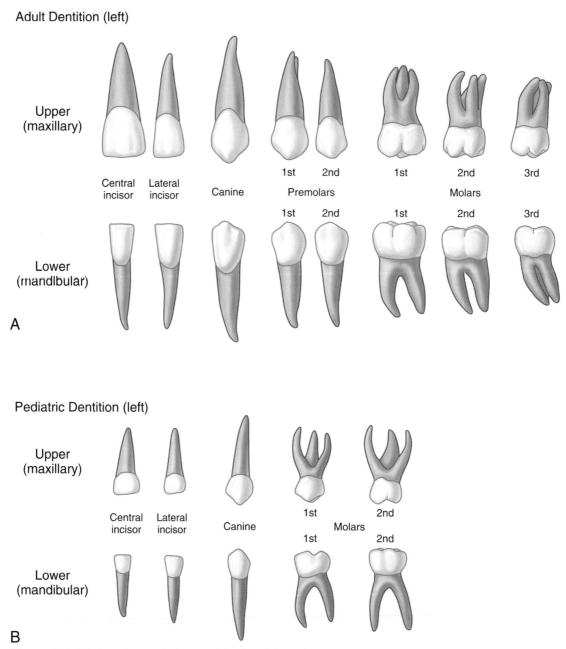

Adult Dentition (left)

Upper (maxillary)

Lower (mandibular)

Central incisor Lateral incisor Canine 1st 2nd Premolars 1st 2nd 3rd Molars

A

Pediatric Dentition (left)

Upper (maxillary)

Lower (mandibular)

Central incisor Lateral incisor Canine 1st 2nd Molars

B

Figure 8–8 (A) There is a total of 32 teeth in the adult. Each quadrant has 1 central incisor, 1 lateral incisor, 1 canine, 2 premolars, and 3 molar teeth. **(B)** There are 20 primary teeth. Each quadrant contains 1 central incisor, 1 lateral incisor, 1 canine, and 2 molar teeth.

Box 8-2 Abnormal Number of Teeth

The number of teeth is determined during embryonic development. The number of teeth can be altered by local factors during development or predetermined by genetic disorders that can affect other structures in addition to the teeth. A condition in which a patient is missing six or less teeth, excluding the 3rd molars, is called **hypodontia**. If more than six teeth are missing (excluding the 3rd molars), the condition is called **oligodontia**. The condition in which a patient has extra or **supernumerary** teeth is called **hyperdontia**. Multiple occurrences of these conditions in a family indicate that the condition is genetically linked, and the patient should be referred for genetic counseling.

not considered a structure of the tooth. The cementum is a component of the **periodontium**, the connective-tissue supporting apparatus of the tooth. The **clinical crown** of the tooth refers to any exposed portion of the tooth in the oral cavity, which can include portions of the root. The interior or **pulp chamber** of the crown contains connective tissue called the **coronal pulp**. The interior chamber of the root is called the **root canal**, which contains the connective tissue that forms the **radicular (root) pulp** (Fig. 8–9). At the apex of each root there is an **apical foramen** that serves as a passageway for nerves, blood vessels, and lymphatic vessels that supply the teeth. Some teeth may display **accessory root canals** on the lateral surface of the root (Fig. 8–9). Because these accessory canals contain nerves, they must be identified and sealed during certain endodontic procedures such as root canals.

Dental clinicians refer to tooth surfaces while examining the teeth for decay or during operative procedures on the tooth. Each tooth has mesial and distal surfaces (Fig. 8–10). The **mesial** surface is directed

Box 8-3 Fused Crowns

As a result of tooth formation, a tooth will occasionally appear to have two crowns. This can result by either **fusion** of two adjacent teeth or by **gemination** in which there is a splitting of the crown of the tooth primordium. It is necessary to study radiographs of the tooth to resolve the difference. Fused teeth will have the normal compliment of roots—that is, fused incisors would have two roots. A tooth resulting from *gemination* would display two crowns with fewer roots—that is, an incisor with two crowns would have one root and not two roots.

toward the anterior midline of the jaw, whereas the **distal** surface is directed away from the midline. The anterior teeth (incisors and canines) have a **facial (labial)** surface that is adjacent to the lips, whereas the posterior teeth (premolars and molars) have a **buccal** surface that face the cheek wall (Fig. 8–10). All mandibular teeth have a **lingual** surface that is

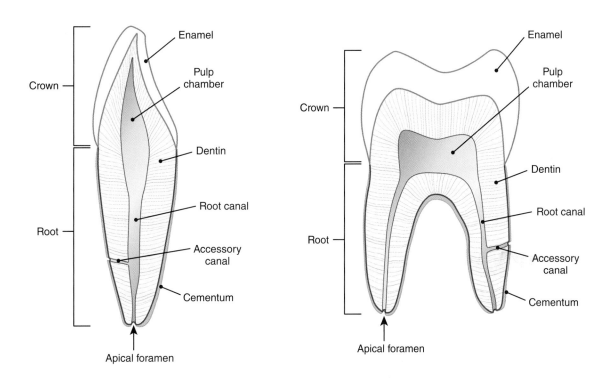

A   B

Figure 8–9 Teeth are composed of an anatomical crown formed by enamel and dentin and a root, which is formed by dentin and covered with cementum. These mineralized tissues protect the connective tissue of the pulp. The pulp chamber is the space of the crown that contains the coronal pulp, whereas the root canal is the comparable space that contains the radicular pulp. Arteries, veins, lymphatic vessels, and nerves gain access to the tooth via the apical foramen. Occasionally, an additional opening along the root called an *accessory root canal* allows additional access to the pulp. **(A)** The incisor and canine teeth have a single cusp and root. **(B)** Molar and premolar teeth have multiple cusps and roots. Each root has a root canal.

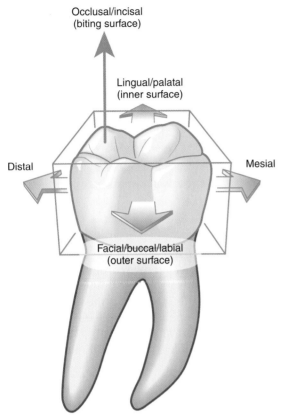

Figure 8–10 The crown of the tooth has five surfaces. The occlusal (incisor) surface serves as the contact point between maxillary and mandibular teeth. The incisors and canines have a labial surface, whereas the premolars and molars have a buccal surface. The lingual surface of the mandibular teeth faces the tongue, whereas the palatal surface of the maxillary teeth is directed toward the hard palate. The mesial surface of the tooth is directed to the median plane, whereas the distal surface is directed posteriorly.

directed toward the tongue, and all maxillary teeth have a **palatal** surface that faces the palate. Finally, the anterior teeth (single cusps) have an **incisal** surface and posterior teeth (multiple cusps) have an **occlusal** surface that come in contact when the arches are closed as in mastication (Fig. 8–10).

Review Question Box 8-3

1. Who has more teeth in the mouth, an adult or a child? Why?
2. What is the difference between the anatomical crown and the clinical crown of a tooth?
3. What is the difference between the pulp chamber and the coronal pulp?
4. What is the difference between the apical foramen and an accessory root canal?

Alveolar Process

The teeth are surrounded by bony extensions of the body of the mandible and maxillae known as the **alveolar processes**. The teeth are attached to the bones of the jaws by a dense layer of connective tissue known as the **periodontal ligament**. The articulation of the roots of the teeth to bone is an example of a *gomphosis*. Recall from Chapter 2 that a gomphosis is a fibrous joint in which a conical structure is attached to bone. The alveolar process is divided into three parts: the cortical plates, the alveolar bone proper (cribriform bone), and the spongiosa. The **cortical plates** are made of a dense, compact bone, which dental clinicians call *cortical bone*. Each tooth is surrounded on its facial surface by an **outer cortical plate** (Fig. 8–11) and on its lingual surface by the **inner cortical plate** (Fig. 8–11). There are no cortical plates separating individual teeth. Directly surrounding the root of the tooth is a layer of bone called the **alveolar bone proper** (inner surface of the socket of the tooth), which is characterized by numerous openings for blood vessels that enter and exit the bone (Fig. 8–12). The alveolar bone proper is also called the **cribriform bone** because of the numerous foramina. In between

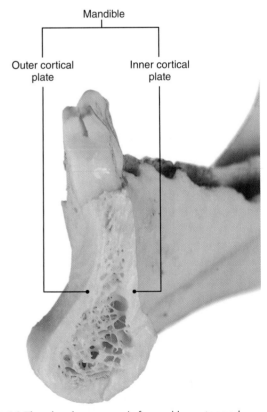

Figure 8–11 The alveolar process is formed by outer and inner cortical plates, which are continuous with the cortical bone of the mandible and maxilla.

the cortical plates and the alveolar bone proper is the **spongiosa**. This layer is formed by thin plates or **trabeculae** of bone (Fig. 8–12). The amount of spongiosa (number of trabeculae) varies on the type of tooth and its position along the mandibular and maxillary arches. As an example, the spongiosa is virtually absent in the mandibular incisors and increases in the molars. This anatomical variation is related to the function of the tooth. The molars (grinding teeth) need more support than the incisors (tearing teeth), and thus the number of trabeculae is greater. All teeth of the maxillary arch have a spongiosa. The spongiosa of the maxillary incisors is prevalent only on their palatal surface and is continuous with the spongy bone of the hard palate. Adjacent teeth are separated by an **interdental septum** (Fig. 8–12), and the roots of a multirooted tooth are separated by an **interradicular septum** (Fig. 8–12). Both septae are composed of the alveolar bone proper and the underlying spongy bone.

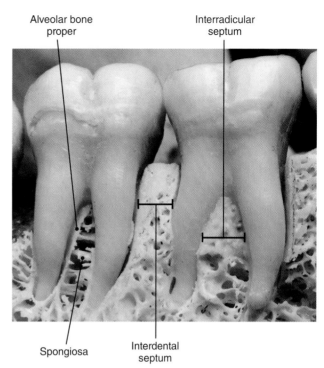

Figure 8–12 The alveolar bone proper, the actual tooth socket, surrounds the root of the tooth. It is supported by the bony plates of the spongiosa. Adjacent teeth are separated by an interdental septum, whereas roots of multiple teeth are separated by the interradicular septum.

Review Question Box 8-4

1. What is the difference between the cortical plates and the alveolar bone proper?
2. Why is a gomphosis a fibrous joint?
3. How can you distinguish the interdental septum from the interradicular septum on a tooth with more than one root?
4. Why does the presence of the spongiosa vary on different teeth?

Clinical Correlation Box 8-1

Mesial Drift

The position of a tooth in its socket can be affected by many conditions, such as crowding of the teeth because of the size of the jaw or external forces on the jaw. As a person ages, the anterior teeth of the mandible have a tendency to become crooked because of the forces of mastication. This condition is called **mesial** or **functional drift**. Pressure on bone causes the bone to be resorbed. While chewing, force is placed on the occlusal and distal surface of the teeth. The lateral pressure causes resorption of the alveolar bone proper on the mesial side of the tooth and the addition of bone on the distal side of the tooth. Orthodontists take advantage of the bone remodeling by placing pressure via orthodontic appliances on bone to straighten teeth.

ORAL CAVITY
Surface Features of the Palate

The roof of the oral cavity is formed by the **hard palate**. The hard palate is divided into the larger, posterior secondary palate and the anterior primary palate. The **secondary palate** is formed by the fusion of the palatine shelves of the maxillary bones during embryological development. The **palatine raphe** is a groove in the midline of the palate that indicates the fusion of the shelves (Fig. 8–13). The **primary palate** is the triangle-shaped, incisor-bearing region of the hard palate. It is characterized by folds of mucosa known as the **transverse palatine folds (rugae)** and the **incisive papilla**, which is a fleshy elevation just posterior to the central incisors (Fig. 8–13). The papilla is very sensitive, because nerves that supply the incisors and the mucosa of the primary palate enter through the incisive canal deep to the papilla. This area is an injection site for local anesthesia of the mucosa of the anterior portion of the hard palate and the palatal gingiva of the incisors (Chapter 18).

Surface Features of the Floor of the Mouth

The floor of the mouth is occupied by the tongue. The region beneath the tongue is called the **sublingual**

Clinical Correlation Box 8-2

Cleft Palates

Clefts in the secondary palate and between primary and secondary palates are the more typical anomalies of the palate. During embryonic development, the medial nasal, lateral nasal, mandibular, and maxillary processes fuse to form the external features of the face. At the same time, the palate is forming internally. Initially, the nasal cavity and oral cavity are continuous. The **palatine shelves**, which are extensions of the maxillary process, are separated by the tongue. As the tongue retracts into the floor of the mouth, the palatine shelves move from a vertical position to a horizontal position and fuse in the midline. Incomplete fusion of the palatine shelves results in a **posterior cleft palate**. The medial nasal process and the palatine shelves also fuse internally. Incomplete fusion of these structures results in either a unilateral or bilateral **anterior cleft palate**.

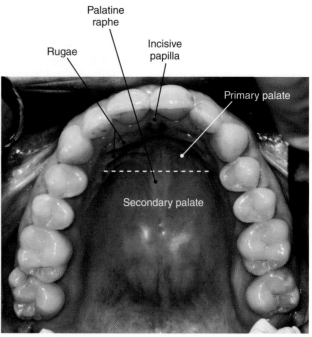

Figure 8–13 The hard palate is divided into the anterior primary palate and the posterior secondary palate. The primary palate is characterized by the incisive papillae and the transverse palatal folds (rugae). The secondary palate is characterized by the palatine raphe, which represents the fusion of the palatine processes of the maxillary bone.

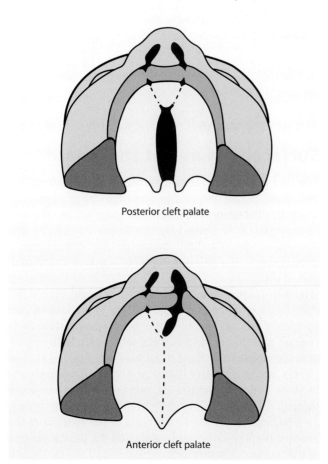

Posterior cleft palate

Anterior cleft palate

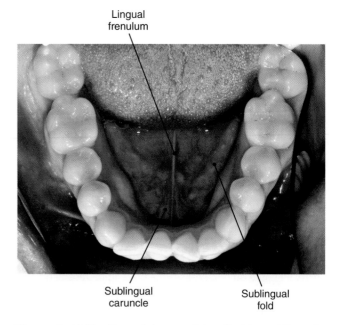

Figure 8–14 The floor of the mouth is called the *sublingual sulcus*. It is characterized by a fold of mucosa, the sublingual fold that covers the sublingual gland. The inferior surface of the tongue is attached to the floor of the mouth by the lingual frenulum. A lingual caruncle is located on each side of the frenulum. The caruncle contains the common opening for the ducts of the submandibular and sublingual glands that release saliva in the oral cavity.

sulcus (Fig. 8–14). Some dental clinicians refer to this area as the **alveolingual sulcus**, which indicates the reflection of the alveolar mucosa onto the inferior surface of the tongue. The **sublingual fold** is a surface feature of the sulcus and is a fold of mucosa that covers the sublingual salivary glands (Fig. 8–14). The tongue is attached to the floor by a fold of mucosa called the **lingual frenulum** (Fig. 8–14). The **sublingual caruncle** is a tuft of mucosa that is located on either side of the frenulum (Fig. 8–14). The caruncle is the location of the shared opening of the submandibular and sublingual salivary glands into the oral cavity. The tongue is divided into two parts: the body (anterior two-thirds) and the root (posterior one-third), by a V-shape groove called the **sulcus terminalis** (terminal sulcus) (Fig. 8–15). Just anterior to the sulcus are 7 to 11 prominent structures called the **vallate papilla** (Figs. 8–15 and 8–16), which contain taste buds. The tongue is divided into right and left halves by the **median sulcus**, a midline groove on the surface of the tongue (Fig. 8–15). The surface of the body of the tongue is covered by numerous papillae, which represent tufts of connective tissue covered by epithelium. The most numerous of these are the **filiform papillae** (Fig. 8–17). They are relatively small projections that assist in the formation of a bolus of food in preparation for swallowing. The larger and less numerous **fungiform papillae** (Fig. 8–17) contain taste buds. The **foliate papillae**, which are actually columnar-like folds of the mucosa (Fig. 8–18), are located on the lateral surface of the tongue and also contain taste buds. The posterior one-third of the tongue is covered by the **lingual tonsils** (Fig. 8–15).

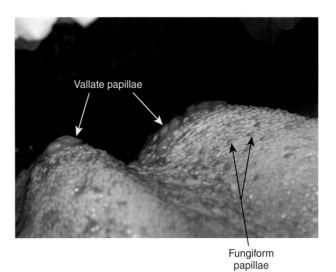

Figure 8–16 The vallate papillae (white arrows) are located anterior to the terminal sulcus, and the fungiform papillae (black arrows) are scattered on the anterior surface of the tongue. Both papillae contain taste buds.

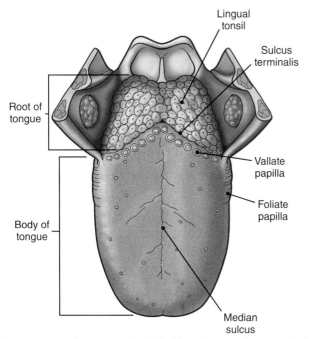

Figure 8–15 The tongue is divided into the anterior two-thirds or body and a posterior one-third or root by the V-shaped terminal sulcus. The median sulcus is a midline groove on the body of the tongue. Seven to eleven vallate papillae are located anteriorly along the terminal sulcus; the foliate papillae are located on the lateral surface.

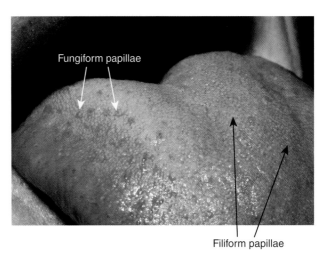

Figure 8–17 The smaller filiform papillae (black arrows) cover most of the surface of the body of the tongue. The papillae do not contain taste buds, but are used to shape the bolus of food in preparation for swallowing. Fungiform papillae (white arrows) are larger than the filiform papillae and are scattered along the surface of the tongue.

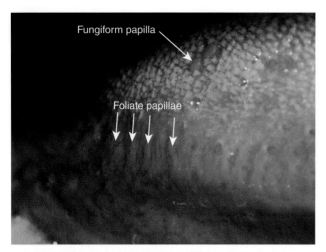

Figure 8–18 The foliate papillae (white arrows) are columnar-like folds on the lateral surface of the tongue, whereas the fungiform papillae are mushroom shaped and scattered on the dorsum of the tongue.

Surface Features of the Lateral Wall

The **pterygomandibular fold** is a vertical fold medial to the ramus of the mandible (Fig. 8–19). The fold is caused by the tightening of the **pterygomandibular raphe**, which is the common connective tissue attachment of the *buccinator* and *superior constrictor muscles* (see Fig. 4–3). The **pterygotemporal depression** is a triangle-shaped region between the mandible and the pterygomandibular fold and is an important landmark for intraoral injections (Chapter 18).

The posterior limit of the oral cavity is the **anterior tonsillar pillars (palatoglossal folds)**. This marks the entrance into the oropharynx. With the mouth open, other structures visible in the oropharynx include the palatine tonsils and the uvula. Recall from Chapter 4 that the *palatine tonsils* are located in between the anterior tonsillar pillars and the **posterior tonsillar pillars (palatopharyngeal folds)**. The **uvula** is the midline structure, which represents the termination of the *soft palate* (see Fig. 4–6).

Review Question Box 8-5

1. What is the difference between the primary and secondary palate?
2. What is the significance of the incisive papilla?
3. What are the differences of the papillae on the surface of the tongue?
4. What are the features of the sublingual sulcus?
5. What are the features of the lateral wall of the oral cavity?

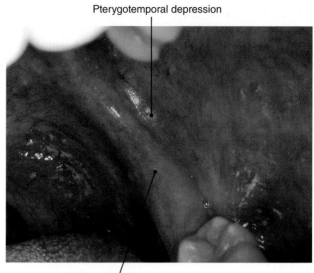

Figure 8–19 The pterygomandibular fold is a taut line of mucosa produced by the tightening of the pterygomandibular raphe when the mouth is opened. The pterygotemporal depression is located between the raphe and the ramus of the mandible. The raphe and depression are landmarks for local anesthesia of the mandible.

MUSCLES OF THE FLOOR OF THE MOUTH

The most superficial muscles that are inferior to the mandible are the anterior and posterior bellies of the digastric muscle. These are considered muscles of the neck, and not the floor of the mouth, but are presented here because of their proximity to the floor of the mouth. The

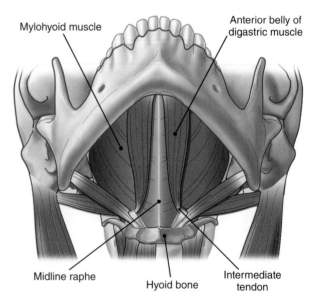

Figure 8–20 The inferior approach to the floor of the mouth reveals the anterior and posterior belly of the digastric muscles. The actual floor is formed by the mylohyoid muscle.

anterior belly of the digastric muscle is located superficial to the mylohyoid muscle (Fig. 8–20). The muscle originates from the **digastric fossa** of the mandible and inserts onto the *intermediate tendon* and the **hyoid bone**. The major functions of the muscle include the elevation of the hyoid bone during swallowing and the depression and retraction of the mandible.

The two muscles that comprise the actual floor of the mouth are the mylohyoid and the geniohyoid muscles. The **mylohyoid muscle** forms a sling that supports the structures of the mouth (Figs. 8–20 and Fig. 8–21). The muscle originates from the **mylohyoid line** (see Fig. 2–23A) of the mandible and courses horizontally toward a linear midline strip of connective tissue called the **midline raphe** (Fig. 8–20). The functions of this muscle include elevating the floor of the mouth and hyoid bone, as well as depressing the mandible. The **geniohyoid muscle** is the deepest of these muscles. The muscle originates on the **mental spine** of the mandible and inserts onto the **body of the hyoid bone** (Fig. 8–21). The direction of the muscle fibers is basically perpendicular to the mylohyoid muscle. The functions of this muscle are to elevate the hyoid bone during swallowing or to depress and retract the mandible when opening the mouth.

Review Question Box 8-6

1. Why is the digastric muscle not considered a part of the floor of the mouth?
2. Why are the digastric, mylohyoid, and geniohyoid muscles considered suprahyoid muscles?

MUSCLES OF THE TONGUE

The tongue is composed of two groups of muscles: the extrinsic muscles of the tongue, which originate outside the tongue, and the intrinsic muscles, which originate inside the tongue. Both extrinsic and intrinsic muscles of the tongue are innervated by the **hypoglossal nerve** (**XII**).

Extrinsic Muscles

The **genioglossus muscle** originates from the *mental spine* and inserts into the dorsum of the tongue and the *body of the hyoid bone* (Fig. 8–22). Its actions are to pull the hyoid bone forward and to protrude the tongue. The second function, protrusion of the tongue, is clinically important because the tongue is used to test for peripheral nerve damage to the **hypoglossal nerve**. The tongue will protrude toward the side of the loss of motor function.

The **hyoglossus muscle** originates from the **hyoid bone** and inserts into the side of the tongue. This muscle depresses the tongue (Fig. 8–22).

The **styloglossus muscle** originates from the **styloid process** of the temporal bone and inserts onto the dorsolateral aspect of the tongue (Fig. 8–22). Its function is to elevate and retract the tongue (Table 8–1).

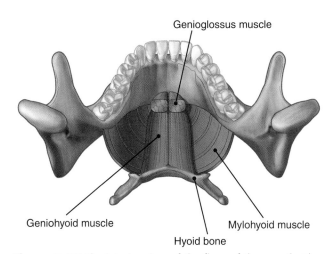

Figure 8–21 The interior view of the floor of the mouth. The genioglossus muscle of the tongue has been cut to expose the geniohyoid muscle, which is attached to the mandible and hyoid bone.

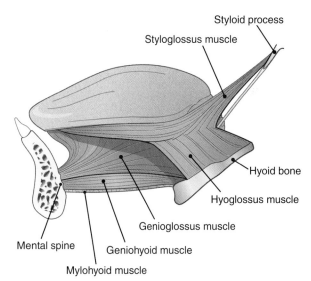

Figure 8–22 There are three extrinsic muscles that contribute to the formation of the tongue. The genioglossus muscle is the largest of these muscles and arises from the mental spine of the mandible. The stylogossus muscle enters the tongue posteriorly from its origin on the styloid process, whereas the hyoglossus muscle arises from the hyoid bone and inserts into the tongue from an inferior direction. Note the relationship of the genioglossus and geniohyoid muscles. Fibers of the mylohyoid muscle are cut in cross section.

TABLE 8-1	Extrinsic Muscles of the Tongue			
Muscle	**Origin**	**Insertion**	**Action**	**Innervation**
Genioglossus	Mental spine	Dorsum of the tongue and the body of the hyoid bone	Protrudes the tongue	Hypoglossal nerve
Hyoglossus	Hyoid bone	Lateral surface of the tongue	Depresses the tongue	Hypoglossal nerve
Styloglossus	Styloid process	Dorsolateral surface of the tongue	Elevates and contracts the tongue	Hypoglossal nerve

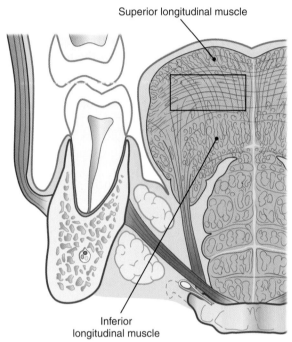

Superior longitudinal muscle

Inferior longitudinal muscle

Figure 8–23 Four groups of intrinsic muscles arise and insert in the tongue. The superior and inferior longitudinal groups are used to curl the tongue superiorly and inferiorly. The transverse and horizontal groups (shown in the box) are used to flatten or narrow the tongue.

Intrinsic Muscles

The intrinsic muscles originate and insert within the tongue. They are divided into **transverse**, **vertical**, and **superior** and **inferior longitudinal muscles** (Fig. 8–23). These muscles shape the tongue. The transverse muscle narrows and elongates the tongue, whereas the vertical muscle flattens and broadens the tongue. The superior longitudinal muscle is used to curl the tongue superiorly, whereas the inferior longitudinal muscle curls the tongue in an inferior direction.

Review Question Box 8-7

1. Why are the muscles of the tongue either extrinsic or intrinsic?
2. How do the functions of the intrinsic and extrinsic muscles of the tongue differ?

SUMMARY

The mouth is divided into the oral vestibule and the oral cavity proper. The oral vestibule is the space between the teeth and the lip and the cheek wall. Major features of the vestibule include the labial frenula, the vestibular fornix, the parotid papilla, and the linea alba. The oral cavity is the space between the teeth that is continuous with the oropharynx, which is located posterior to the anterior tonsillar pillars. The hard palate forms the roof of the oral cavity, whereas the floor is formed by the mylohyoid and geniohyoid muscles covered by the mucosa of the sublingual sulcus. Within the sulcus, the lingual frenulum attaches the tongue to the floor of the mouth. The lingual caruncles are located on the sides of the frenulum and contain the common opening of the sublingual and submandibular salivary glands into the oral cavity. The sublingual gland is located deep to the sublingual fold on the floor of the mouth. The anterior two-thirds of the tongue protrudes into the oral cavity. Its dorsal surface is covered by specialized papillae that contain taste buds. The extrinsic muscles of the tongue originate from outside of the oral cavity, whereas the intrinsic muscles originate and insert within the tongue.

There are 20 primary and 32 secondary teeth. Although features of individual teeth differ, all teeth are composed of a crown and a root system. The crown is formed by dentin and enamel, which surround the connective tissue of the coronal pulp. The connective tissue of the radicular pulp is surrounded by dentin. The number of cusps and roots depends on the location and function of the teeth. The incisors are the cutting teeth with a single cusp and root. Premolars and molars grind food and have multiple cusps and roots.

The teeth are attached to the alveolar processes of the mandible and maxilla by the periodontal ligament. The alveolar process is made of outer and inner cortical plates and the alveolar bone proper (actual socket of the tooth) separated by varying amounts of spongy bone dependent on the location of the tooth in the jaw. Adjacent teeth are separated by the interdental septae, whereas the roots are separated by the interradicular septae. The alveolar bone and tooth complex is surrounded by gingiva. The mucosa of the attached gingiva is tightly bound to the bone or the tooth.

The interdental papilla is the tent-shaped gingiva between adjacent teeth. In between the contact points of the teeth is the col. The tooth is separated from the free gingiva by the gingival sulcus.

The pterygomandibular fold and pterygotemporal depression lie medial to the ramus of the mandible. These structures are important landmarks for intraoral injection.

Two groups of muscles form the tongue. The styloglossus, genioglossus, and hyoglossus muscles are the extrinsic muscles that originate from bones and generally control gross movements of the tongue. The intrinsic muscles originate and insert into the tongue and control finer movements of the tongue, such as curling or flattening of the tongue. Both extrinsic and intrinsic muscles are innervated by the hypoglossal nerve (XII).

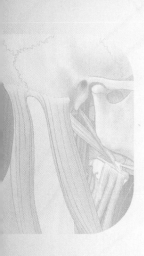

LEARNING LAB
Exercises for review, practice, and study

Laboratory Activity 8-1

Identifying Surface Features of the Vestibule and the Oral Cavity

Objective: Intraoral examinations require the dental hygienist to determine if there are any changes in the surface features of the vestibule and oral cavity that may indicate disease. In this exercise, you will examine the surface features of your mouth.

Materials Needed: Adequate lighting and a small mirror. *For further consideration:* Some structures are more easily identifiable on another individual using a dental mirror, but should only be undertaken in a supervised dental setting. Thus, some of the structures discussed in the chapter will not be included in this exercise.

Step 1: Begin this exercise by studying the structures in the oral vestibule. Part your lips as if making a smile or grin.

- Verify that the *vestibule* is a space located between the cheek walls, lips, and the teeth, which can be subdivided into *buccal* and *labial vestibules*.
- Identify the *vestibular fornix*, a V-shaped groove where the labial and buccal mucosae reflect onto the surface of the mandible and maxillary bones.
- Pull down the lower lip and identify the *lingual frenulum* as a fold of mucosa that attaches the lip to the mandible.
- Now elevate the upper lip and identify the frenulum of the upper lip.

Step 2: Now examine the mucosa that covers the mandible.

- Observe that the *alveolar mucosa* is the darker colored surface on the alveolar process next to the vestibular fornix. The lighter pink-colored surface is the *gingiva*.
- Identify the *mucogingival line* that separates these two regions of the mucosa.
- The gingiva is divided into the *attached gingiva*, which is adherent to the bone, and the *free gingiva*, which forms the free margin of the gingiva.
- Note that there is a *sulcus* that separates the free gingiva from the attached gingiva. The depth of this sulcus is normally 1 to 3 mm. Greater depths are an indication of periodontal disease.
- The tent-shaped region between adjacent teeth is called the *papillary gingiva*.

Step 3: Now open your mouth and examine the oral cavity. Start by raising your tongue and observe the structures associated with the inferior surface of the tongue.

- Identify the *lingual frenulum*, which attaches the tongue to the floor of the mouth, and the *lingual caruncles*, which are located on the surfaces of the frenulum.
- The area under the tongue is called the *sublingual sulcus* and is characterized by a fold of mucosa called the *sublingual fold*. In some individuals, the sublingual gland can be identified by gentle palpation of the fold.

Step 4: Observe the dorsal surface of the tongue.

- Identify the *lingual groove* that bisects the tongue.
- Protrude your tongue and realize that this represents the *body* of the tongue.
- The *root* of the tongue is separated from the body by the V-shaped *terminal sulcus*.
- Identify the 7 to 11 large *vallate papillae*, which are aligned along the sulcus. Next examine the surface of the body of the tongue.
- The roughened surface is produced by the lingual papillae; the *filiform papillae* are the most numerous. The *fungiform papillae* are larger and are scattered along the surface. The *foliate papillae* are located along the lateral surface of the tongue in the vicinity of the terminal sulcus. These columnar folds are not well developed in humans and may be difficult to observe.
- Now identify the *anterior tonsillar pillars*, which mark the posterior limit of the oral cavity.

Step 5:   Continue your examination with the hard palate.

- The hard palate is bisected by the *palatine raphe*.
- Observe that the *primary palate* is the anterior portion of the palate that contains the incisors.
- Look for the horizontal folds of the mucosa that are called *rugae* by dental clinicians.
- Identify the *incisive papillae*, as a small tuft of the mucosa just posterior to the central incisors. This area of the mucosa is extremely sensitive.
- The remainder of the hard palate is called the *secondary palate*. Its surface can be flat or display a moundlike shape.

Step 6:   This exercise concludes with identifying structures along the lateral wall of the oral cavity.

- Locate the *pterygomandibular fold*, which is located posterior to the molars. The fold is produced by the stretching of the *pterygomandibular raphe* deep to the fold. The superior constrictor is located deep to the mucosa posterior to the fold, and the buccinator muscle is located deep to the mucosa anterior to the fold.
- Look for a triangle-shaped depression between the pterygomandibular fold and the ramus of the mandible. This is the *pterygotemporal depression* and is the injection site for the inferior alveolar nerve block.

For Discussion or Thought:

1. *Realize that understanding the normal surface features of the oral cavity and vestibule is necessary for recognizing changes that may occur by pathological conditions.*

2. *What changes would suggest inflammation?*

Learning Activity 8-1

Floor of the Mouth—External View

Match the numbered structures with the correct terms listed to the right.

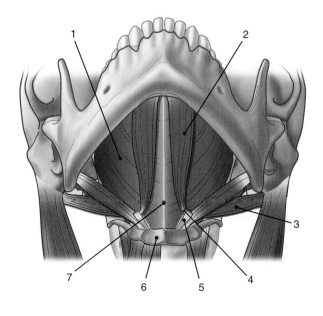

_____ Anterior belly of the digastric muscle

_____ Connective tissue sling

_____ Hyoid bone

_____ Intermediate tendon

_____ Midline raphe

_____ Mylohyoid muscle

_____ Posterior belly of the digastric muscle

Learning Activity 8-2

Floor of the Mouth—Internal View

Match the numbered structures with the correct terms listed to the right.

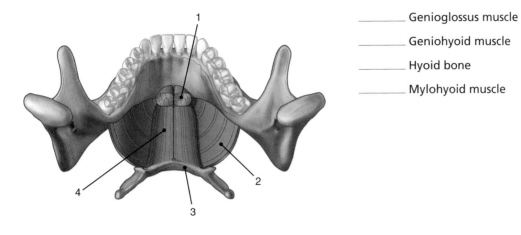

_____ Genioglossus muscle

_____ Geniohyoid muscle

_____ Hyoid bone

_____ Mylohyoid muscle

Learning Activity 8-3

Tongue—Sagittal View

Match the numbered structures with the correct terms listed to the right.

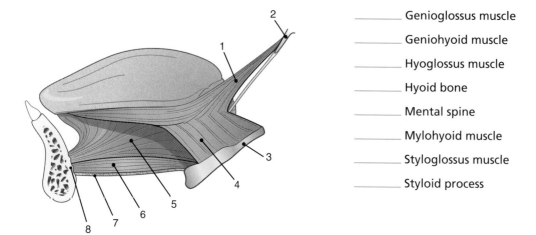

_____ Genioglossus muscle

_____ Geniohyoid muscle

_____ Hyoglossus muscle

_____ Hyoid bone

_____ Mental spine

_____ Mylohyoid muscle

_____ Styloglossus muscle

_____ Styloid process

9

Salivary Glands

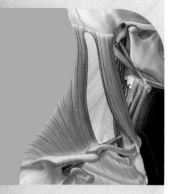

Objectives

1. Distinguish between extrinsic and intrinsic salivary glands.
2. Discuss the major functions of saliva.
3. Discuss the gross anatomical structure, location, anatomical relationships, and duct system of the extrinsic salivary glands.

Overview

How often have you said, "That smells so good that it makes my mouth water?" The water is saliva, which is formed and released by salivary glands both inside and outside of the mouth. Although two of the primary functions of saliva are to moisten food for swallowing and to initiate the digestion of carbohydrates, the nondigestive functions are very important to the dental hygienist. Saliva cleanses the mouth and contains antibodies that help establish an environment hostile to bacterial growth. The saliva also contains ions that help prevent the demineralization of the teeth and enzymes that reduce the time needed to clot blood.

INTRODUCTION TO THE SALIVARY GLANDS

The salivary glands are divided into two groups according to their location either within the walls or outside the walls of the mouth. The **intrinsic** (*minor*) salivary glands are rather small glands that are located within the walls of the oral cavity and vestibule. They are generally named according to their locations: buccal glands are

found in the cheek wall, labial glands are located in the superior and inferior lips, palatine glands are present in the hard palate and the soft palate, and the anterior gland and the posterior lingual gland are contained within the tongue. Others are named after individuals: the glands of von Ebner, which are located under the vallate papillae, and the glands of Blandin-Nühn, which are situated on the inferior (ventral) tip of the tongue. Although the intrinsic salivary glands only secrete 5% of the saliva, their functioning is very important in moistening the mouth and retaining dentures.

The most familiar salivary glands are the large **extrinsic** (*major*) glands located outside of the oral cavity, which includes the parotid, submandibular, and sublingual glands. Approximately 95% of the watery secretion, known as **saliva**, forms within these glands and is carried to the oral cavity by a complex system of ducts. In this chapter, the structure and relationships of the extrinsic salivary glands will be presented.

FUNCTIONS OF SALIVA

Saliva functions in a variety of ways. Because saliva is a fluid, it cleanses and moistens the mouth, which helps prevent bacteria from sticking onto the surface of the teeth and the mucosa. Dental hygienists need to understand that individuals with dry mouth (**xerostomia**) are more prone to periodontal disease. Saliva cleanses the taste buds, thus enhancing the sensation of taste. Saliva contains ions that regulate pH. Maintaining a neutral pH limits bacterial growth. Calcium and phosphate ions in the saliva help maintain the chemical balance in favor of the formation of hydroxyapatite crystals. Saliva also contains amylase (an enzyme) that digests carbohydrates and antibodies that bind to foreign antigens and facilitates their destruction. Furthermore, saliva contains enzymes that clot the blood faster than if the blood was exposed to air. Although saliva is generally thought of as being a fluid, it contains varying amounts of mucus, which can be used to coat the surface of foods to make them easier to swallow.

Review Question Box 9-1

1. What is the difference between intrinsic and extrinsic salivary glands?
2. Which functions of saliva require a chemical action?

STRUCTURE OF THE EXTRINSIC SALIVARY GLANDS

Parotid Gland

The **parotid gland** is the largest of the three extrinsic or major salivary glands; however, the pair of glands produces only about 30% of the saliva. Each gland is covered by a tough fibrous capsule, which is a continuation of the investing fascia of the neck. The gland is described as being triangular in shape with its base facing the zygomatic arch and its apex directed inferiorly and posteriorly to the angle of the mandible (Fig. 9–1). The large excretory duct of the gland is called **Stensen's duct** by clinicians. The parotid duct crosses over

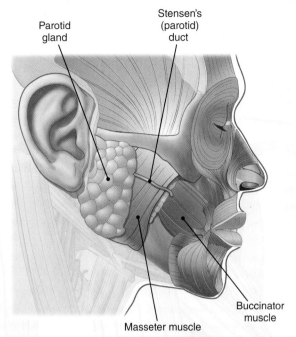

Figure 9–1 The parotid gland is triangular shaped with its base toward the zygomatic arch, and its apex near the angle of the mandible. The parotid duct (Stensen) crosses the masseter muscle and penetrates the buccinator muscle to reach the oral cavity.

the **masseter muscle** and then pierces the **buccinator muscle** to enter the oral vestibule (Fig. 9–1). The duct opens onto a small mound of tissue, the **parotid papilla**, which is located on the cheek wall opposite the second molar (see Fig. 8–4).

The gland is bounded anteriorly by the ramus of mandible, posteriorly by the mastoid process of the temporal bone, inferiorly by the posterior belly of the digastric muscle, and medially by a sagittal plane drawn through the styloid process.

Three major structures pass through the parotid gland. These include (1) the **external carotid artery**, which supplies blood to the deep face and superficial temporal region; (2) the **retromandibular vein**, which drains blood from the deep face and superficial temporal region (Fig. 9–2); and the five branches of the **facial nerve** (**VII**), which supply the muscles of facial expression. The branches are named according to their regional location as the **temporal**, **zygomatic**, **buccal**, **marginal mandibular**, and **cervical nerves** (Fig. 9–3).

Review Question Box 9-2

1. What are the boundaries of the parotid gland?
2. How does the duct of the parotid gland reach the oral cavity?
3. What structures pass through the parotid gland?

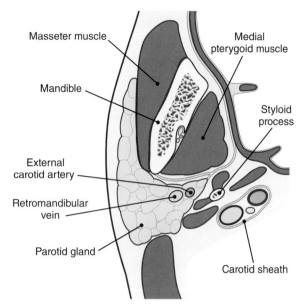

Figure 9–2 Cross section of the parotid bed. The masseter muscle is located on the lateral surface of the mandible and the medial pterygoid muscle is found on its medial surface. The deep portion of the parotid gland extends medially toward the styloid process. The retromandibular vein and external carotid artery pass through the deep portion of the gland.

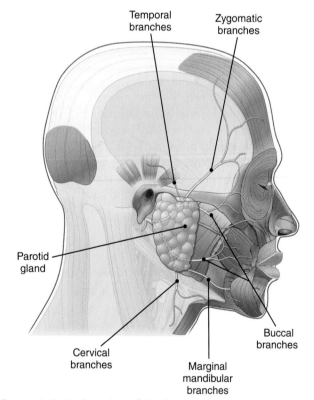

Figure 9–3 Five branches of the facial nerve pass through the gland to innervate the muscles of facial expression.

Submandibular Gland

The **submandibular gland** is the second largest of the extrinsic (major) salivary glands and produces approximately 60% of the saliva. A major portion of the gland is located inferior to the mandible in the **submandibular triangle**. Recall that this triangle is a subdivision of the anterior cervical triangle and is bordered by the anterior belly of the digastric muscle, the posterior belly of the digastric muscle, and the body of the mandible (Fig. 9–4). The *submandibular gland* is surrounded by the investing fascia of the neck and is separated from the oral cavity by the **mylohyoid muscle**, which forms the floor of the mouth.

The submandibular gland is composed of a body and an uncinate process. The *body* of the gland is located in the submandibular triangle inferior to the mylohyoid muscle (Fig. 9–4). The **uncinate process** is a U-shaped extension of the gland that curves around the free edge of the mylohyoid muscle to reach the posterior aspect of the floor of the mouth (Fig. 9–5). The excretory duct of the submandibular gland, which is called **Wharton's duct** by clinicians, extends from the uncinate process and courses along the floor of the mouth to join the main duct of the sublingual gland. The duct terminates on the **sublingual caruncle** lateral to the **lingual frenulum** (Fig. 9–5).

Several **submandibular lymph nodes** lie adjacent to the gland (Fig. 9–4). Enlargement of these nodes can indicate inflammation or cancer in the oral cavity and superficial face (Chapter 12). The **facial artery** enters the submandibular triangle deep to the posterior belly of the digastric muscle and courses posterior to the submandibular gland en route to the face. The **facial vein**, on the other hand, passes anterior to the gland to reach the face (Fig. 9–4).

Review Question Box 9-3

1. What is the relationship of the submandibular gland to the mylohyoid muscle?
2. What is the course of the submandibular duct in the oral cavity?

Sublingual Gland

The almond-shaped **sublingual gland** is the smallest of the extrinsic (major) salivary glands. The gland secretes approximately 5% of the total volume of saliva.

The sublingual gland is located in the floor of the mouth and is covered on its surface by a fold of mucosa known as the **sublingual fold**. The gland contains a single major duct that clinicians call **Bartholin's duct**.

Figure 9–4 The body of the submandibular gland is located in the submandibular triangle along with submandibular lymph nodes. The facial artery and vein pass through the triangle to gain access to the face. The gland is separated from the oral cavity by the mylohyoid muscle.

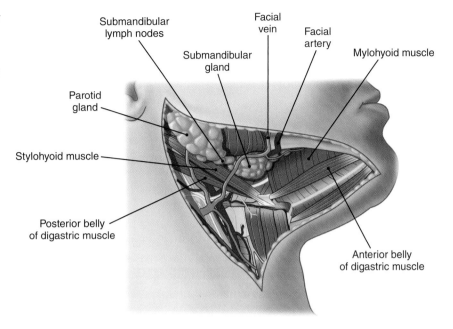

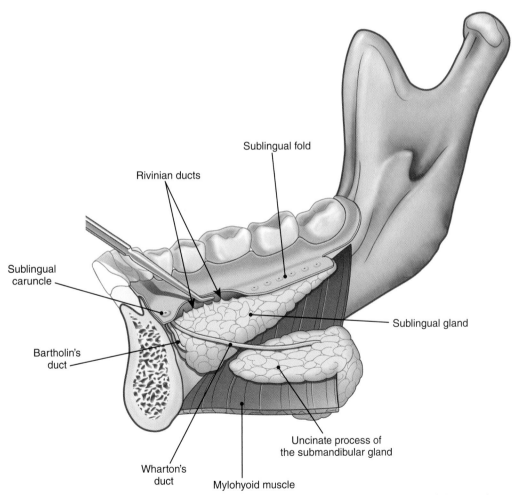

Figure 9–5 The uncinate process of the submandibular gland is located in the floor of the mouth along with the sublingual gland. The duct (Wharton's) of the submandibular gland and the major duct (Bartholin's) of the sublingual gland join to empty into the sublingual caruncle. The minor ducts (Rivinian) of the sublingual gland empty along the sublingual fold.

This duct joins the submandibular duct (Wharton's duct) to empty through a small opening on the sublingual caruncle lateral to the lingual frenulum (Fig. 9–5). In addition, 2 to 12 minor ducts, which clinicians call **Rivinian ducts**, empty into openings on the sublingual fold (Fig. 9–5).

Review Question Box 9-4

1. What is the location of the sublingual glands?
2. How do the ducts of the sublingual gland empty into the oral cavity?

Clinical Correlation Box 9-1

Salivary Gland Disorders

There are generally three types of disorders associated with salivary glands: *obstruction*, *infection*, and *tumors*. These disorders more commonly affect the parotid and the submandibular glands.

The ducts of the salivary glands can be obstructed by a stone, which is clinically called a **sialolith**. The stones can block the flow of saliva into the oral cavity. Patients will complain of a dry mouth (*xerostomia*) and tenderness in the region of the gland due to swelling of the gland.

Infections of the salivary glands can be either viral or bacterial. **Mumps** is a viral infection, which can be painful because of the enlargement of the gland within its thick fascial covering. Bacterial infections can develop because of an obstruction of the duct system, as well as poor dental hygiene.

Tumors of the salivary glands can be either benign or malignant. Growth of the tumor may infringe upon branches of the facial nerve, which can lead to paralysis of the muscles of facial expression that are innervated by affected branches.

SUMMARY

Salivary glands are classified according to their size and location. The extrinsic (major) salivary glands are relatively large glands located outside of the walls of the mouth, whereas the intrinsic (minor) salivary glands are small and located within the walls of the oral cavity and vestibule. Saliva is a watery fluid that contains enzymes, clotting factors, ions, antibodies, and varying amounts of mucus. The fluid component of saliva cleanses the surface of the teeth, crevices in the walls of the oral cavity, and the taste buds. The amylase enzyme begins the digestion of carbohydrates. The ions help maintain the proper balance of calcium ions and the neutral pH of the saliva. The antibodies reduce the amount of bacteria, whereas the clotting factors reduce the clotting time of blood (blood clots faster). A decrease in salivary secretion increases the chances for periodontal disease.

The parotid gland, which is the largest salivary gland, is located between the ramus of the mandible and the ear. Stensen's duct crosses the masseter muscle and penetrates the buccinator muscle to empty onto the parotid papillae on the buccal wall opposite the second molar. The facial nerve, retromandibular vein, and external carotid artery pass through gland and can be affected by diseases of the gland. The body of the submandibular gland is located in the submandibular triangle, whereas the uncinate process lies on the superior surface of the mylohyoid muscle. Wharton's duct exits the uncinate process and empties into an opening on the sublingual caruncle. The sublingual gland (smallest) lies beneath the sublingual fold in the floor of the mouth. Multiple Rivinian ducts empty on the surface of the fold, whereas Bartholin's duct joins Wharton's duct to empty onto the sublingual caruncle.

LEARNING LAB
Exercises for review, practice, and study

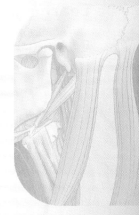

Laboratory Activity 9-1

Palpation of the Major Salivary Glands

Objective: Palpation of the salivary glands is a part of the routine dental examination. In this exercise, you will use yourself as a model to locate the major salivary glands.

Materials Needed: A mirror and gauze. *Optional:* Gloves and a dental mirror.

Step 1: Begin your study by palpating the area between the ramus of the mandible and inferior to the external auditory meatus. This is the location of the most superficial portion of the parotid gland. Swelling and tenderness in this area could indicate infection within the gland.

- Palpate the *masseter muscle* on the ramus of the mandible. Confirm the presence of the muscle by lightly biting down on your teeth and feeling for the contraction of the muscle.
- Attempt to identify the *parotid* or *Stensen's duct*, which crosses over the masseter muscle and penetrates the buccinator muscle to empty on the parotid papilla. Some individuals can palpate the duct along the anterior border of the masseter muscle and the ramus of the mandible.
- The *parotid papilla* is located on the buccal wall of the vestibule, opposite the second molar. You can visualize this with a dental mirror or by palpating with your finger along the surface of the buccal wall.

Step 2: Now palpate under the mandible in the *submandibular triangle* for the body of the submandibular gland. In older individuals, the gland may extend beyond the borders of the digastric muscles. Again, local swelling and tenderness can indicate inflammation of the gland.

- Identify the *sublingual caruncles* on either side of the lingual frenulum, which attaches the tongue to the floor of the mouth.
- Look for a small opening or *punctum* on the surface of the caruncles. This represents the common opening of the ducts for the submandibular and sublingual salivary glands. What are the clinical names for these ducts? If you said that the submandibular duct is called *Wharton's duct* and the sublingual duct is *Bartholin's duct*, you are correct.
- Dry the area of the caruncle with gauze or tissue paper. You should be able to detect drops of saliva passing through the opening on the caruncle.

Step 3: Now locate the sublingual fold on the floor of the mouth.

- With your finger or tongue, gently press along the fold. Some individuals may be able to palpate portions of the sublingual gland. Realize that swelling and tenderness in this area can indicate infection of the gland or other pathology of the floor of the mouth.
- Wipe the surface of the sublingual fold with gauze or tissue paper. You should see small droplets of saliva arising off the surface of the sublingual fold indicating the openings of the Rivinian ducts along the fold.

For Discussion or Thought:

1. *What is the clinical significance of the test for the flow of saliva from the openings of the salivary glands in the mouth?*

Learning Activity 9-1

Relationships of the Parotid Gland

Match the numbered structures with the correct terms to the right.

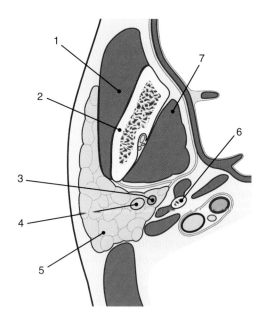

_____ External carotid artery

_____ Mandible

_____ Masseter muscle

_____ Medial pterygoid muscle

_____ Parotid gland

_____ Retromandibular vein

_____ Styloid process

Learning Activity 9-2

Relationships of the Submandibular Gland

Match the numbered structures with the correct terms to the right.

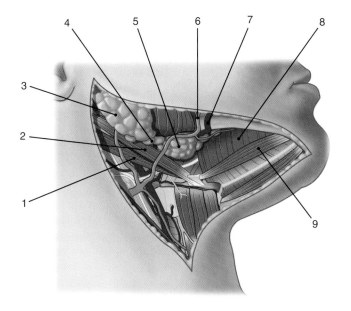

_____ Anterior belly of the digastric muscle

_____ Facial artery

_____ Facial vein

_____ Mylohyoid muscle

_____ Parotid gland

_____ Posterior belly of the digastric muscle

_____ Stylohyoid muscle

_____ Submandibular gland

_____ Submandibular lymph nodes

Learning Activity 9-3

Relationships of the Sublingual and Submandibular Glands

Match the numbered structures with the correct terms to the right.

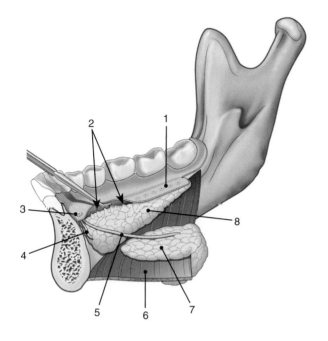

_____ Bartholin's duct

_____ Mylohyoid muscle

_____ Rivinian ducts

_____ Sublingual caruncle

_____ Sublingual fold

_____ Sublingual gland

_____ Uncinate process

_____ Wharton's duct

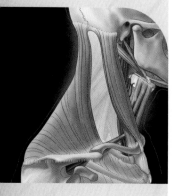

chapter

10

Fascial Spaces and the Spread of Infection

Objectives

1. Explain the concept of fascial spaces and describe the fascial layers of the neck.
2. Identify the boundaries and contents of the fascial spaces of the floor of the mouth and describe the possible infection pathways through the spaces.
3. Trace the pathway of infection from the oral cavity into the neck.

Overview

What does the term "angina" mean to you? The most common answer is that angina is the severe chest pain associated with a heart attack caused by a lack of oxygen to the heart. Actually, angina refers to spasmodic, suffocating, strangling pain. Angina associated with chest pain is a diminutive form of *angina pectoris*. However, the term *angina* is used to describe a very painful, life-threatening condition caused by the spread of infection from the floor of the mouth into the neck—that is, infection from an abscessed tooth. The infection can spread behind the trachea, which can cause the suffocation. Therefore, the term *angina* refers to the feeling of strangling. If the spread of the infection is not impeded, the infection can spread to the chest. How can this happen? In this chapter, you will study how connective tissue spaces in the oral cavity connect with similar spaces in the neck that allow the spread of infection.

INTRODUCTION TO FASCIAL SPACES AND THE SPREAD OF INFECTION

Fascia is a fibrous sheath of connective tissue that encases muscles, blood vessels, nerves, and organs. In essence, fascia subdivides the body into compartments. These compartments can be mechanisms for supporting organs or they can serve as conduits that allow structures to pass from one region of the body to another. In the head and neck, the compartments, as well as the potential **fascial spaces** in between the compartments, prevent structures from sticking to each other and allow movement of organs such as the trachea and esophagus during swallowing. The fascial spaces are clinically important because the spaces can either isolate or facilitate the spread of infection. Of particular interest to the dental hygienist is the communication of the fascial spaces of the floor of the mouth to the spaces of the neck. This continuity of the fascial spaces allows **odontogenic** (arising from the tooth) infections

to spread into the **mediastinum** (the portion of the thorax that contains the heart).

FASCIAE OF THE NECK

As in all regions of the body, the neck is covered by a layer of skin that is connected to underlying structures by connective tissue. The skin is divided into two layers: the epidermis and the dermis. The epidermis is formed by epithelium, whereas the dermis is formed by connective tissue. An additional layer of connective tissue, which is called the *hypodermis*, lies deep to the dermis and attaches the skin to the underlying structures. In gross anatomy, the hypodermis is called the **superficial fascia.** Unlike other regions, the superficial fascia of the neck contains skeletal muscle, namely the *platysma muscle* (Figs. 10–1A and 10–2), which was discussed in Chapter 5 as a muscle of facial expression. The next layer, which is called **deep fascia**, is more complex. This layer subdivides the neck into a series of tubes within a tube. The outer tube is a musculofascial

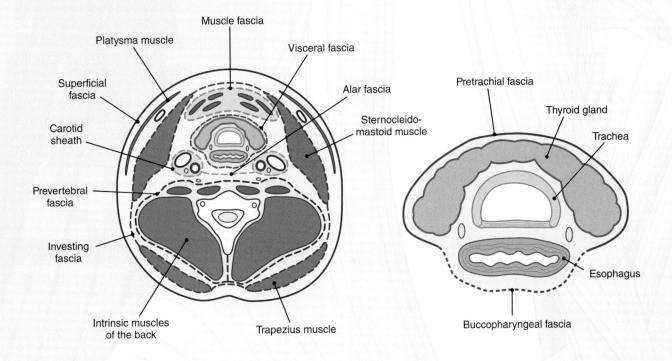

A

B

Figure 10–1 (A) A cross section of the neck inferior to the larynx reveals that it is divided by layers of fascia. The platysma muscle lies within the superficial fascia. An outer musculofascial collar is formed by the investing fascia that encircles the neck and encloses the trapezius and sternocleidomastoid muscles. The muscle fascia covers the infrahyoid muscles. The carotid sheath encloses blood vessels and nerves, whereas the prevertebral fascia surrounds the intrinsic muscles of the neck. The alar fascia is located in between the carotid sheaths. **(B)** The visceral fascia encloses the thyroid gland, trachea, esophagus, and nerves within the visceral compartment. The pretracheal fascia is the portion of visceral fascia that covers the thyroid gland and trachea, whereas the buccopharyngeal fascia lies on the posterior surface of the esophagus.

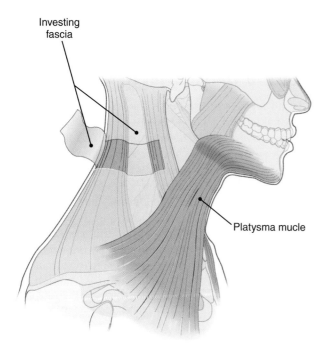

Investing fascia

Platysma mucle

Figure 10–2 The platysma muscle lies within the superficial fascia under the skin. The investing fascia forms a connective tissue collar that surrounds the neck. The superior border is a plane parallel to the inferior border of the mandible, whereas the inferior border parallels the clavicle.

collar surrounding the entire neck that contains smaller tubular compartments of blood vessels, nerves, viscera, and muscle (Fig. 10–1A).

Deep Fascia

The terminology used to discuss the deep fascia can be confusing because the deep fascia is described as being formed by three layers: (1) a superficial layer called the *investing fascia*, (2) a middle layer of *visceral fascia* and *muscular fascia*, and (3) a deep layer called the *prevertebral fascia*. In turn, these layers can be divided into sublayers. It is not important for the dental hygienist to understand the origin of the fascial layers, but to understand that the fascia divides the neck into compartments and that infection can spread within a compartment or the connective tissue spaces between them.

The outermost, superficial layer of the deep fascia is called the **investing fascia** (not hypodermis) because it forms a layer that surrounds the neck like a collar (Figs. 10–1A, 10–2, and 10–3). Starting at the posterior surface of the neck, the investing fascia attaches along the median plane from the external occipital protuberance to the spinous processes of the cervical vertebrae. Superiorly, the fascia courses anteriorly on an imaginary line along the mastoid process of the temporal bone and the body of the mandible. Inferiorly, the investing fascia is attached to the acromion, the clavicle, and the

manubrium (Fig. 10–2). Inferior to the hyoid bone, the fascia splits to surround the sternocleidomastoid and trapezius muscles (Fig. 10–1A) then fuses to form the roof of the posterior cervical triangle (Chapter 3), and finally splits once again to attach onto the anterior and posterior surfaces of the manubrium (Fig. 10–2). Thus, the investing fascia forms the roof for both the anterior and posterior triangles of the neck. Superior to the hyoid bone, the investing fascia covers the submandibular and submental triangles and their contents (Fig 10–3).

The middle layer of the deep fascia is subdivided into muscular and visceral components. The **muscle fascia** surrounds the infrahyoid muscles (Fig. 10–1A), namely the omohyoid, sternohyoid, sternothyroid, and thyrohyoid muscles (discussed in Chapter 3). The visceral component is called the **pretracheal fascia**. This layer surrounds the thyroid gland, trachea, pharynx, and esophagus (Figs. 10–1B and 10–3). The portion of the fascia on the posterior surface of the pharynx is specifically called the **buccopharyngeal fascia** (Fig. 10–1B). As you will see later in the chapter, this fascial layer can serve as a pathway for the spread of infection.

The innermost layer of the deep fascia surrounds the intrinsic muscles of the neck and is called **prevertebral fascia** (Fig. 10–1A). The **alar fascia**, which is a derivative of the prevertebral fascia, is located in a potential space between the vertebral column and the pharynx (Figs. 10–1A and 10–3) and is discussed in more detail later in the chapter.

The **carotid sheath** is a composite of several fascial layers, and its derivation is beyond the scope of this book. It encloses the common carotid and internal carotid arteries, the internal jugular vein, the vagus nerves, and the deep cervical lymph nodes (Fig. 10–1A). The sheath extends from the base of the skull to the root of the neck and blends with the connective tissue of the great vessels of the heart.

Review Question Box 10-1

1. What is the difference between superficial fascia and the outermost, superficial layer of the deep fascia?
2. What fascial layer surrounds the infrahyoid muscles?
3. What is the difference between the pretracheal and buccopharyngeal fascia?
4. What fascial layer surrounds the intrinsic muscles of the neck?

FASCIAL SPACES RELATED TO THE FLOOR OF THE MOUTH

The relationship between the apices of the roots of the teeth to the insertion of the **mylohyoid muscle** onto the **mylohyoid line** of the mandible is critical to the

Figure 10-3 Layers of the deep cervical fascia.

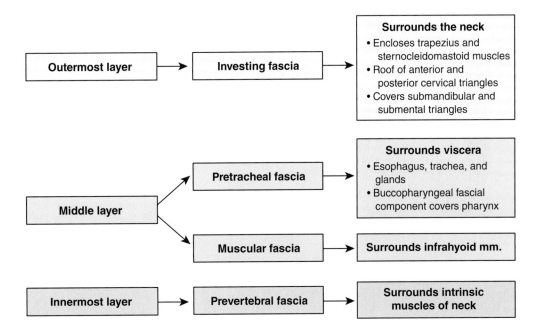

understanding of the potential spread of infection from an abscessed tooth. Infection from the roots of the teeth located superior to the insertion of the mylohyoid muscle will spread into the floor of the mouth. Infection from the roots of teeth that extend inferior to the insertion of the muscle (that is, second and third molars) spread into the submandibular space, which is located outside of the oral cavity (Fig. 10-4).

Sublingual Space

The **sublingual space** is the compartment bordered by the mucosa of the floor of the mouth and the mylohyoid muscle (Fig. 10-5A). Several important structures that lie within this space can be affected by the spread of pus from an abscess of the incisors, canines, premolars, and first molars. These structures include the sublingual gland, the duct of the submandibular gland, the lingual artery and nerve, and the hypoglossal nerve.

The posterior border of the mylohyoid muscle is free, that is, it is not attached to bone (Fig. 10-5B). This allows infection from the floor of the mouth to spread into the spaces posterior and lateral to the mylohyoid muscle.

Submandibular Space

The **submandibular space** is bordered by the investing fascia of the neck, the mylohyoid muscle, the inferior border of the mandible, and the anterior and posterior bellies of the digastric muscle (Fig. 10-6). Major structures in this space include the submandibular gland,

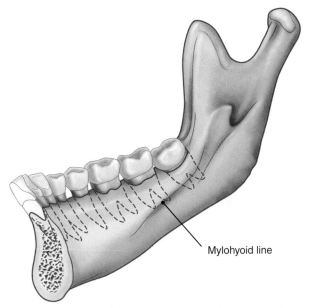

Figure 10-4 The position of the apices of the roots to the attachment of the mylohyoid muscle to the mylohyoid line of the mandible determines the spread of infection into the fascial space of the mouth. Infections of the first molar, premolars, canine, and incisors will spread into the floor of mouth, whereas infection from second and third molars spread inferior to the muscle.

submandibular lymph nodes, and the facial artery and veins. Because the apices of the roots of the second and third molars are located inferior (superficial) to the attachment of the mylohyoid muscle, infection from these teeth can spread into the submandibular space.

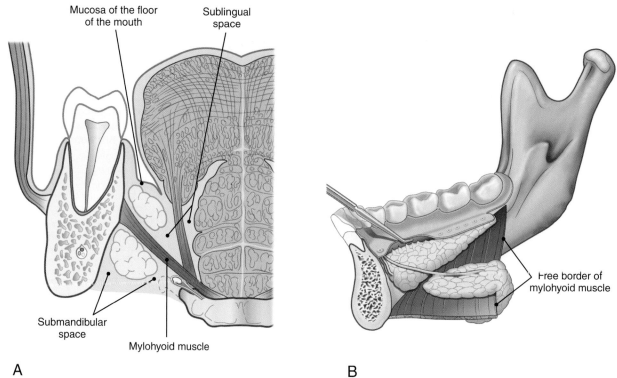

A   B

Figure 10–5 (A) The sublingual space is bounded by the mucosa of the floor of the mouth and the mylohyoid muscle, whereas the submandibular space lies inferior to the mylohyoid muscle. **(B)** The free border of the mylohyoid muscle allows infection to spread posteriorly into other fascial spaces.

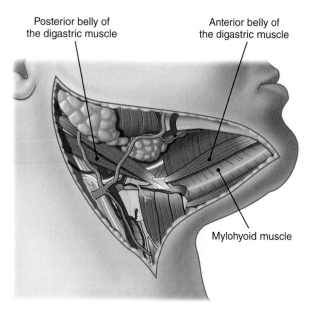

Figure 10–6 The submandibular space is bordered by the anterior and posterior bellies of the digastric muscle and the inferior border of the body of the mandible. The floor is formed by the mylohyoid muscle, and the roof is formed by cervical investing fascia that has been removed to visualize underlying structures.

Submental Space

The **submental space** lies between the two anterior bellies of the digastric muscles and the hyoid bone and is bordered superficially by the investing fascia (forms the roof) of the neck, and on its deep surface (forms the floor) by the mylohyoid muscle (Fig. 10–7). Infection from the incisor teeth drains into this space.

Review Question Box 10-2

1. What is the difference between the submental space and the submental triangle; and the submandibular space and the submandibular triangle?
2. What are the boundaries of the sublingual space?
3. What role does the mylohyoid muscle have in the spread of infection from an abscessed tooth?

LATERAL PHARYNGEAL SPACE

Infections from the floor of the mouth can gain access to the **lateral pharyngeal space** after spreading beyond the posterior margin of the mylohyoid muscle (Figs. 10–8

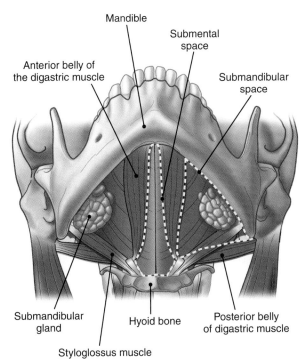

Figure 10–7 The submental space is bordered by the anterior bellies of the digastric muscles and the hyoid bone. The floor is the mylohyoid muscle, and the roof is the cervical investing fascia. Note the close relationship of the submandibular and submental space, which allows the spread of infection between these two spaces.

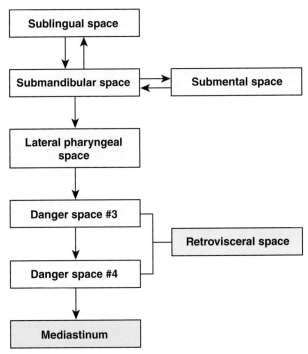

Figure 10–8 Progression of odontogenic infection to the mediastinum.

and 10–9). This space is shaped like an inverted cone. It is located between the *pharyngeal wall* medially, the *medial pterygoid muscle* on the surface of the mandible laterally, and the *prevertebral fascia* posteriorly. The space contains the styloid process and the carotid sheath and its contents (Fig 10–9).

RETROVISCERAL SPACE OF THE NECK

Once infection reaches the lateral pharyngeal space, it can spread down the back of the neck through the **retrovisceral space** (Figs. 10–8 and 10–9). This space is located between the vertebral column and the visceral compartment of the neck. The space is bordered superiorly by the *base of the skull*, inferiorly by the **root of the neck** (Fig. 10–9), laterally by the *carotid sheaths* (Fig. 10–1A), posteriorly by the *prevertebral fascia*, and anteriorly by the *buccopharyngeal fascia* (Figs. 10–1A, 10–9, and 10–10).

This space is divided by a linear layer of *alar fascia* oriented in a frontal plane. The alar fascia is attached superiorly to the *base of the skull*, laterally to the *carotid sheath*, and anteriorly to the *buccopharyngeal fascia* at the root of the neck. The space between the alar fascia and the buccopharyngeal fascia is called the **retropharyngeal space** or **danger space #3** (Fig. 10–10). This space is continuous with the lateral pharyngeal space superior to the hyoid bone, but is closed inferiorly by the fusion of the alar fascia with the buccopharyngeal fascia. Infection in this space causes swelling of the neck and difficulty in breathing (Fig 10–8). **Danger space #4** is located between the alar fascia and the prevertebral fascia (Fig. 10–10). This space is closed superiorly by the skull and is continuous inferiorly with the thorax. Swelling in this area can cause difficulty in swallowing and breathing.

Review Question Box 10-3

1. What is the difference between the lateral pharyngeal space and the retrovisceral space?
2. What is the difference between danger space #3 and danger space #4?
3. Compare the pathways of infection from the first mandibular premolar and the second mandibular molar teeth into danger space #3.
4. How can an infection spread from danger space #3 into danger space #4?
5. What can happen if an infection spreads into danger space #4?

Clinical Correlation Box 10-1

Ludwig's Angina

Ludwig's angina is a bilateral swelling of the *submental, sublingual,* and *submandibular spaces*. It is commonly formed by the abscess of the apices of the teeth. The pus penetrates the lingual plates of the mandibular teeth and gains access to either the sublingual space or the submandibular space, depending on the relationship of the root apices to the mandibular attachment of the mylohyoid muscles. Because the roots of the second and third molars extend inferiorly beyond the attachment, infection spreads into the submandibular space. Because of the anatomical relationship of the submental, sublingual, and submandibular spaces, infection

can spread in either direction in these spaces. The patient presents with extreme hardness to the floor of the mouth and has difficulty swallowing (**dysphagia**). The tongue is elevated and can be pushed to one side. Infection can then spread into the lateral pharyngeal space and cause an indurated (hardened) swelling of the neck. If not treated, the infection can advance into the danger spaces of the neck, which can result in asphyxiation (suffocation), which is life threatening. Further spread into the thorax can cause **mediastinitis** (inflammation of the mediastinum). The mediastinum is the region between the lungs that contains such vital organs as the heart, trachea, esophagus, thymus gland, and lymph nodes.

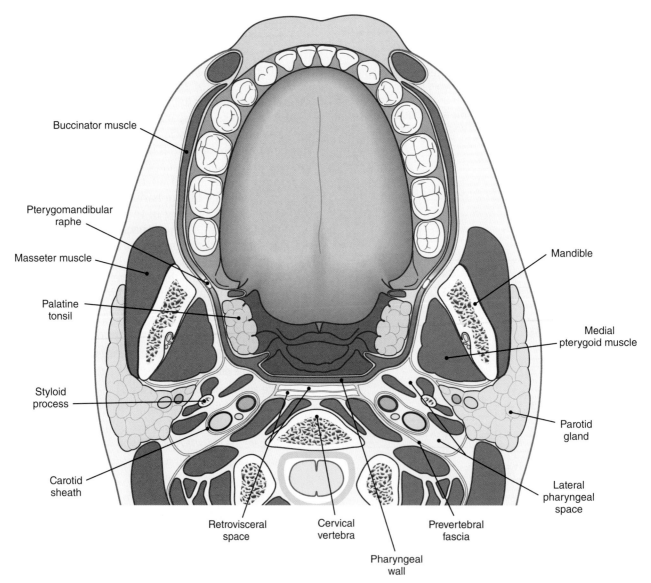

Figure 10–9 Horizontal section through the mouth just superior to the occlusal plane. The lateral pharyngeal space is located posterior to the mandible and lies in between the medial pterygoid muscle and the pharyngeal wall. The space contains the styloid process and the carotid sheath. The retrovisceral space lies between the cervical vertebrae and the pharynx. It is divided by the alar fascia.

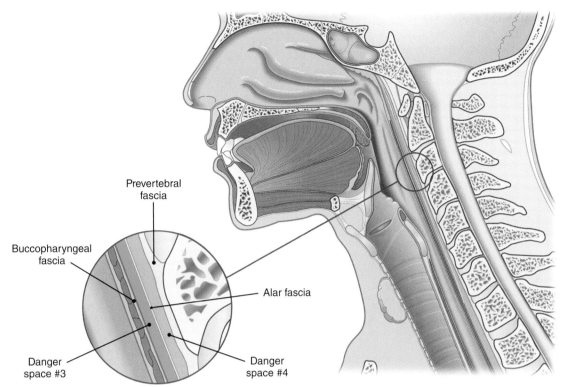

Figure 10–10 Sagittal section through the neck. The retrovisceral space is located between the buccopharyngeal fascia and prevertebral fascia. The space is divided into two danger spaces by the alar fascia, which is a sheet of connective tissue that lies in a frontal plane extending from the base of the skull to the root of the neck. Danger space #3 or retropharyngeal space is located between the buccopharyngeal fascia and the alar fascia and is continuous superiorly with the lateral pharyngeal space. Danger space #4 lies between the alar and prevertebral fasciae and is continuous inferiorly with the mediastinum.

SUMMARY

The neck is divided into compartments and spaces by the various layers of the deep fascia. The investing fascia is the outermost layer that surrounds the trapezius and sternocleidomastoid muscles. The middle layer is divided into a muscular layer that surrounds the infrahyoid muscles and the pretracheal fascia, which encircles the visceral structures of the neck. The portion of the pretracheal fascia that covers the pharynx is called the buccopharyngeal fascia. The prevertebral fascia is the innermost layer of the deep fascia that encases the intrinsic muscles of the neck. The carotid sheath is a combination of the various layers of the deep fascia. The floor of the mouth is divided into three fascial spaces by the mylohyoid muscle. The sublingual space lies superior to the mylohyoid muscle, whereas the submandibular and submental spaces are located inferior to the muscle. Infection can spread through these spaces because they are confluent at the posterior border of the mylohyoid muscle. Infection from the spaces of the floor of the mouth can spread into the lateral pharyngeal space that lies between the pterygoid muscles and the pharyngeal wall. Infection can then spread into the retrovisceral space, which is located posterior to the visceral compartment. This space is bordered anteriorly by the buccopharyngeal fascia, laterally by the carotid sheath, superiorly by the base of the skull, posteriorly by the prevertebral fascia, and inferiorly by the mediastinum. The alar fascia divides the retrovisceral space into danger spaces #3 and #4. Infection from the lateral pharyngeal space can spread into danger space #3 between the buccopharyngeal fascia and the alar fascia. Infections in the neck are life threatening because of suffocation and possible spread into the mediastinum.

Learning Activity 10-1

Submandibular and Sublingual Space

Match the numbered structures with the correct terms listed to the right.

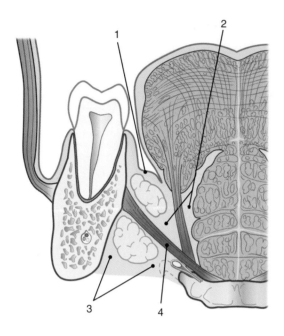

_____ Mucosa of the floor of the mouth

_____ Mylohyoid muscle

_____ Sublingual space

_____ Submandibular space

Learning Activity 10-2

Lateral Lingual Space

Match the numbered structures with the correct terms listed to the right.

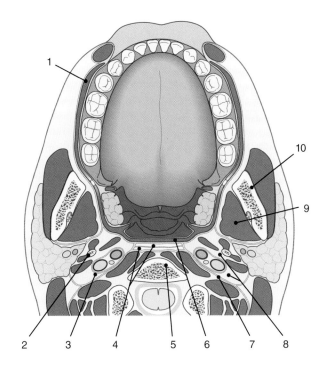

_____ Buccinator muscle

_____ Carotid sheath

_____ Cervical vertebra

_____ Lateral pharyngeal space

_____ Mandible

_____ Medial pterygoid muscle

_____ Pharyngeal wall

_____ Prevertebral fascia

_____ Retrovisceral space

_____ Styloid process

chapter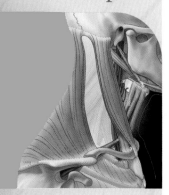

11

Vascular Supply of the Head and Neck

Objectives

1. Define the circulatory system and distinguish between the cardiovascular system and the lymphatic system.
2. Identify the chambers of the heart and the great vessels entering and exiting the heart and trace the flow of blood passing through the heart via the systemic and pulmonary circulations.
3. Identify the major branches of the subclavian artery and external carotid artery and trace the distribution from branches of these vessels that supply blood to the head and neck.
4. Describe the formation of the superficial veins of the head and neck and distinguish their pattern of drainage.
5. Describe the drainage pattern of the deep veins of the face through the pterygoid plexus and discuss the relationship of the superficial veins of the face, the pterygoid plexus, and the cavernous sinus.

Overview

Blood carries nutrients from the digestive system and oxygen from the lungs to the body tissues. In addition, hormones are released into the blood that regulate the functioning of the organ systems. Carbon dioxide is released into the blood and is exchanged for oxygen in the lungs, whereas other metabolic wastes are routed to the kidney for excretion. The heart serves as a pump that helps produce the pressure required to circulate the blood through the vessels that connect to organ systems. The circulation of blood is critical to life. Barely a day goes by in which there are advertisements on television, the radio, or Internet for medications to prevent heart disease by reducing the amount of cholesterol that can form plaque on the inside of the arteries and reduce the blood supply to the heart. The dental hygienist must understand the risk in treating patients with cardiovascular disease. The hygienist must also realize that poor circulation not only affects the heart, but also affects the tissues within the oral cavity. Thus, it is important to learn the basic structure of the heart and the circulation of blood through the heart and body tissues.

INTRODUCTION TO THE VASCULAR SUPPLY OF THE HEAD AND NECK

The circulatory system transports blood throughout the body. It is subdivided into two components: the cardiovascular system and the lymphatic system. The **cardiovascular system** is formed by the heart, arteries, veins, and capillaries that distribute and collect blood from the body tissues. Exchange of nutrients and gases (oxygen and carbon dioxide) occur in capillaries that connect the arterial supply to the venous return. The **lymphatic system** collects fluids and proteins that escape from the cardiovascular system. The fluid, which is clear to white in color, is called **lymph**. Lymph is filtered by lymph nodes that are situated at various points before the fluid is returned to the blood–vascular system. The system includes other organs, such as the spleen, thymus, and tonsils, all of which form lymphocytes. These cells play an important role in the immune system. The focus in this chapter is the distribution and return of blood from the head and neck, whereas Chapter 12 will discuss the distribution of the lymph nodes.

THE STRUCTURE OF THE HEART

The heart is composed of two muscular pumps that lie side by side. Each pump has one chamber for receiving blood, the **atrium**, and one chamber that pumps blood, the **ventricle** (Fig. 11–1). The right side of the heart has a role in the **pulmonary circulation**, whereas the left side is involved in the **systemic circulation**. The *right atrium* receives deoxygenated blood from the body and moves the blood into the right ventricle. Contraction of the *right ventricle* pumps the blood into the pulmonary trunk and its branches, the pulmonary arteries, to reach the lungs. Once oxygenated in the lungs, pulmonary veins return the oxygenated blood to the *left atrium* of the heart, which then flows into the *left ventricle*. The left ventricle contracts and pumps the oxygenated blood into the aorta for distribution to the body (Fig. 11–2). The separation of the ventricles by the **interventricular septum** (Fig. 11–1) and the atria by the **interatrial septum** prevents the mixing of oxygenated and deoxygenated blood.

The right atrium and the right ventricle are separated by the **tricuspid valve**, whereas the left atrium and left ventricle are separated by the **mitral valve** or **bicuspid valve** (Fig. 11–1). While the heart is in its resting stage or **diastole**, the valves are open and blood flows from the atria into the ventricles assisted by contraction of the muscles of the atrium. During **systole**, the contractions of the ventricles close the valves, thus preventing the reflux of blood from the ventricles into the atria. The cusps of the valves are attached by tendinous cords

 Box 11-1 Comparison of Arteries and Veins

Arteries and veins accompany each other in their course of distribution through the body. The vessels can be distinguished grossly by their size relative to the thickness of their walls. Arteries tend to be round with thick walls and a relatively small lumen compared to veins. A vein has a thin wall and a large lumen as compared to arteries. Veins are usually larger than their companion arteries and the walls generally collapse without the presence of blood. Blood vessels are formed by three layers or tunics (t.) of tissue that are adapted to the function of the vessels. The **tunica adventitia** is the outermost layer of connective tissue that surrounds the vessels. This layer is thicker in veins than arteries. The **tunica media** is formed by smooth muscle and is usually thicker in arteries than in veins. The thicker walls of arteries are required because of the blood pressure needed to distribute the blood to the tissues. The blood pressure within the arteries is controlled by the **sympathetic nervous system**. The **tunica intima** is the innermost layer of epithelium specifically called **endothelium**. Exchange of nutrients and gases occur in the blood **capillaries**, which are comprised essentially of endothelium. Blood pressure in the capillaries and the venous system is much lower than in the arteries. To overcome the forces of gravity, the veins have valves, which are folds in the t. intima. Contraction of skeletal muscles surrounding the veins forces blood toward the heart. As the muscles relax, the blood flows in a retrograde fashion because of gravity. The backflow of blood causes the valves to close, thus preventing the blood to flow below the valves. Obstruction of blood flow can cause veins to enlarge and form **varicose** veins. Increased pressure in both arteries and veins can cause a local dilation of the vessel called an **aneurysm**. Rupture of an aneurysm of the aorta can be deadly, whereas rupture of small vessels in the brain can cause a **stroke**, which can result in temporary or permanent loss of function.

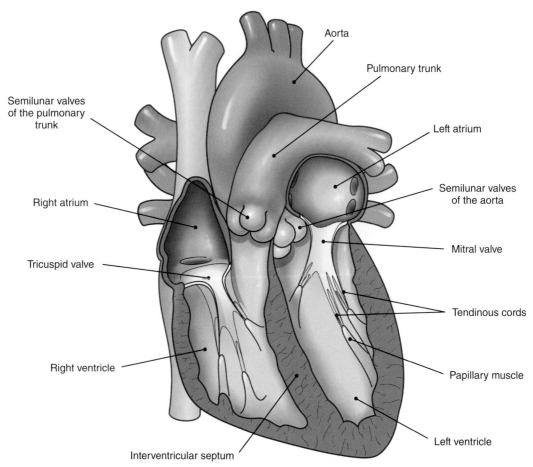

Figure 11–1 The heart is designed to pump blood to the lungs and body simultaneously without mixing oxygenated and deoxygenated blood. The atria of the heart receive blood from the lungs and body tissues, whereas the ventricles pump the blood to the body via the aorta and to the lungs by the pulmonary trunk. The tricuspid and mitral valves separate the atria and ventricles to prevent backflow of blood from the ventricles into the atria. The pulmonary trunk and aorta contain semilunar valves that prevent the backflow of blood from these vessels when the heart is relaxed. Mixing of oxygenated and deoxygenated blood between the ventricles is prevented by the interventricular septum. A similar septum separates the atria, but is hidden from view by the pulmonary trunk and aorta.

to **papillary muscles** on the walls of the ventricle (Fig. 11–1). Contraction of these muscles pulls tension on the cord, thus controlling the closure of the valves. Blood passing through valves that do not close properly cause a rushing sound called a **murmur**.

The outflow tracts of the ventricles—the pulmonary trunk on the right side and the aorta on the left side—also contain valves that prevent the reflux of blood back into the heart during diastole (Fig. 11–1). The structure of these valves will be discussed in the next section.

Review Question Box 11-1

1. What chambers of the heart contract during systole?
2. What cardiac valves open during diastole?
3. Why are the atria and ventricles separated by a septum?

THE GREAT VESSELS

The **great vessels** are the primary arteries and veins of the heart. The arteries include the following:

a. Pulmonary trunk and arteries
b. Ascending aorta and aortic arch
c. Brachiocephalic trunk
d. Left common carotid artery
e. Left subclavian artery

The primary veins are as follows:

a. Left and right brachiocephalic veins
b. Superior and inferior vena cavae
c. Pulmonary veins

Arteries are defined as blood vessels that carry blood *away from* the heart, whereas veins carry blood *to* the heart. The arteries that carry blood to the lungs arise from the heart as the **pulmonary trunk**. The pulmonary trunk

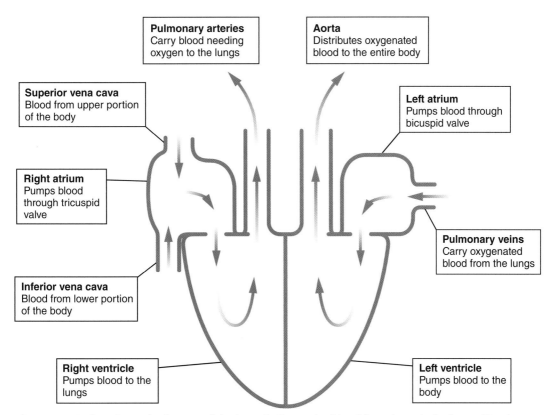

Pulmonary arteries
Carry blood needing
oxygen to the lungs

Aorta
Distributes oxygenated
blood to the entire body

Superior vena cava
Blood from upper portion
of the body

Left atrium
Pumps blood through
bicuspid valve

Right atrium
Pumps blood
through tricuspid
valve

Pulmonary veins
Carry oxygenated
blood from the lungs

Inferior vena cava
Blood from lower portion
of the body

Right ventricle
Pumps blood to the
lungs

Left ventricle
Pumps blood to the
body

Figure 11–2 The schematic diagram of the heart indicates the blood flow through the heart. Blood enters the right atrium via veins from the upper and lower regions of the body. Deoxygenated blood enters the right ventricles and exits the pulmonary trunk to reach the lungs. Oxygenated blood is returned to the left atrium by the pulmonary veins. The blood flows into the left ventricle and exits through the aorta to be distributed to the body tissues.

divides into right and left **pulmonary arteries** (Figs. 11–3 and 11–4) that carry deoxygenated blood to the lungs, whereas the **aorta**, the vessel that supplies blood to the rest of the body, carries oxygenated blood. The aorta ascends a short distance and arches from the right to the left (Figs. 11–3 and 11–4). The first branch of the **aortic arch** is called the **brachiocephalic trunk or artery**. The brachiocephalic trunk extends superiorly for a short distance and bifurcates into the right **subclavian artery** and the right **common carotid artery** (Fig. 11–5). The next branches of the aortic arch are the **left common carotid artery** followed by the **left subclavian artery** (Fig. 11–3).

The heart is supplied by the right and left **coronary arteries**, which are branches of the **ascending aorta** (Fig. 11–3). During systole, blood is forced out of the heart into the aorta. As the heart relaxes during diastole, blood flow back into the heart is prevented by the **semilunar valve**. Unlike the atrioventricular valves, there are no cusps attached to papillary muscles. The semilunar valve is formed by three small valvules that are semilunar in shape (Fig. 11–1). As blood flows back toward the heart, blood collects on the surface of the valves, forcing them to close together and thus allowing blood to flow into the coronary arteries. A similar valve found in the pulmonary trunk prevents backflow into the right ventricle.

Venous blood from the systemic circulation is returned to the *right atrium* of the heart via the inferior and superior vena cavae. The **inferior vena cava** returns blood from the lower limbs and trunk, whereas the **superior vena cava** returns blood from the upper limbs, neck, and head (Figs. 11–3 and 11–4). The superior vena cava is formed by the right and left **brachiocephalic veins** (Fig. 11–3). As the name implies, these veins collect blood from the brachium or arm via the **subclavian vein** as well as the head by the **internal jugular vein** (Fig. 11–3). Oxygenated blood from the pulmonary circulation is returned to the heart via the pulmonary veins that empty into the **left atrium** (Figs. 11–3 and 11–4).

Review Question Box 11-2

1. What arteries are the first branches of the aorta?
2. What is the difference between the atrioventricular valves and the semilunar valves?
3. What is the difference between the brachiocephalic trunk and the brachiocephalic veins?
4. Into what chambers does blood enter into the heart?

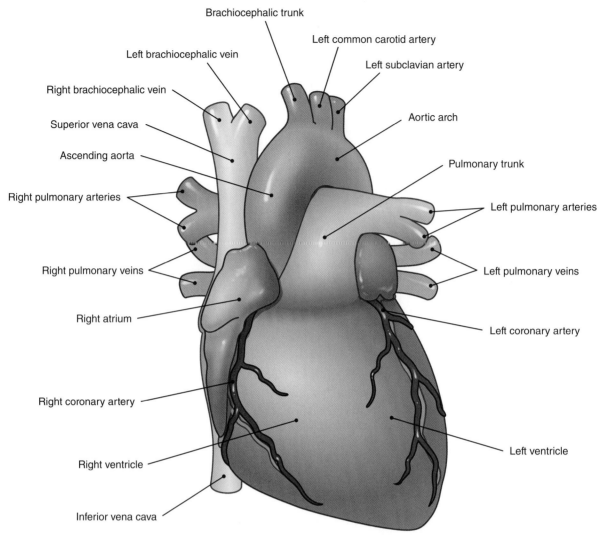

Brachiocephalic trunk

Left common carotid artery

Left brachiocephalic vein

Left subclavian artery

Right brachiocephalic vein

Superior vena cava

Aortic arch

Ascending aorta

Pulmonary trunk

Right pulmonary arteries

Left pulmonary arteries

Right pulmonary veins

Left pulmonary veins

Right atrium

Left coronary artery

Right coronary artery

Left ventricle

Right ventricle

Inferior vena cava

Figure 11–3 Anterior view of the heart. The superior and inferior venae cavae, the aorta and its branches, and the pulmonary trunk and its branches are called the *great vessels* of the heart. From right to left, the branches of the aorta are the brachiocephalic trunk, the left common carotid artery, and the left subclavian artery. Because of embryological development, the right common carotid and subclavian arteries are branches of the brachiocephalic trunk. The right and left coronary arteries are branches of the ascending aorta. These vessels supply oxygenated blood to the musculature of the heart. Lack of oxygen to the heart by the narrowing of the vessels can lead to a heart attack.

Subclavian Arteries

En route to the upper extremities, the *right* and *left subclavian arteries* extends several branches into the anterior and posterior triangles of the neck (Chapter 3). These vessels supply blood to the muscles of the neck and back, as well as the thoracic wall, the thyroid gland (**inferior thyroid artery**), brain (**vertebral artery**), and other structures not discussed in this textbook (Fig. 11–5). Recall from your study of the skull (Chapter 2), that the *vertebral artery* ascends in the neck through the transverse foramina of the cervical vertebrae and enters the skull through the foramen magnum. Within the skull, the two vessels fuse to form the basilar artery that supplies blood to the brain (Chapter 13). The subclavian artery extends over the

first rib to form the axillary (armpit) artery, which continues into the arm as the brachial artery and its branches.

Review Question Box 11-3

1. What major structures of the head and neck are supplied by branches of the subclavian artery?

Carotid Arteries

After branching from the brachiocephalic trunk on the right side and the aortic arch on the left side, the left and right *common carotid arteries* enter into the **carotid**

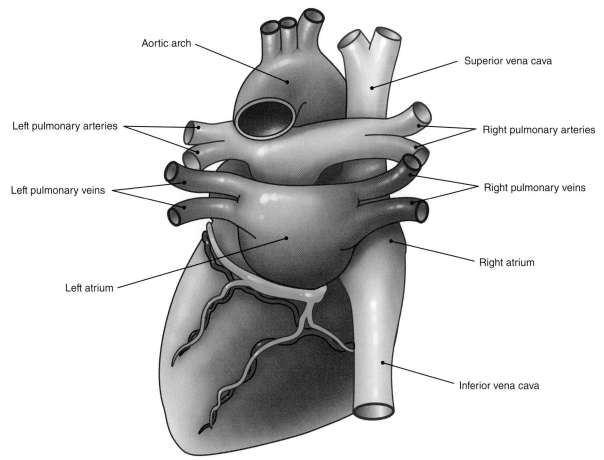

Aortic arch

Left pulmonary arteries

Left pulmonary veins

Left atrium

Superior vena cava

Right pulmonary arteries

Right pulmonary veins

Right atrium

Inferior vena cava

Figure 11–4 Posterior view of the heart shows the inflow of the pulmonary veins into the left atrium and the superior and inferior vena cavae into the right atrium. The aortic arch crosses over the pulmonary arteries to reach the right side of the body.

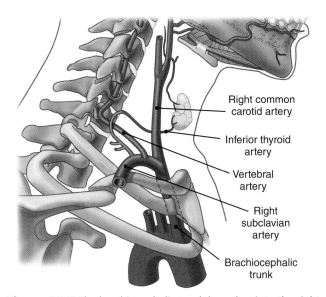

Right common carotid artery

Inferior thyroid artery

Vertebral artery

Right subclavian artery

Brachiocephalic trunk

Figure 11–5 The brachiocephalic trunk branches into the right common carotid artery and the right subclavian artery. Several branches diverge from the subclavian artery in the neck. The inferior thyroid artery supplies blood to the thyroid gland, and the vertebral artery enters the vertebral column to reach the skull to supply blood to the brain. The subclavian artery ends after crossing the first rib and continues inferiorly as the axillary and brachial arteries, which supply blood to the upper extremity.

triangle (Fig. 11–6A and B). Recall from Chapter 3 that the carotid triangle is a subsidiary of the anterior triangle of the neck and is bordered by the sternocleidomastoid muscle, the superior belly of the omohyoid muscle, and the posterior belly of the digastric muscle. Within the carotid triangle, the common carotid artery bifurcates (divides into two parts) at the level of the thyroid cartilage into the **external** and **internal carotid arteries** (Fig. 11–6A and B). The internal carotid artery does not branch in the neck; it will be discussed as a component of the vertebral–basilar–carotid system that supplies blood to the brain (Chapter 13).

As the external carotid artery courses through the neck, five branches diverge into the carotid triangle. The most inferior branch of the external carotid is the **superior thyroid artery** (Fig. 11–6A and B). This artery courses inferiorly to supply blood to the thyroid gland. As the vessel descends, the superior thyroid artery called the **superior laryngeal artery** branches from the vessel to supply portions of the larynx (Fig. 11–6A and B). Superiorly, the next major branch is the **lingual artery**, which travels a short distance anteriorly, then passes deep to the **hyoglossus muscle** to reach the oral cavity (Fig. 11–6A and B). This artery supplies blood to the tongue and the floor of the mouth.

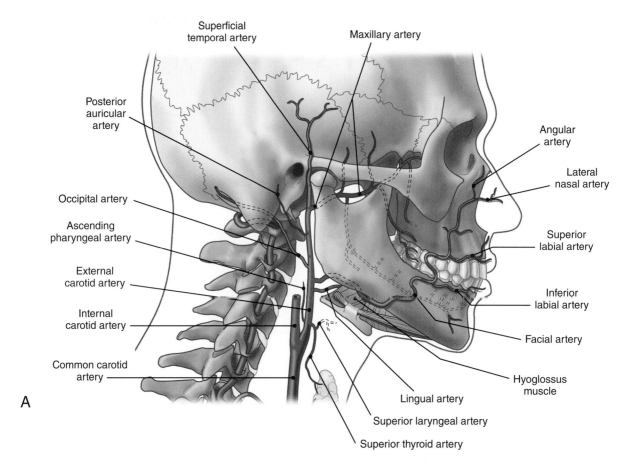

A

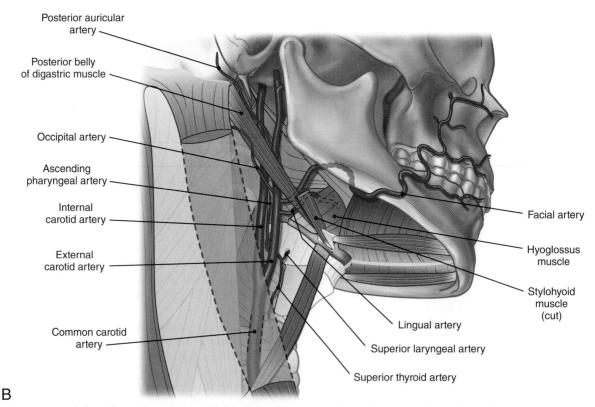

B

Figure 11–6 (A) An illustration of the major branches of the external carotid artery in the neck and face. **(B)** Within the carotid triangle, the common carotid artery divides into the internal and external carotid arteries. The internal carotid artery has no branches in the neck. The external carotid artery has five branches that supply blood to the thyroid gland, the larynx, the pharynx, the occipital region, the tongue, and the face. The lingual artery passes deep to the hyoglossus muscle to reach the tongue. As the facial artery passes through the submandibular triangle to reach the face, it extends branches to the submandibular gland, lips, and side of the nose, then terminates as the angular artery medial to the eyelids. After leaving the triangle, the external carotid artery sends a small branch to the ear and terminates as the maxillary and superficial temporal arteries.

The next major branch, the **facial artery**, courses through the submandibular triangle deep to the submandibular gland to reach the inferior border of the mandible and the superficial face. This artery supplies blood to the submandibular gland, the submental region, and the skin and muscles of the face (Fig. 11–6A and B). Upon reaching the corners of the mouth, the facial artery sends *inferior* and *superior* **labial artery** branches to the upper and lower lips. As it ascends along the side of the nose, the artery sends an **lateral nasal artery** branch to the ala of the nose, and terminates as the **angular artery** at the medial commissure (where the upper and lower eyelids join) of the eye (Fig. 11–6A).

Two other branches of the external carotid are the **occipital artery**, which supplies blood to the back of the neck, and the **ascending pharyngeal artery**, which supplies blood to the muscles of the pharynx (Fig. 11–6A and B).

After branching in the carotid triangle, the external carotid artery leaves the triangle by passing deep to the posterior belly of the digastric. At this point, the **posterior auricular artery** branches from the main vessel to supply blood to the ear. The external carotid then terminates as two arteries: the **maxillary artery** and the **superficial temporal artery** (Fig. 11–6A and B). The superficial temporal artery supplies blood to the region superficial to the temporal bone, whereas the maxillary artery is a second source of arterial blood supply to the face. It will be discussed in more detail in the next section.

Review Question Box 11-4

1. What are the branches of the external carotid artery in the carotid triangle and the areas that are supplied by these branches?
2. Why is the posterior auricular artery not located in the carotid triangle?
3. What are the terminal branches of the external carotid artery?

Maxillary Artery

After branching from the external carotid artery, the *maxillary artery* passes deep to the ramus of the mandible to reach the infratemporal fossa (Fig. 11–6A). For descriptive purposes, the artery is divided into three parts by the **lateral pterygoid muscle**; the branches are summarized in Figure 11–7. The first part lies proximal to the lateral pterygoid muscle—that is, between the ramus of the mandible and the posterior border of the muscle. The second portion lies either superficially or deep to the lateral pterygoid muscle, whereas the third portion lies distal to

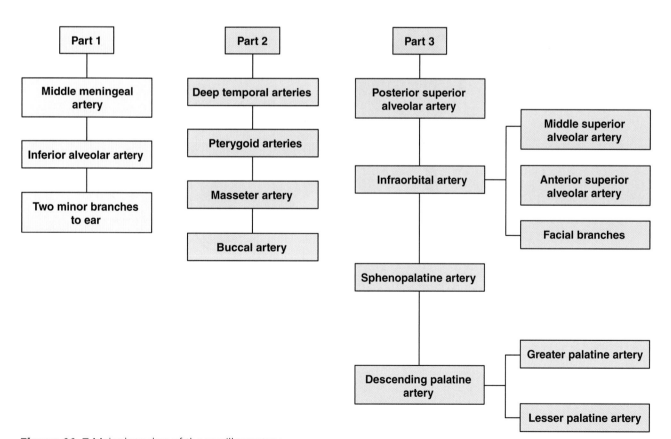

Figure 11–7 Major branches of the maxillary artery.

the anterior border of the muscle Fig. 11–8). The maxillary artery is extremely important because its branches supply blood to the dura mater of the brain, the muscles of mastication, both the maxillary and mandibular teeth, and the nasal cavity. The branches most important to the dental hygienist are discussed in the next section.

Branches of Part 1

The **middle meningeal artery** ascends in the infratemporal fossa and enters into the foramen spinosum to reach the interior of the skull (Figs. 11–8 and 11–9). The artery divides into several branches, which supply blood to the dura mater and the bones of the skull. An accessory meningeal artery may be present but is of lesser significance and will not be detailed.

The **inferior alveolar artery** enters into the **mandibular foramen** on the medial surface of the mandible and supplies all of the mandibular teeth (Fig. 11–8). Upon reaching the **mental foramen**, a branch exits through the foramen as the **mental artery** to supply blood to the chin. The terminal portion of the inferior alveolar artery

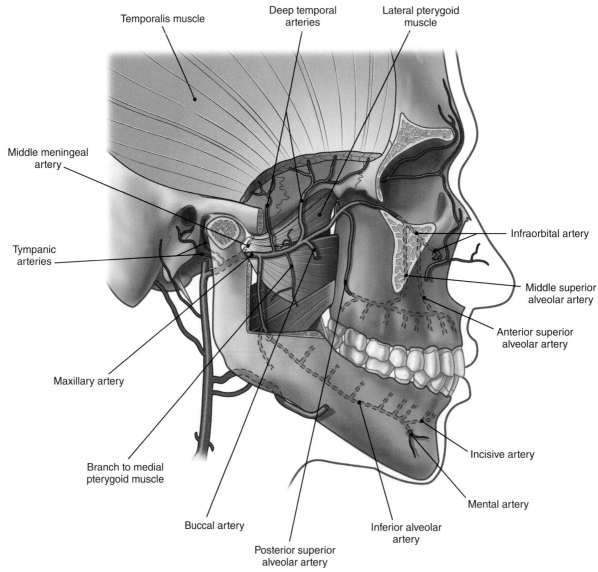

Figure 11–8 In the infratemporal fossa, the maxillary artery is divided into three parts according to the relationship to the lateral pterygoid muscle. The first part, which is proximal to the muscle, extends branches that supply blood to the dura and the mandibular teeth. The inferior alveolar artery supplies blood to the molar and premolar teeth and terminates as the mental and incisive arteries. The incisive artery supplies blood to the canine and incisor teeth. The second part of the artery lies on either the superficial or deep surface of the muscle. Branches of the second part supply blood to the muscles of mastication and the cheek wall. The third part, which lies distal to the muscle, extends branches that supply blood to the molar teeth and a branch that enters the orbit where it sends branches to the remaining teeth and terminates on the surface of the face.

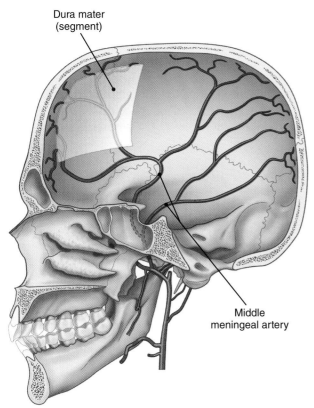

Dura mater
(segment)

Middle
meningeal artery

Figure 11–9 Sagittal view of the cranial cavity. A segment of dura mater has been left on the bone and the remainder has been removed. The middle meningeal artery enters the skull and supplies blood to the dura mater, which covers the brain.

within the mandibular canal beyond the mental foramen is called the **incisive artery** and supplies blood to the canine and incisor teeth (Fig. 11–8).

There are two minor tympanic branches to the ear, but the dental hygienist does not encounter them.

Branches of Part 2

The anterior and posterior **deep temporal arteries** course deep to the temporalis muscle, which they supply (Fig. 11–8).

The **pterygoid arteries** supply blood to the medial and lateral pterygoid muscles (Fig. 11–8).

The **masseteric artery** courses through the mandibular notch to supply blood to the masseter muscle.

The **buccal artery** arises between the superior and inferior heads of the lateral pterygoid muscles and on the superficial surface of the buccinator to supply blood to this muscle (Fig. 11–8).

Branches of Part 3

The **posterior superior alveolar artery** enters the maxilla by a foramen of the same name and supplies blood to the posterior maxillary teeth (Fig. 11–8).

The **infraorbital artery** courses in the infraorbital groove along the floor of the orbit. While passing through the floor of the orbit, it gives off the **middle** and **anterior superior alveolar arteries** that supply blood to the remainder of the maxillary teeth (Fig. 11–8).

The **sphenopalatine artery** enters into the nasal cavity via the **sphenopalatine foramen** and supplies blood to the nasal septum and lateral wall of the nasal cavity (Fig. 11–10).

The **descending palatine artery** passes through the greater palatine canal and branches into the **greater** and **lesser palatine arteries** (Fig. 11–10). These vessels gain access to the surface of the palate via the greater and lesser palatine foramina (Chapter 2), respectively. The greater palatine artery courses anteriorly along the hard palate to reach the **incisive canal**, where it anastomoses with arterial branches from the nasal cavity. The lesser palatine artery courses posteriorly to supply blood to the soft palate (Fig. 11–10).

Review Question Box 11-5

1. What divides the maxillary artery into three parts?
2. How does the branching pattern of the inferior alveolar and superior alveolar arteries from the maxillary artery differ?
3. What structures are supplied by the second part of the maxillary artery?
4. How do the orbit, palate, and nasal cavity receive their blood supply?

VENOUS DRAINAGE

The venous drainage of the head and neck is by veins that form the **external jugular vein** and *internal jugular vein*. The distributions of these veins are roughly comparable to the distribution of the external and internal carotid arteries. As you will see, these two venous systems are connected and infection from the face and teeth can possibly spread to more critical areas such as the brain.

From both anatomical and functional viewpoints, it is important to remember some fundamental differences between the arterial and venous systems. First, arteries carry blood away from the heart. Therefore, all arteries have their origin from either the pulmonary trunk or the aorta. Arteries are discussed in terms of branching from these main trunks that terminate in the tissues. Veins begin in the tissues and carry blood back to the heart. Smaller veins join to form larger veins, which eventually combine to form either the inferior or superior vena cava that return the blood to the heart.

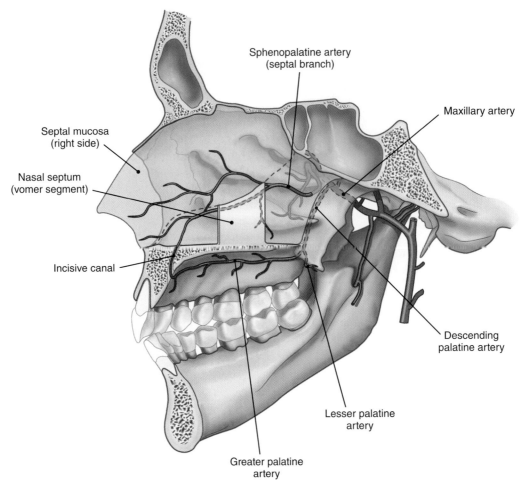

Figure 11–10 In the sagittal view of the nasal cavity, the bony septum has been removed except for a small portion of the vomer. The mucosa on the right side of the septum is intact. The sphenopalatine artery which is a branch of the maxillary artery, enters the nasal cavity and supplies portions of the nasal cavity. The septal branch courses along the nasal septum between the bone and the mucosa and then enters the incisive canal to reach the palate. The descending palatine artery descends and terminates as the greater palatine artery (to the hard palate) and the lesser palatine artery (to the soft palate).

External and Internal Jugular Veins

To understand how the *external jugular vein* forms, it is necessary to understand the drainage of blood into the **retromandibular vein**, which contributes to its formation. As the name implies, the vein lies behind (retro to) the ramus of the mandible. It is not visible because it lies within the parotid gland. The **superficial temporal vein** and the **maxillary vein** form the *retromandibular vein* (Figs. 11–11 and 11–12). These two veins drain the same regions that their companion arteries supply. Near the inferior border of the mandible, the retromandibular vein divides into anterior and posterior divisions (Figs. 11–11 and 11–12). The *posterior division* joins the posterior auricular vein, which drains the region around the ear to form the *external jugular vein* (Figs. 11–11 and 11–12). The external jugular vein crosses superficially over the **sternocleidomastoid muscle** and penetrates the investing fascia on the roof of the posterior triangle of the neck. The blood vessel passes deep to the clavicle to drain into the **subclavian vein** (Fig. 11–11). Many individuals have an **anterior jugular vein** that is found in the midline of the neck (Fig. 11–11). This vein starts in the submental region, courses inferiorly, and travels deep to the sternocleidomastoid muscle to empty into the external jugular vein.

The *anterior division* of the retromandibular vein combines with the **facial vein**, which drains the face, to form the **common facial vein** (Figs. 11–11 and 11–12). This vein passes deep to the sternocleidomastoid muscle to empty into the *internal jugular vein* (Fig. 11–12). The formation of the internal jugular vein takes place at the base of the skull by the union of the sigmoid and inferior petrosal dural sinuses that drain the brain. The details of the venous drainage of the brain will be discussed in Chapter 13.

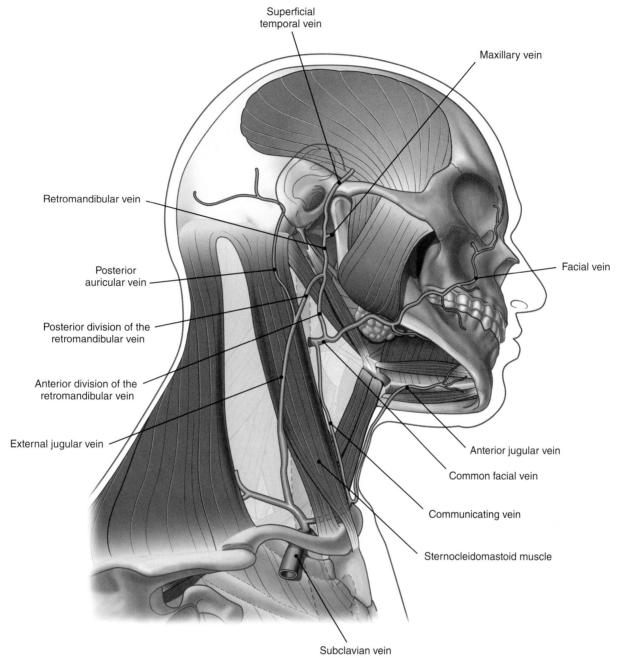

Figure 11–11 The retromandibular vein is formed by the union of the superficial temporal and maxillary veins. The retromandibular vein divides into anterior and posterior divisions. The posterior division joins the posterior auricular vein to form the external jugular vein. The external jugular vein descends superficially to the sternocleidomastoid muscle to empty into the subclavian vein. The anterior division combines with the facial vein to form the common facial vein, which crosses deep to the sternocleidomastoid muscle to empty into the internal jugular vein. The anterior jugular vein, when present, drains the submental region and empties into the subclavian vein. The common facial and the anterior jugular veins are often connected by an unnamed vein that parallels the anterior border of the sternocleidomastoid muscle.

The internal jugular vein receives tributaries from the pharyngeal, the lingual, the facial, and the thyroid veins. The internal jugular and the subclavian veins empty into the *brachiocephalic vein.* The left and right brachiocephalic veins join to form the *superior vena cava* (Fig. 11–3).

One final note: The superficial veins are variable and do not always follow the pattern described. Frequently, the anterior jugular vein is connected to the common facial vein by a large communicating vein (Fig. 11–11), and sometimes the external jugular vein may be absent.

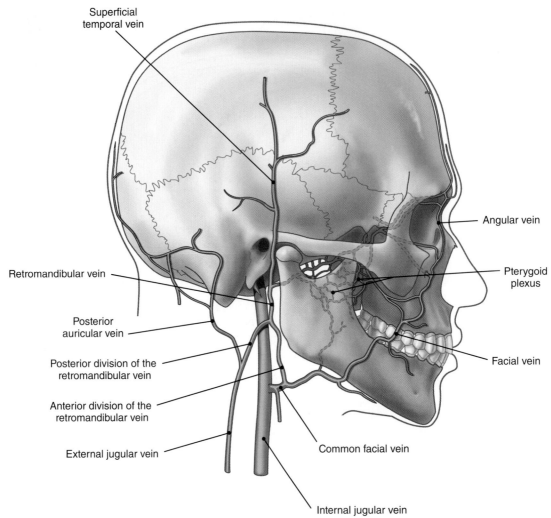

Figure 11–12 The internal jugular vein begins at the base of the skull and receives the common facial vein, which is formed by the anterior division of the retromandibular and common facial veins. The formation of the external jugular vein by the posterior division of the retromandibular vein and posterior auricular vein is also shown.

1. What venous structures form the retromandibular vein?
2. What venous structures form the common facial vein?
3. What is the structural difference between the external jugular and internal jugular veins?
4. Into what venous structures do the external jugular and internal jugular veins drain?

Pterygoid Plexus of Veins

The **pterygoid plexus** of veins is a system of branching veins within the *infratemporal fossa* (Fig. 11–13). The fossa contains the muscles of mastication, the maxillary artery and its branches, and the nerves that supply blood to the tongue, the floor of mouth, and all of the mandibular teeth. The plexus drains blood from regions supplied by the maxillary artery to include the following:

a. Muscles of mastication
b. Maxilla
c. Mandible
d. Dura mater of the brain
e. Face
f. Orbit
g. Nasal cavity

The pterygoid plexus drains into the *maxillary vein*; as mentioned before, this vein joins the superficial temporal vein to form the retromandibular vein (Figs. 11–11 and 11–12).

The plexus is of clinical importance because it has connections with the **cavernous sinus** within the cranial cavity (Fig. 11–13). Because of these connections, it is possible that an infection of dental origin can spread into the cranial cavity. The plexus also has connections with

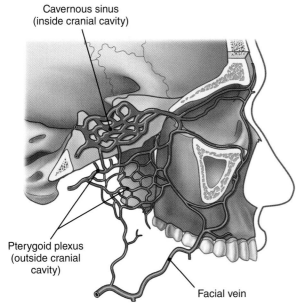

Cavernous sinus
(inside cranial cavity)

Pterygoid plexus
(outside cranial
cavity)

Facial vein

Figure 11–13 The pterygoid plexus is located in the infratemporal fossa and drains the same regions as the maxillary artery. Its location makes it vulnerable to damages by needle puncture during intraoral injections for local anesthesia of mandibular and maxillary teeth. The cavernous sinus, which has connections to the pterygoid plexus, is a venous structure in the middle cranial fossa, which surrounds the pituitary gland. Infections can pass from the pterygoid plexus to the cavernous sinus. The facial artery is valveless and has connections to both the pterygoid plexus and the cavernous sinus. Thus, infections from the face can also spread into the cavernous sinus and pterygoid plexus.

the *facial vein* that could allow an infection on the surface of the face to reach the pterygoid plexus and spread to more internal structures (Fig. 11–13). Secondly, the pterygoid plexus is subject to trauma during oral nerve blocks of the posterior superior alveolar and inferior alveolar nerves. Trauma to the plexus, such as a blow to the face or an aberrant needle during intraoral injections,

can cause a hematoma, which is visible as a large purple (unoxygenated blood) swelling on the cheek wall.

Review Question Box 11-7

1. Why are the veins of the deep face called the *pterygoid plexus*?
2. Why are connections of the pterygoid plexus to the cavernous sinus and the veins of the face important?
3. The pterygoid plexus is a tributary of what vein?

Clinical Correlation Box 11-1

Danger Zone of the Face
The *danger zone of the face* is a triangle-shaped area in which the drainage of blood can flow from the superficial face into the cavernous sinus or the pterygoid plexus. The apex of the triangle begins at a point in the median plane between the eyebrows, and its sides pass laterally along the ala of the nose to the corners of the mouth. The base of the triangle is the inferior border of the upper lip. The facial vein originates near the medial angle of the eye and courses inferolaterally along the face to the submandibular triangle. Along its path, it receives tributaries from the nose and lips. In addition, the facial vein connects with the ophthalmic veins in the orbit, which drain into the cavernous sinus, then joins the deep facial vein, which empties into the pterygoid plexus. In the upright position, gravity causes the blood in the facial vein to flow toward the heart. However, the facial vein is valveless. Thus, while lying down, or if there is a blood clot (thrombosis) in the facial vein, blood can flow in a retrograde direction into either the cavernous sinus or pterygoid plexuses. If an infection should reach the cavernous sinus, the consequences can be severe.

Clinical Correlation Box 11-2

Bacteremia and Sepsis
The peripheral blood is considered a sterile environment free of bacteria. On occasions, bacteria can enter the bloodstream through damaged blood vessels that can occur with infections such as pneumonia or infections of the urinary tract, surgical procedures, and dental procedures. **Bacteremia** is the presence of bacteria in the blood. The presence of bacteria is generally transient, because the body's immune system will remove the bacteria. However, it is possible for bacteria to become localized in certain organs such as the kidney and cause damage. Bacteria also have a tendency to collect around artificially placed devices, such as joint replacements, catheters, and heart valves and can

be released into the bloodstream. Patients recovering from surgery or joint replacement, or who have a depressed immune system may be given antibiotics as a precaution before a dental procedure, including routine dental hygiene procedures. If the blood is overwhelmed by bacterial growth, the bacteria can spread systemically leading to a life-threatening condition known as **sepsis**. Sepsis occurs with a systemic inflammatory response triggered by the release of chemicals by the immune system to fight an infection. Sepsis is characterized by a drop in blood pressure, which results in shock, and function of major organs such as the kidney, lungs, and central nervous system are suppressed.

SUMMARY

The circulatory system is comprised of the cardiovascular and lymphatic systems. The cardiovascular system is composed of the heart and blood vessels that distribute blood to—and collect blood from—the tissues of the body. The lymphatic system is comprised of vessels that collect fluids and proteins that escape the blood vessels. The lymphatic system returns the fluid in the form of lymph back to the general circulation. The heart is a pump comprised of four chambers, two atria, and two ventricles. For the pulmonary circulation, the atrium on the right side collects deoxygenated blood from the body and transfers the blood during diastole to the right ventricle. During systole, the right ventricle pumps the blood through the pulmonary trunk and arteries to reach the lungs to exchange carbon dioxide for oxygen. Oxygenated blood is returned to the left atrium heart via the pulmonary veins and is transferred into the left ventricle. For the systemic circulation, the left ventricle pumps the blood into the aorta and its primary branches to be distributed to the body. Blood is collected by veins that drain into the superior vena cava that empties into the right atrium. The direction of blood flow through and from the heart are regulated by valves separating the atria and ventricles and valves that separate the right ventricle from the pulmonary trunk and the left ventricle from the aorta.

The first branches of the ascending aorta are the coronary arteries, which supply blood to the heart. The aorta then arches from the right to left and is called the aortic arch. Three branches arise from the arch, in order, the brachiocephalic trunk, the left common carotid artery, and the left subclavian artery. The right subclavian and common carotid arteries are branches of the brachiocephalic trunk. Two important branches of the subclavian artery are the vertebral artery, which supplies blood to the brain, and the inferior thyroid artery, which supplies a portion of the thyroid gland. The common carotid artery divides into the internal carotid artery and the external carotid artery. The internal carotid artery supplies blood to the brain, whereas branches of the external carotid artery in the neck supply blood to the pharynx, larynx, thyroid gland, face, and tongue. Its maxillary branch supplies blood to the muscles of the temporal and infratemporal fossae, the dura mater, the mandibular and maxillary teeth, the orbit, the hard and soft palates, and the nasal cavity.

Regional veins coalesce to form larger veins that eventually drain into the superior vena cava and inferior vena cava, which return blood to the right atrium. In the head and neck, the retromandibular vein collects venous blood from the superficial temporal vein and the maxillary vein. The retromandibular vein divides into an anterior division and a posterior division. The posterior division contributes to the formation of the external jugular vein, which empties into the subclavian vein. The anterior division joins the facial vein to form the common facial vein, which empties into the internal jugular vein. The internal jugular vein and subclavian vein merge to form the brachiocephalic vein. The left and right brachiocephalic veins form the superior vena cava.

The pterygoid plexus of veins collects blood from the same areas supplied by the maxillary artery; the pterygoid plexus is connected to the superficial veins of the face and to the cavernous sinus within the skull. The vessels can be mechanisms of spreading infection from the superficial and deep face to interior structures of the skull.

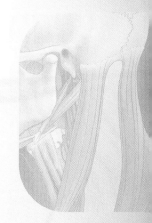

LEARNING LAB
Exercises for review, practice, and study

Laboratory Activity 11-1

Tracing Blood to and From Structures of the Head

By tracing a drop of blood from the heart to structures of the head and its return to the heart, you will understand not only the pathways of the arterial and venous flow, but also the name of the blood vessels. Use the following pathway for the pulmonary circulation, starting with the right atrium as a guide for this exercise.

Right atrium → right ventricle → pulmonary trunk → right and left pulmonary arteries → lungs → right and left pulmonary veins → left atrium → left ventricle

Beginning at the arch of the aorta, trace a drop of blood to the muscles of mastication, to the muscles of facial expression, and to the mandibular and maxillary incisors on the right side of the body.

Determining Arterial Pathways

Step 1: Using Figures 11–3 and 11–5 as a guide, first consider what the common pathway to all these structures from the heart is. Does your common pathway include the following sequence?

Aortic arch → brachiocephalic trunk → right common carotid artery → right external carotid artery

Step 2: Realize at this point that the blood diverges to reach its target organ.

Step 3: Use Figure 11–6 to follow the distributing arteries of the external carotid artery to the areas they supply.

Muscles of mastication. For the muscles of mastication, the sequence continues with the right maxillary artery → individual branches to each muscle.

Muscles of facial expression. Blood reaches the muscles of facial expression via the right facial artery.

Mandibular incisors. Blood reaches the incisors through the right maxillary artery → right inferior alveolar artery → right incisive artery. How would the blood flow to the right maxillary incisors be different?

Step 4: Recall that the maxillary teeth are supplied by three different arterial branches: the posterior superior alveolar, middle superior alveolar, and anterior superior alveolar arteries. For the right maxillary incisors, blood passes into the right maxillary artery → right infraorbital artery → right anterior superior alveolar artery → dental branches.

How would the pathway change if the structures were on the left side? If you said that blood would flow from the aortic arch into the left common carotid artery, then into the left external carotid artery, you are correct. Check your answers with the pathways in the following illustration.

Answer Key to The Arterial Pathways

Arterial Supply to the Muscles of Mastication

Aortic arch → brachiocephalic trunk → right common carotid artery → right external carotid artery → right maxillary artery → branches to each muscle

Arterial Supply to the Muscles of Facial Expression

Aortic arch → brachiocephalic trunk → right common carotid artery → right external carotid artery → right facial artery → branches to each muscle

Arterial Supply to the Mandibular Incisors

Aortic arch → brachiocephalic trunk → right common carotid artery → right external carotid artery → right maxillary artery → right inferior alveolar artery → right incisive artery → dental branches

Arterial Supply to the Maxillary Incisors

Aortic arch → brachiocephalic trunk → right common carotid artery → right external carotid artery → right maxillary artery → right infraorbital artery → right anterior superior alveolar artery → dental branches

179

Determining The Venous Return

The venous return is a little more complex. The veins that drain the peripheral structures have the same names as the artery; however, these vessels converge to form the pterygoid plexus.

Step 1:   Using Figure 11–12, look for similarities in the drainage pattern.

Mandibular incisors.   For the mandibular incisors, blood passes through the right incisive vein → right inferior alveolar vein → right pterygoid plexus → right maxillary vein → right retromandibular vein.

Maxillary incisors.   For the maxillary incisors, blood passes through the right anterior superior alveolar vein → right infraorbital vein → right pterygoid plexus → right maxillary vein → right retromandibular vein.

Muscles of mastication.   The veins of the muscles of mastication on the right also drain into the right pterygoid plexus → right maxillary vein → right retromandibular vein.

   The retromandibular vein divides into an anterior and a posterior division, which means there are two alternate pathways to the heart.

Step 2:   Use Figure 11–12 to determine the two pathways. The posterior division empties into the right external jugular, and the sequence continues as the right subclavian vein → right brachio-cephalic vein → right superior vena cava → right atrium. For the anterior division, the sequence continues as the right common facial vein → internal jugular vein → right brachiocephalic vein → right superior vena cava → right atrium.

Step 3:   The blood from the facial muscles do not empty into the retromandibular vein, but into the facial vein. How does this change the direction of the blood flow?

   Right facial vein → right common facial vein → internal jugular vein → right brachiocephalic vein → right superior vena cava → right atrium.

   How would the pathways change if the structures were on the left side? If you said that blood flow would be the same, except for being on the left side, you are correct. Check your answers with the pathways in the answer key below.

Answer Key for The Venous Return

Right Mandibular Incisors

Dental branches → incisive vein → inferior alveolar vein → pterygoid plexus → maxillary vein → retromandibular vein → alternate pathways through anterior or posterior divisions of the retromandibular vein

(1) Anterior division → common facial vein → internal jugular vein → brachiocephalic vein → superior vena cava → right atrium

(2) Posterior division → external jugular vein → subclavian vein → brachiocephalic vein → superior vena cava → right atrium

Venous Return From the Right Maxillary Incisors

Dental branches → anterior superior alveolar vein → infraorbital vein → pterygoid plexus → maxillary vein → retromandibular vein → alternate pathways through the anterior or posterior divisions of the retromandibular vein in the previous answer

Venous Return for the Muscles of Mastication

Muscular branches → pterygoid plexus → maxillary vein → retromandibular vein → alternate pathways through the anterior or posterior divisions of the retromandibular vein as described earlier

Venous Return for the Muscles of Facial Expression

Muscular branches → facial vein → common facial vein → internal jugular vein → brachiocephalic vein → superior vena cava → right atrium

Learning Activity 11-1

Heart—Anterior View

Match the numbered structures with the correct terms listed below.

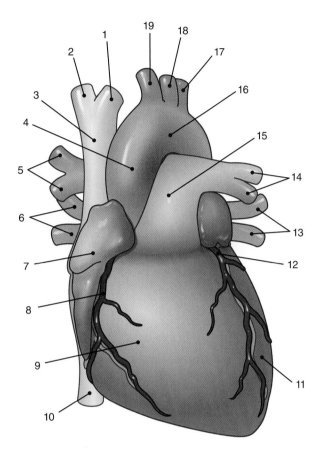

_____ Aortic arch

_____ Ascending aorta

_____ Brachiocephalic trunk

_____ Inferior vena cava

_____ Left brachiocephalic vein

_____ Left common carotid arteries

_____ Left coronary artery

_____ Left pulmonary artery

_____ Left pulmonary veins

_____ Left subclavian artery

_____ Left ventricle

_____ Pulmonary trunk

_____ Right atrium

_____ Right brachiocephalic vein

_____ Right coronary artery

_____ Right pulmonary arteries

_____ Right pulmonary veins

_____ Right ventricle

_____ Superior vena cava

Learning Activity 11-2

Major Branches of the Carotid Artery

Match the numbered structures with the correct terms listed below.

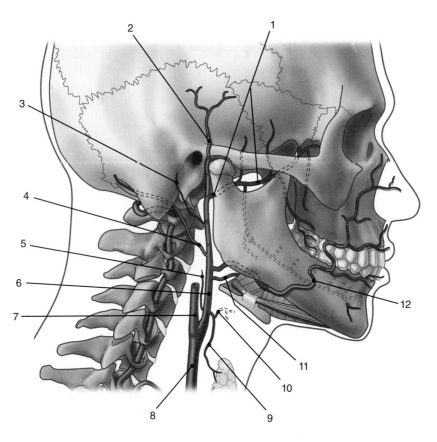

_____ Ascending pharyngeal artery

_____ Common carotid artery

_____ External carotid artery

_____ Facial artery

_____ Internal carotid artery

_____ Lingual artery

_____ Maxillary artery

_____ Occipital artery

_____ Posterior auricular artery

_____ Superior laryngeal artery

_____ Superficial temporal artery

_____ Superior thyroid artery

Learning Activity 11-3

Carotid Arteries in the Carotid Triangle

Match the numbered structures with the correct terms listed below.

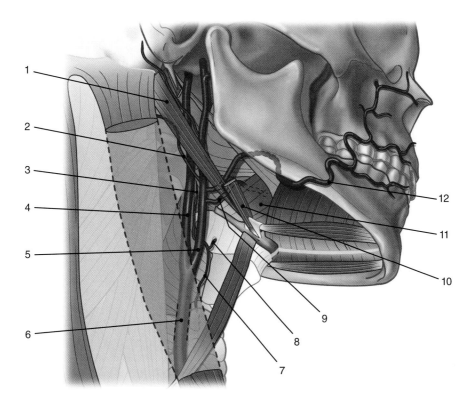

_____ Ascending pharyngeal artery

_____ Common carotid artery

_____ External carotid artery

_____ Facial artery

_____ Hyoglossus muscle

_____ Internal carotid artery

_____ Lingual artery

_____ Occipital artery

_____ Posterior belly of the digastric muscle

_____ Stylohyoid muscle

_____ Superior laryngeal artery

_____ Superior thyroid artery

Learning Activity 11-4

Maxillary Artery—Lateral View

Match the numbered structures with the correct terms listed below.

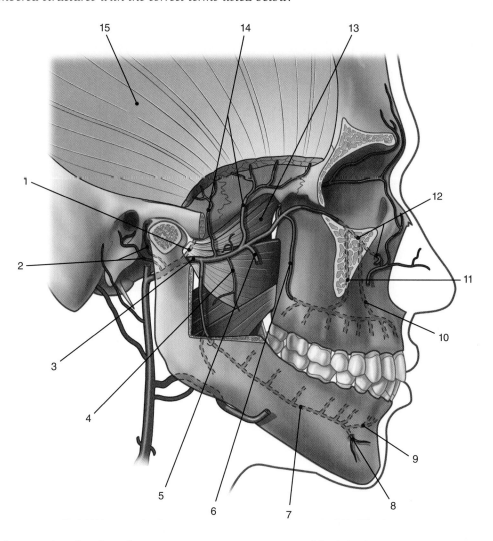

_____ Anterior superior alveolar artery

_____ Buccal artery

_____ Deep temporal arteries

_____ Incisive artery

_____ Inferior alveolar artery

_____ Infraorbital artery

_____ Lateral pterygoid muscle

_____ Maxillary artery

_____ Mental artery

_____ Middle meningeal artery

_____ Middle superior alveolar artery

_____ Posterior superior alveolar artery

_____ Pterygoid branches

_____ Temporalis muscle

_____ Tympanic branches

Learning Activity 11-5

Veins of the Neck

Match the numbered structures with the correct terms listed below.

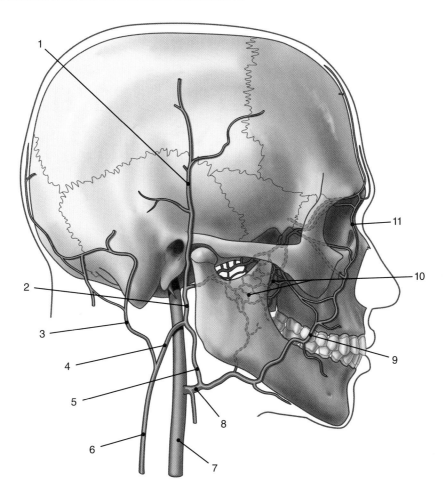

_____ Angular vein

_____ Anterior division of the retromandibular vein

_____ Common facial vein

_____ External jugular vein

_____ Facial vein

_____ Internal jugular vein

_____ Posterior auricular vein

_____ Posterior division of the retromandibular vein

_____ Pterygoid plexus

_____ Retromandibular vein

_____ Superficial temporal vein

chapter 12

Lymphatic Drainage of the Head and Neck

Objectives

1. Discuss the functions of the lymphatic system.
2. Discuss the function of lymph nodes and the clinical significance of the lymph nodes.
3. Identify the location of the major lymph nodes that drain the face and neck and discuss their areas of drainage.

Overview

As mentioned in the previous chapter, fluids and proteins lost at the capillary beds are returned to the circulation as lymph. The lymph is carried in vessels similar to veins that are connected to a series of lymph nodes, comparable to beads on a string. The lymph nodes filter the lymph before it is returned into the venous system. Lymph nodes also produce antibodies to some foreign substances. In areas that are inflamed from bacterial infection or cancer, bacteria and cancer-containing cells can enter the lymphatic system and spread to other parts of the body. Both dentists and dental hygienists have learned the importance of examining patients' lymph nodes for the spread of infection as well as the presence or spread of oral cancers in the head and neck.

INTRODUCTION TO THE LYMPHATIC DRAINAGE OF THE HEAD AND NECK

The **lymphatic system** is a subdivision of the circulatory system that is composed of the lymphatic vessels and organs, which include the lymph nodes, spleen, thymus, and tonsils. Unlike the cardiovascular system, which carries blood to and from the heart, the lymphatic system is unidirectional. The lymphatic system returns to the venous system extracellular fluid and proteins that are lost during circulation. This proteinaceous fluid, which is called **lymph**, is clear to white in color. Lymph is collected by capillaries similar in structure to blood capillaries. The capillaries join to form larger vessels, **lymphatic vessels**, which resemble veins. The lymph is filtered of debris by the lymph nodes that are situated at various points along the vessels before returning to the general circulation.

The lymph organs form and circulate cells called **lymphocytes**, which are needed as part of the body's defense system against invading foreign substances (**antigens**). The system also forms and circulates **antibodies**, which help neutralize specific types of antigens.

LYMPH NODES

The **lymph nodes** filter lymph and are the organs that form both lymphocytes and antibodies. The lymph nodes are organized in chains of tiny kidney bean–shaped structures linked by lymphatic vessels (Fig. 12–1). These chains follow the general drainage pattern of the venous system. Lymph is first collected by **lymphatic capillaries**, which are similar to—but not the same as—the capillaries of the cardiovascular system (Fig. 12–2).

Several capillaries merge to form *lymphatic vessels* (Fig. 12–2). Like veins, the walls of the vessels are thin and contain valves to prevent the retrograde flow of lymph. Lymph enters the lymph nodes via afferent lymphatic vessels, which are located along their convex surface, and the fluid percolates through the organ (Fig. 12–3). As the lymph passes through the organ, debris is removed from the fluid. The cleansed lymph exits through efferent lymphatic vessels located at the hilum (Fig. 12–3) of the node (concave surface). The efferent lymphatic vessels then continue to the next lymph node. Along their pathway, the vessels drain

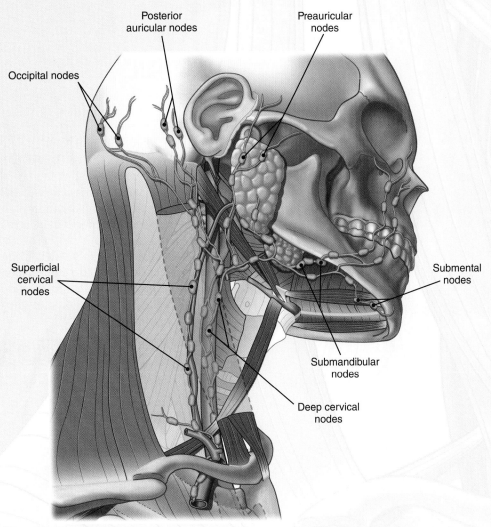

Figure 12–1 Lymph nodes are organized in chains of kidney bean–shaped structures connected by lymphatic vessels. The superficial lymph nodes drain into the superficial cervical lymph nodes, whereas the deeper lymph nodes empty in the deep cervical lymph nodes. All lymph from the head and neck lymph nodes eventually empties into the deep cervical lymph nodes. The fluid then returns to the general circulation through the venous system.

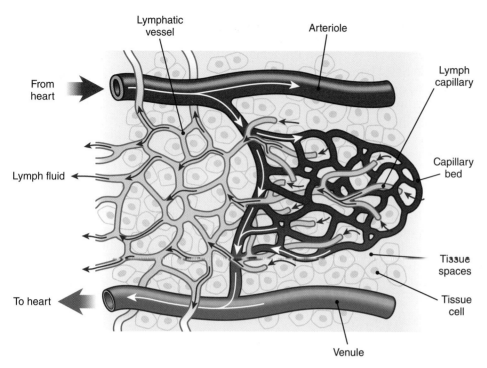

Figure 12–2 Blood enters the capillaries via the arterioles and is returned to the heart by venules, which form larger veins. Proteinaceous fluid that escapes general circulation is collected as lymph via lymph capillaries that are intertwined with the capillaries of the cardiovascular system. The lymphatic capillaries join to form lymphatic vessels.

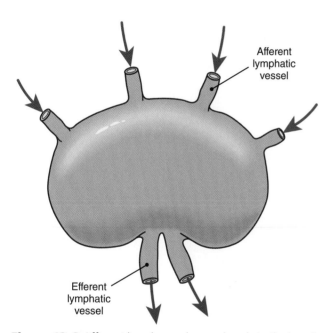

Figure 12–3 Afferent lymph vessels carry lymph to the lymph nodes. The fluid percolates through the nodes and is filtered of the debris. The filtered lymph leaves the nodes at the hilum via the efferent lymph vessels, which course to the next lymph node in the chain.

nodes are protective in function, infection and cancer can easily spread from one portion of the body to another through the lymphatic channels.

Palpation of lymph nodes in the neck, under the mandible, and around the ear is a very important component of a proper oral examination by a dental clinician. Enlargement of lymph nodes can be a clinical indicator of disease. Usually, enlarged lymph nodes that are soft and painful indicate an infection, whereas nodes that are hard and painless indicate cancer. Knowing the flow of the lymphatic drainage can help determine the site of infection. As an example, the enlargement of the nodes under the chin can indicate an infection in the medial portion of the lower lip or the tip of the tongue.

Review Question Box 12-1

1. What is the difference between an antigen and an antibody?
2. How are lymph capillaries different from blood capillaries?
3. What are the functions of lymph nodes?
4. What is the difference between afferent and efferent lymphatic vessels?
5. What does enlargement of lymph nodes indicate?

lymphatic capillaries from the surrounding tissues. The vessel (now an afferent lymphatic vessel) enters into the next lymph node, and the debris is removed. This cleansing process from one lymph node to another continues until the efferent vessels form larger **lymphatic trunks** that empty into the venous system. Although the lymph

NODES OF THE HEAD AND NECK

The lymph nodes are named according to the region of drainage. The following paragraphs describe some regional nodes of clinical interest to the dental hygienist.

The **preauricular nodes** are located superficial to the parotid gland and anterior to the ear. These nodes drain the forehead, the lateral scalp, the lateral portion of the eyelids, and the anterior aspect of the ear. The **posterior auricular nodes** are located behind the ear, and the **occipital lymph nodes** are situated at the back of the head (Fig. 12–1). This group of regional lymph nodes empty into the **superficial cervical lymph nodes**, which follow the course of the external jugular vein (Fig. 12–4).

The **submental lymph nodes** are located in the submental triangle underneath the chin. These nodes drain the tip of the tongue, the central region of the floor of the mouth, the central incisors, and the medial portion of the lower lip. These nodes drain into the **submandibular lymph nodes**, which are located within the submandibular triangle deep to the submandibular gland (Fig. 12–1). Superficially, the submandibular nodes drain the medial portion of the eyelids, the nose, the cheek, the upper lip, and lateral portions of the lower lip. They also drain the gingiva and all maxillary teeth, the gingiva and mandibular teeth that are not drained by the submental lymph nodes (canines, premolars, and molars), as well as the lateral surface of the tongue. The submandibular nodes empty directly into the **deep cervical lymph nodes**.

These deep nodes follow the course of the **internal jugular vein**.

As a general rule, the superficial nodes drain into the *superficial cervical lymph nodes*. The superficial cervical lymph nodes can be palpated on the surface of the sternocleidomastoid muscle. The deeper lymph nodes, as well as the superficial cervical lymph nodes, drain into the deep cervical lymph nodes that are located along the internal jugular vein. The *deep cervical lymph nodes* are considered to be the final common pathway of lymph drainage for much of the head and neck before joining the larger lymphatic trunks that empty directly into the venous system.

Review Question Box 12-2

1. Which lymph nodes drain into the superficial cervical lymph nodes and which drain into the deep cervical lymph nodes?
2. On what blood vessel are the superficial cervical lymph nodes located?
3. On what blood vessel are the deep cervical lymph nodes located?

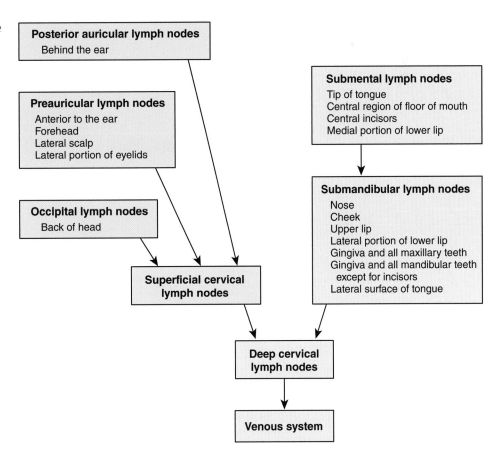

Figure 12–4 Lymphatic drainage in the head and neck.

Box 12-1 Supraclavicular Lymph Nodes

Even though the supraclavicular lymph nodes do not drain lymph from the head and neck regions, the dental hygienist who performs head and neck exams for lymph nodes must be aware of their presence. The nodes are located in the supraclavicular triangle located laterally to where the clavicle joins the sternum (sternoclavicular joint). The right supraclavicular lymph node drains the area that contains the heart (mediastinum), the lungs, and the esophagus. The node on the left side filters lymph from the thorax and abdomen.

SUMMARY

Lymph nodes are the organs of the lymphatic system that filter lymph, form lymphocytes, and synthesize antibodies. Lymph is composed of fluids and proteins that are lost from the systemic circulation at the capillary beds. The fluids and proteins are collected by lymphatic capillaries that join together to form larger lymphatic vessels. Afferent lymphatic vessels direct lymph toward the lymph node, where the fluid is normally cleansed of debris, and leave the nodes through efferent lymphatic vessels. These vessels will collect lymph from other capillaries and carry the lymph to another lymph node, where the cleansing process is continued. Bacteria, viruses, and cancer cells that are not removed by a lymph node can spread to other lymph nodes and eventually into the cardiovascular system where they can spread to other parts of the body. Palpating lymph nodes in the head and neck can indicate regional infection or cancer and help determine the spread of the disease.

LEARNING LAB

Exercises for review, practice, and study

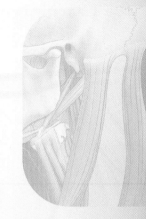

Laboratory Activity 12-1

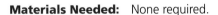

Examination of the Lymph Nodes of the Head and Neck

Objective: In this exercise, you will use yourself as a model to examine the lymph nodes of interest to the dental hygienist by palpation with your index and middle fingers. Normal lymph nodes are generally impalpable; however, it is not unusual to encounter very small, soft, pliable nodes. Infected nodes tend to be enlarged, soft, and painful to the touch. Cancerous nodes generally are enlarged, hard, and painless. Also, cancerous nodes tend to stick to underlying structures and are rigid.

Materials Needed: None required.

Step 1: Start your examination by attempting to palpate the *occipital lymph nodes* located along the superior nuchal line on the posterior surface of the skull. Use the fingers of both hands and lightly touch the area in a circular motion. Compare the left side from the right side and note any difference.

Step 2: Continue the examination by palpating the *posterior auricular lymph nodes* superficial to the mastoid process posterior to the ear.

Step 3: Continue anteriorly by moving your fingers onto the surface of the parotid gland and palpate the *preauricular lymph nodes*.

Step 4: Next, examine underneath the inferior border of the mandible in the *submandibular triangle* for *submandibular lymph nodes* and continue along the border in the *submental triangle* for the *submental lymph nodes*.

Step 5: Now turn your attention to the cervical lymph nodes.

- The *superficial cervical lymph nodes* can be palpated as they cross superficial to the *sternocleidomastoid muscle* following the path of the external jugular vein.
- The *deep cervical lymph nodes* course along the internal jugular vein deep to the sternocleidomastoid muscle. To palpate these nodes, turn your head and relax your sternocleidomastoid muscle on the side to be examined. Curl your fingers and gently (this could cause some discomfort) palpate under the anterior border of the sternocleidomastoid muscle.

Step 6: Lastly, palpate in the hollow area above the clavicle just lateral to the attachment of the clavicle and the sternum for the *supraclavicular lymph nodes*. Swelling in these nodes can indicate inflammation or cancer from the abdomen and thorax.

For Discussion or Thought:

1. *What conclusions can be made if you are unable to palpate lymph nodes during an examination for lymph nodes?*

Learning Activity 12-1

Lymphatic Drainage of the Head and Neck

Match the numbered structures with the correct terms listed to the right.

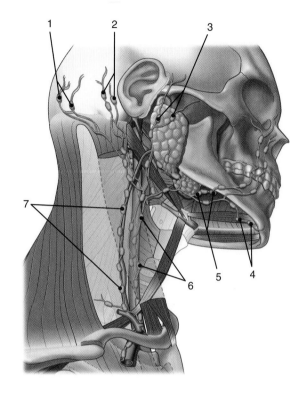

_____ Deep cervical lymph nodes

_____ Occipital lymph nodes

_____ Posterior auricular nodes

_____ Preauricular nodes

_____ Submandibular lymph nodes

_____ Submental lymph nodes

_____ Superficial cervical lymph nodes

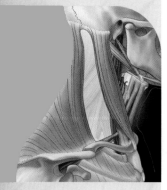

chapter

13

Brain and Spinal Cord

Objectives

1. Discuss the subdivision of the nervous system according to its structure and function.
2. Identify the meningeal coverings of the brain; explain how they contribute to the structure and function of the dural sinuses.
3. Identify the lobes, major gyri, sulci, and fissures of the cerebrum and describe their general functions.
4. Identify the vessels and describe the arterial supply to the brain.
5. Discuss the formation and flow of cerebral spinal fluid from the ventricular system to its drainage into the dural sinuses.
6. Identify the external surface features of the spinal cord.

Overview

Expressions such as "he has all the brains in the family" or "she is the brain of the class" equate the brain to the degree of intelligence. This is partially correct. In addition, our personality, our emotions, and our ability to plan and problem solve are also attributes of the brain. Our brain controls our movements, our ability to speak, and all bodily functions that sustain life via connections with the brain stem and the spinal cord. Our brain allows us to distinguish general sensations, such as pain and temperature, and the special sensations that allow us to see, smell, taste, hear, and maintain equilibrium. Injury to the brain by physical trauma, stroke, or illness can permanently impair bodily functions depending on the scope of the damage. No one can dispute the importance of the brain and the spinal cord, but what is the clinical significance of these organs to the dental hygienist? A stroke (lack of blood flow to a part of the brain) can cause paralysis in the muscles of facial expression, atrophy to muscles of the tongue, a decrease in salivary flow, and difficulty opening and closing the mouth. Dental hygienists will also encounter patients with various physical disabilities because of neurological

194

injuries that do not necessarily affect the mouth, but will affect patients' ability to get in and out of the dental chair and their comfort during the dental examination. Stroke victims usually have difficulty speaking or understanding what you are saying. The dental hygienist's knowledge of the structure and function of the brain and spinal cord will help in understanding their patients' medical conditions.

INTRODUCTION TO THE BRAIN AND SPINAL CORD

The nervous system is composed of two major subdivisions: the **central nervous system (CNS)** and the **peripheral nervous system (PNS)**. The CNS is composed of the **brain** and **spinal cord**, whereas the PNS is composed of the **cranial** and **spinal nerves**, which innervate the peripheral structures of the body such as muscles, glands, and sensory receptors. The fibers of the sensory neurons of the PNS convey stimuli from the environment to the spinal cord, which is then relayed to the brain for processing. Sensory neurons in the brain distinguish the general sensations of pain, temperature, touch, pressure, proprioception (movement), and tickle, as well as the special senses of hearing, taste, smell, equilibrium, and vision. Motor neurons located in the cerebrum, which are called *upper motor neurons*, regulate motor activities by stimulating **lower motor neurons** of the cranial nerves and the ventral horn of the spinal cord. Other neurons function in perceptive activities such as emotion, personality, memory, judgment, critical thinking, and reasoning, whereas others form centers for the control of respiration, heart rate, speech, endocrine secretion, and other autonomic functions. In this chapter, the basic gross structure and function of the brain and spinal cord are presented, whereas Chapter 14 will discuss the motor and sensory pathways between the brain and spinal cord.

THE MENINGES

The brain is covered by a three-layer protective cover called the **meninges** (singular: **meninx**). The outermost meninx is the **dura mater** (meaning "hard mother"), which is tough and fibrous (Figs. 13–1A and B). The middle meningeal layer is the **arachnoid mater**, which is more delicate than the dura (Fig. 13–1B). The innermost meninx, the **pia mater**, cannot be separated from the brain (Fig. 13–1B). Between the arachnoid and pia is the **subarachnoid space**. The subarachnoid space contains threadlike fibers (spiderweb) and **cerebral spinal fluid**, which acts as a shock absorber protecting the brain from trauma.

1. How does the pia mater differ from the arachnoid mater?
2. What is located in the subarachnoid space?

Clinical Correlation Box 13-1

Meningitis

Meningitis is an inflammation of the meninges that can be caused by bacteria and viruses. Bacterial meningitis is extremely serious. An individual with meningitis generally exhibits progressively severe headaches, fever, sensitivity to light, and a stiff neck. If not properly treated, the inflammation can result in death.

THE BRAIN

The brain is formed by the paired cerebral hemispheres or cerebrum, the diencephalon, the brain stem, and the cerebellum.

Cerebrum

The **cerebrum** is the largest component of the brain. Its surface is characterized by a series of convoluted ridges of neural tissue that are separated by grooves. Each ridge is called a **gyrus**, and the groove in between is a **sulcus**. The cerebrum is divided into lobes by deeper grooves called **fissures**. The cerebrum is divided into two **cerebral hemispheres** by the **longitudinal fissure** located in the midline on the superior surface of the brain and are separated by a fold of dura called the **falx cerebri**. (See the section on dural sinuses in this chapter.)

Each cerebral hemisphere is divided into four lobes that are visible from the surface. The names of the lobes correspond to the bone that covers them. The more anterior **frontal lobe** is separated from the **parietal lobe** by the transversely oriented **central sulcus** (Fig. 13–2). The parietal lobe is separated from the **temporal lobe** by the **lateral fissure** (Fig. 13–2) and is separated from the

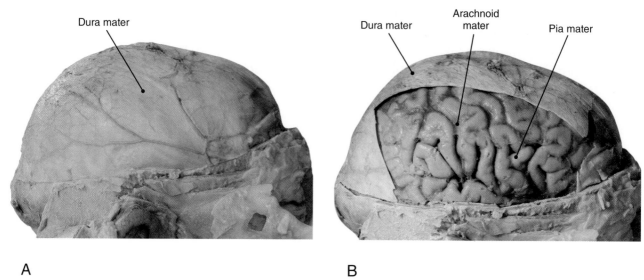

A

B

Figure 13–1 (A) The dura mater is the tough meningeal cover that attaches to the skull. **(B)** Reflection of the dura reveals the delicate arachnoid mater. A portion of the arachnoid has been removed to access the subarachnoid space, which is filled with cerebral spinal fluid. The pia mater is an inseparable layer attached directly to the brain.

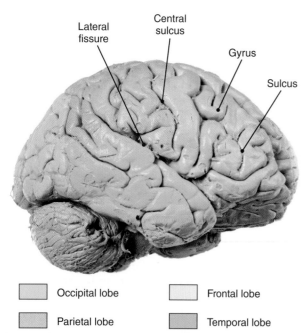

Occipital lobe   Frontal lobe

Parietal lobe   Temporal lobe

Figure 13–2 The surface of the cerebrum is characterized by convolutions of brain tissue, called the *gyri* (singular: *gyrus*), which are separated by grooves called *sulci* (singular: *sulcus*). The frontal, parietal, and temporal lobes are separated by the central sulcus and the lateral fissure. The occipital lobe is separated from the parietal lobe on the external surface by an imaginary dashed line corresponding to the parieto-occipital fissure on the medial surface.

occipital lobe by the **parieto-occipital fissure**, which is best seen in sagittal sections of the brain (Fig. 13–3). The cerebral hemispheres are joined by a large bundle of crossing fibers called the **corpus callosum**, which allows communication between the two hemispheres (Fig. 13–3).

The cerebral hemispheres surround the two **lateral ventricles**, which contain cerebral spinal fluid. The ventricles are separated by a membrane of tissue known as the **septum pellucidum** (Fig. 13–3).

The cerebrum plans and executes motor movements and processes all sensory information to a conscious level. Our personalities, emotions, and ability to problem solve and think are all functions of the cerebrum. The neurons responsible for these functions are located in the gyri of the various lobes of the cerebral hemispheres. Although the functions of the brain are complex, there are some well-defined areas associated with loss of function because of strokes or disease.

Review Question Box 13-2

1. What separates the frontal lobe and the parietal lobe?
2. What separates the parietal lobe from the temporal lobe?
3. What separates the occipital lobe from the parietal lobe?
4. What is the function of the corpus callosum?

Frontal Lobe

The *frontal lobe* contains four gyri: the precentral gyrus, superior frontal gyrus, middle frontal gyrus, and inferior frontal gyrus.

The **precentral gyrus** is the **primary motor area** that controls all the major body movements (Fig. 13–4). In addition, the **frontal eye fields** control eye movements, whereas **Broca's area** or the **motor speech area**, controls speech. The motor speech area is located in the dominant hemisphere (left hemisphere for right-handed individuals) on the lower part of the inferior frontal gyrus just above

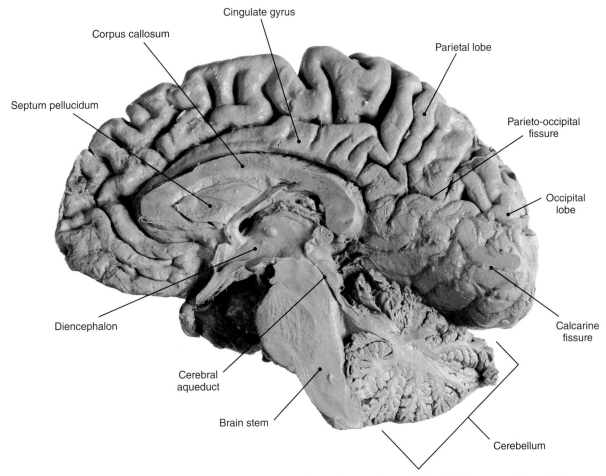

Cingulate gyrus

Corpus callosum

Parietal lobe

Septum pellucidum

Parieto-occipital
fissure

Occipital
lobe

Diencephalon

Calcarine
fissure

Cerebral
aqueduct

Brain stem

Cerebellum

Figure 13–3 A section through the median plane shows the cerebrum, diencephalon, brain stem, and cerebellum. The cerebrum surrounds the two lateral ventricles, which are separated by the membranous septum pellucidum. The parieto-occipital fissure separates the occipital and parietal lobes. The primary visual gyri (orange areas) are separated by the calcarine fissure. The cingulate gyrus, which forms the limbic lobe, lies on the surface of the corpus callosum, which connects the two cerebral hemispheres.

the lateral fissure (Fig. 13–4). This area controls the production of speech and is susceptible to damage by strokes. Patients with deficits in this area know what they want to say, but have difficulty saying the words. Other regions of the frontal lobe are association areas that are involved in memory, reasoning, judgment, intelligence, critical thinking, emotions, and personality.

Parietal Lobe

The **primary sensory area** is located within the **postcentral gyrus** of the *parietal lobe* (Fig. 13–4). This area is concerned with general sensations from the body such as pain, temperature, touch, and proprioception. As in the precentral gyrus, there is regional representation in the neurons receiving sensory information.

Occipital Lobe

The primary function of the *occipital lobe* is to process visual information. The gyri that surround the **calcarine fissure** collectively form the **primary visual cortex**,

Box 13-1 Mapping of Cortex

The regions of the body are specifically mapped to the localization of the neurons in the cortex (outer region of an organ). For example, the legs and feet are located on the medial surface of the precentral gyrus facing the longitudinal fissure, whereas the face and hands are on the lateral surface. In addition, the number of neurons dedicated to regions of the body is variable. The hands, face, lips, and mouth are supplied by more neurons than the trunk, which essentially means that we have greater motor control of our hands, face, and head than our trunk.

which is best seen in sections through the median plane (Fig. 13–3). Basic shapes and colors are perceived in the primary visual cortex, but are interpreted as specific objects—that is, something round is a ball, the sun, or the moon in regions known as association areas.

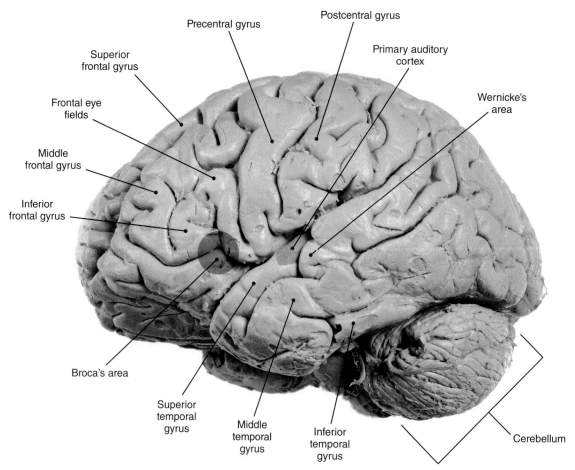

Figure 13–4 The lateral view of the left cerebral hemisphere shows that the frontal lobe is divided into the superior, middle, and inferior gyri, and the precentral gyrus. The precentral gyrus is the primary motor area. Additional specialized motor centers include Broca's area and the frontal eye fields. The postcentral gyrus is a feature of the parietal lobe and is the main sensory area. The temporal lobe is formed by the superior, middle, and inferior temporal gyri and functions in hearing. Wernicke's area of the middle temporal gyrus is associated with language.

Clinical Correlation Box 13-2

Broca Aphasia

Individuals with **Broca's aphasia** have difficulty speaking fluently, but can comprehend what is being said to them. These individuals have difficulty turning a thought into a sequence of meaningful words. They speak slowly and have difficulty forming words. Their speech pattern is described as *telegraphic*, in that they leave out nonessential words as when sending a telegraph message or shorthand for taking notes. Individuals often become frustrated with the inability to say what they are thinking.

Temporal Lobe

The *temporal lobe* is composed of the superior, middle, and inferior temporal gyri. Its main function is to process auditory information. One area susceptible to stroke, **Wernicke's area** (Fig. 13–4), is associated with language

and comprehension. Patients affected by a stroke in this area can form the words, but have difficulty in recalling the words they would like to say. The inferior temporal gyrus has been linked to higher levels of visual processing, such as object recognition and recognition of faces.

Clinical Correlation Box 13-3

Wernicke's Aphasia

Individuals with **Wernicke's aphasia** have problems understanding language, as opposed to speaking. Depending on the severity of the aphasia, patients may have difficulty understanding what is being said and may have difficulty reading and writing. Even though they can speak fluently, they use nonsense words and sentences. As an example, "we went to grandma's house drove small airplane baked shoes." Some use words that seem appropriate, but are used incorrectly, such as "a dog walks on its feet."

Limbic Lobe

The **limbic lobe** is hidden from view and is best seen in a sagittal view of a bisected brain. The lobe is formed predominately by the **cingulate gyrus**, which lies on the surface of the corpus callosum. The lobe is part of the limbic system, which controls emotions (Fig. 13–3).

Review Question Box 13-3

1. What is the difference in function between the precentral and postcentral gyrus?
2. What differences occur in a stroke involving Broca's versus Wernicke's area?
3. What is meant by the primary visual area versus visual association areas?
4. What gyrus is the major component of the limbic system?
5. What would be affected by a stroke in the limbic system?

Diencephalon

The **diencephalon** lies deep in the brain between the cerebrum and the brain stem (Fig. 13–3). It is composed of the thalamus, hypothalamus, and the epithalamus.

The **thalamus** is a bilateral structure that surrounds the third ventricle (Fig. 13–5A). The thalamus is structurally and functionally complex. Of particular interest to the dental hygienist is its role as a relay station for many sensory modalities on their route to the sensory areas in the cerebral cortex. (This will be discussed in Chapter 14.)

The **hypothalamus** (below the thalamus) can be identified on the inferior surface of the brain by a pair of rounded eminences called the **mammillary bodies**, in addition to the infundibulum and the optic chiasm (Fig. 13–5B). The mammillary bodies are associated with memory related to olfaction. The **infundibulum** (pituitary stalk) connects the pituitary gland to the ventral surface of the hypothalamus. The hypothalamus regulates the autonomic nervous system in that it controls such bodily functions as temperature, water and electrolyte balance, sleep, hunger, and reproduction. The **pineal gland** is the major structure of the **epithalamus** (above the thalamus). The gland produces melatonin, a hormone that is involved in the control of daily rhythms (Fig. 13–5A).

Review Question Box 13-4

1. What is the difference in functions of the thalamus, hypothalamus, and epithalamus?

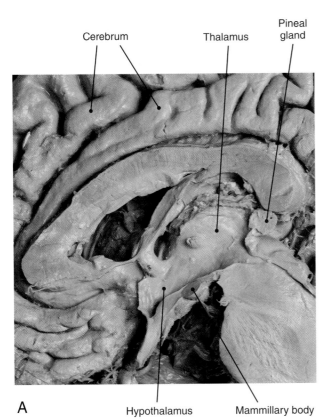

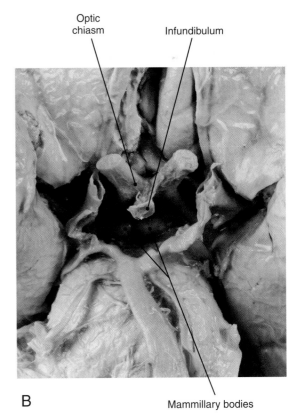

Figure 13–5 The diencephalon lies directly under the cerebrum. **(A)** In sagittal section, the thalamus appears as a bulge in the wall of the third ventricle. The epithalamus, which is identified by the presence of the pineal gland, lies superior and posterior to the thalamus. The hypothalamus lies anterior and inferior to the thalamus. **(B)** Ventral view of the diencephalon. The hypothalamus is composed of the optic chiasm, the infundibulum of the pituitary gland, and the mammillary bodies.

Cerebellum

The **cerebellum**, which is divided into two lobes, is located posterior and inferior to the occipital and parietal lobes (Fig. 13-3). The cerebellum receives sensory input from the semicircular canals of the vestibular apparatus in the middle ear and from muscles. The cerebellum coordinates balance, equilibrium, and smooth movements of the skeletal muscular system.

Brain Stem

The **brain stem** is composed of the **midbrain, pons,** and **medulla oblongata** (Fig. 13-6). It contains the nuclei of the cranial nerves, nerve tracts that travel to and from the cerebral cortex, and centers that regulate the respiratory and circulatory systems.

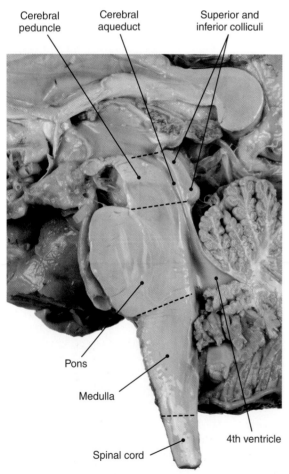

Cerebral peduncle

Cerebral aqueduct

Superior and inferior colliculi

Pons

Medulla

Spinal cord

4th ventricle

Figure 13–6 The midbrain, pons, and medulla are viewed in the median plane. The midbrain is composed of the superior and inferior colliculi, the cerebral aqueduct, and the cerebral peduncles. The basilar portion of the pons appears as a bulge between the midbrain and medulla. The fourth ventricle lies between the cerebellum and the pons and medulla.

 Box 13-2 Reticular Formation

Within the brain stem, there is a network of nuclei and fiber tracts that form the reticular formation. The reticular formation, which is one of the oldest phylogenic structures of the brain, contains centers that control respiratory and heart rate. Because the reticular formation also generates impulses that keep the cerebrum awake and alert, it is called the *reticular activating system*. Sleep results from a decreased activity of the reticular formation, and dysfunction can lead to a coma or unconsciousness.

Midbrain

The *midbrain* is located in between the diencephalon and the pons. The roof is characterized by two pairs of spherical eminences that are called colliculi (Fig. 13-6). The **superior colliculus** serves as a reflex center for head, eye, and body movements in response to visual stimuli, whereas the **inferior colliculus** is the reflex center related to movements from auditory stimuli. The floor is formed by the two **cerebral peduncles**, which are fiber bundles descending from the cerebral cortex (Fig. 13-6). These fibers synapse with lower motor neurons of the cranial nerves and the spinal cord. Internally, a small canal, the **cerebral aqueduct**, separates the colliculi and the cerebral peduncles. This canal is frequently called the **aqueduct of Sylvius** and contains cerebral spinal fluid (Figs. 13-3 and 13-6).

Pons

The *pons* is located just caudal to the midbrain. It is easily recognized by its bulblike protrusion on the anterior surface (Fig. 13-6). The basal portion of the pons contains information that is being relayed from the cerebral cortex to the cerebellum. In this way, the cerebrum tells the cerebellum what movements it wants the cerebellum to coordinate. The dorsal portion of the pons contains cranial nerve nuclei, as well as ascending and descending tracts from the brain and spinal cord. The pons is separated from the cerebellum by the **fourth ventricle**, which also contains cerebral spinal fluid (Fig. 13-6).

Medulla Oblongata

The *medulla oblongata* is the most caudal portion of the brain stem (Fig. 13-6). The *medulla*, as it is generally called, also contains cranial nerve nuclei and ascending and descending tracts from the brain and spinal cord. The motor fibers form the pyramidal tracts, which appear as linear elevations on the ventral surface of the brain stem. This area of the brain stem contains the cardiac and respiratory centers, which regulate the heart and breathing rates. The caudal part of the fourth ventricle lies on the surface of the medulla (Fig. 13–6).

Review Question Box 13-5

1. What is the functional difference between the superior and inferior colliculi?
2. What is the functional relationship between the pons and cerebellum?
3. What is the relationship of the fourth ventricle to the pons and medulla?
4. Why would major trauma to the medulla be life threatening?

ARTERIAL SUPPLY TO THE BRAIN

Many areas of the body, including the brain, have a dual blood supply. This is very important, because a loss of blood supply to the brain could lead to diminished function or death. The brain is supplied by the vertebrobasilar system and the internal carotid system of arteries. The **vertebral artery** is a branch of the subclavian artery (see Fig. 11–5). The left and right vertebral arteries ascend in the foramina of the transverse processes of the cervical vertebrae to reach the ventral surface of the brain stem where they join to form the single **basilar artery** (Fig. 13–7). The **internal carotid artery** is a terminal branch of the **common carotid artery** and enters the skull through the carotid canal (Fig. 13–7).

Two important arteries branch off the vertebral artery prior to the formation of the basilar artery. The **posterior inferior cerebellar arteries** arise laterally from the vertebral arteries to supply that portion of the cerebellum. Medially, a branch from each vertebral artery joins to form the **anterior spinal artery**, which is found in the ventral median fissure of the spinal cord (Fig. 13–7).

The first major branch of the basilar artery is the paired **anterior inferior cerebellar artery**. Next, several smaller **pontine branches** are followed by the next major paired branch, the **superior cerebellar artery**. The basilar artery terminates by splitting into the left and right **posterior cerebral arteries**. These arteries supply the entire occipital lobe and the inferior portion of the temporal lobe (Fig. 13–8).

After entering the skull through the carotid canal, the internal carotid artery terminates as two main arteries, the **anterior cerebral** and the **middle cerebral arteries**, which supply their respective areas of the cerebrum. The left and right anterior cerebral arteries are joined by the very short **anterior communicating artery** (Fig. 13–7).

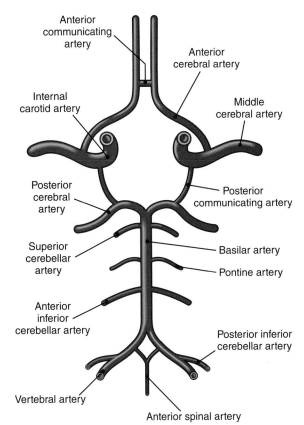

Figure 13–7 The brain is supplied by two sources: the internal carotid artery and the vertebral artery. The vertebral artery supplies branches to the spinal cord and cerebellum and fuses, forming the basilar artery. It extends branches to the pons and cerebellum before terminating as the posterior cerebral arteries. The anterior cerebral, anterior communicating, and posterior communicating branches of the internal carotid artery join the posterior cerebral arteries of the basilar artery to form the circle of Willis.

The anterior cerebral arteries supply the medial surface of the cerebrum and the superior border of the frontal and parietal lobes (Fig. 13–8). The **posterior communicating artery** branches off the internal carotid artery just before its terminal bifurcation (Fig. 13–7). This vessel joins the internal carotid artery to the posterior cerebral artery. These connections form a circle of blood vessels, the **circle of Willis**, around the optic chiasm, mammillary bodies, and the base of the infundibulum of the pituitary gland (Fig. 13–7).

The middle cerebral artery does not contribute to the formation of the circle of Willis, but is very important because it supplies a large area of the cerebrum. The artery supplies most of the lateral surface of the cerebrum that includes portions of the frontal, parietal, and temporal lobes (Fig. 13–8). Realize that a massive stroke could affect the postcentral and precentral gyri, which would affect both motor and sensory functions.

Review Question Box 13-6

1. What vessels branch from the vertebral artery before they form the basilar artery?
2. What are the terminal branches of the basilar artery?
3. What branch of the internal carotid artery is not included in the circle of Willis?
4. What part of the body and its function would be affected by a stroke of the middle cerebral artery along the precentral gyrus?

DURAL SINUSES

The veins of the brain empty into specialized venous channels within the dura called the **dural sinuses**. These sinuses are located in the dural folds that separate components of the brain. The *falx cerebri* separates the two cerebral hemispheres and the **tentorium cerebelli** separates the occipital lobes of the cerebrum from the cerebellum (Fig. 13–9). Large dural sinuses, such as the **sigmoid sinus**, can leave depressions on the floor of the cranial cavity (Fig. 13–10). All venous blood empties into the **internal jugular vein**.

Box 13-3 Venous Return

The superior border of the falx cerebri contains the *superior sagittal sinus*, whereas the inferior border next to the corpus callosum contains the *inferior sagittal sinus*. Venous blood from these sinuses flow into the *straight sinus* located at the junction of the falx cerebri with the tentorium cerebelli. A small *occipital sinus* is found in the falx cerebelli. These sinuses empty into a common area on the posterior surface of the brain known as the *confluens of sinuses*. The confluens is drained by the paired *transverse sinuses* located in the border of the tentorial cerebelli, which are attached to the skull. The transverse sinuses empty into the *sigmoid sinuses*, which empty into the *internal jugular vein*.

The superior sagittal and cavernous sinuses are clinically relevant. The **superior sagittal sinus** collects cerebral spinal fluid from the subarachnoid space and blood from the superficial veins of the cerebrum. (See the section on cerebral spinal fluid in this chapter.) Shearing of a cerebral vein as it enters the dural sinus can cause bleeding in the subdural space (subdural hematoma). This can cause permanent damage in the area under

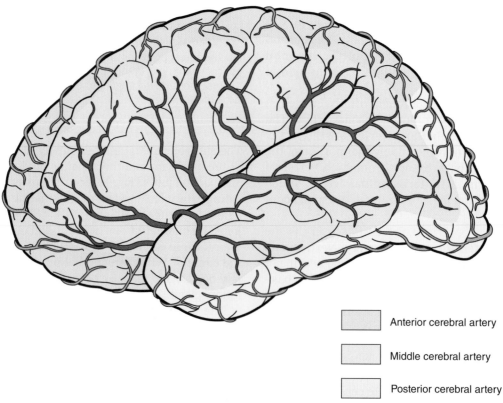

☐ Anterior cerebral artery

☐ Middle cerebral artery

☐ Posterior cerebral artery

Figure 13–8 The anterior cerebral artery supplies the superior margin and medial aspect of the frontal and parietal lobes. The middle cerebral artery supplies most of the lateral surface of the cerebrum to include the precentral and postcentral gyri. The posterior cerebral artery supplies the occipital lobe and inferior margin of the temporal lobe.

Figure 13–9 The falx cerebri and tentorium cerebelli are major folds of the dura mater, and they contain dural venous sinuses.

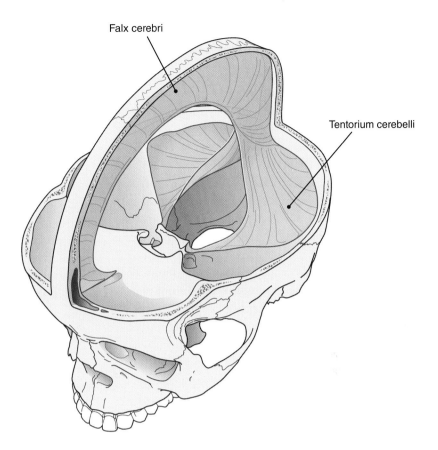

Falx cerebri

Tentorium cerebelli

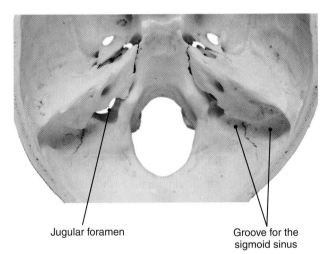

Jugular foramen

Groove for the sigmoid sinus

Figure 13–10 The sigmoid sinus is an example of a dural sinus that forms a groove in the surface of floor of the cranial cavity as it exits the jugular foramen.

pressure from the swelling. The **cavernous sinuses** are two interconnected venous structures that are located on either side of the sella turcica (Fig. 13–11). Several important nerves and blood vessels are located in the walls of the sinuses (Fig. 13–11). The cavernous sinuses also receive tributaries from the external face and the pterygoid plexus (Chapter 11). Infections of the cavernous sinus can have severe effects on the orbit and, if not controlled, can cause death.

Review Question Box 13-7

1. What are the locations of the dural sinuses?
2. What venous structure located outside the skull receives blood from the dural sinuses?
3. What is the danger of a blood clot in the cavernous sinus?

CEREBRAL SPINAL FLUID

Cerebral spinal fluid (CSF) is a clear, colorless fluid that is secreted by specialized vascular structures known collectively as the *choroid plexus*. CSF has a different protein and electrolyte content than plasma and functions to protect and lighten the weight of the central nervous system. Components of the **choroid plexus** can be found in the lateral, third, and fourth ventricles (Fig. 13–12).

The *lateral ventricles* are C-shaped epithelial-lined spaces that are surrounded by the lobes of the cerebrum. The main portion of the ventricle, which is located between the parietal lobes, is called the *body*. Extensions of the ventricle, which are called *horns*, are located in the frontal, occipital, and temporal lobes. The **anterior horns** extend into the frontal lobes, whereas the **lateral horns** extend into the temporal lobe, and the **posterior horns** extend into the occipital lobe (Fig. 13–13). The bodies of the two lateral ventricles are separated in the midline by a membrane of tissue called the *septum*

Cavernous Sinus Thrombosis

The *cavernous sinus* is one of several venous channels found within the dura mater of the cranial cavity. The sinus lies along the floor of the middle cranial cavity lateral to the sella turcica. It is connected to the superficial veins of the face and the pterygoid plexus of veins in the infratemporal fossa. The sinus can become inflamed from infections arising from the superficial face and the pterygoid plexus. The swelling of the sinus slows the blood flow, which can contribute to the formation of a blood clot (thrombosis). In addition to receiving venous blood from the orbit, nerves that control eye moments and open the upper lid pass through the walls of the cavernous sinus. The internal carotid artery also courses through the cavernous sinus and sends a branch to the retina. Signs of **cavernous sinus thrombosis** include severe headaches with fever, bulging eyes and eyelids due to edema, inability to move the eyeball, drooping eyelids, dilated pupils, and even blindness. Because it has vascular connections to other dural sinuses, infection can spread to other portions of the brain and result in death.

pellucidum (Fig. 13–12). CSF produced in the lateral ventricles flows into the third ventricles through a pair of openings known as the **interventricular foramen** (of Monroe) (Fig. 13–12).

The **third ventricle** is surrounded by the structures of the thalamus (Fig. 13–12). The CSF flows from the third ventricle into the *cerebral aqueduct* (of *Sylvius*) located

in the midbrain and then into the rhomboid-shaped fourth ventricle (Fig. 13–12). The floor of the fourth ventricle is formed by the pons and the medulla and is overlaid by the cerebellum (Fig. 13–12). The CSF then flows through openings in the walls of the fourth ventricle to reach the subarachnoid space and circulates around the brain and spinal cord.

CSF is constantly being formed, and thus the fluid is returned to the peripheral blood circulation to prevent an increase in intracranial pressure on the neural tissue, which could damage the brain. CSF returns to the peripheral circulation by passing through tufts of capillary-like structures called **arachnoid granulations**, which are found in the *superior sagittal sinus* (Fig. 13–14).

Review Question Box 13-8

1. What is the difference between the choroid plexus and the arachnoid granulations?
2. Trace the flow of cerebral spinal fluid from the lateral ventricle to the superior sagittal sinus.

SPINAL CORD

In the adult, the spinal cord extends within the vertebral canal from the foramen magnum to approximately the second lumbar vertebra. As in the brain, the spinal cord is covered by the three meninges (Figs. 13–15A and B). However, unlike the brain, the *dura mater* is not attached to bone. An **epidural space**, which contains fat and blood vessels, separates the vertebrae from the spinal cord. A narrow **subdural space** separates the dura from the underlying *arachnoid mater*. The arachnoid mater is

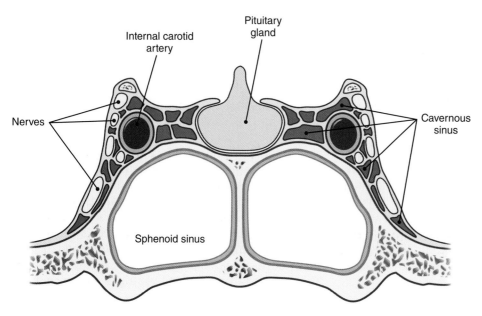

Figure 13–11 The cavernous sinuses lay on either side of the pituitary gland, which is located in the sella turcica. The walls of the sinus contain several nerves that supply structures of the orbit. The internal carotid artery passes through the cavernous sinus en route to the inferior surface of brain.

Hydrocephalus

Hydrocephalus (water in the head) is the enlargement of the ventricles of the brain caused by obstruction of the flow of cerebral spinal fluid. The obstruction usually occurs in narrowed channels such as the interventricular foramen or the cerebral aqueduct. Depending on the intracranial pressure, the brain can be pushed onto the bones of the skull, which could cause severe damage to the brain tissue. In infants whose fontanels are not fully closed, the cranium can become enlarged by the increase in intracranial pressure.

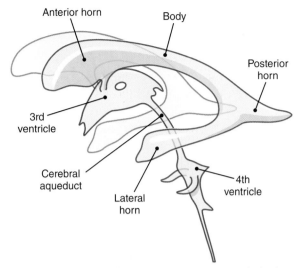

Figure 13–13 A cast of the ventricular system with the brain tissue removed. The lateral ventricles are composed of a body and smaller horns that extend into the frontal (anterior horn), occipital (posterior horn), and temporal lobes (lateral horn). The continuity of the lateral, third, and fourth ventricles via the interventricular foramen and cerebral aqueduct are shown.

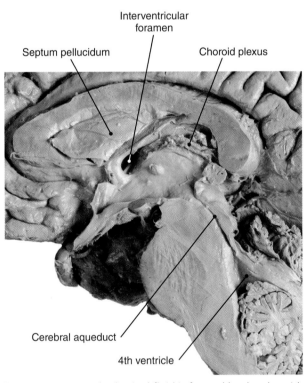

Figure 13–12 Cerebral spinal fluid is formed by the choroid plexus in the ventricles. The fluid flows from the lateral ventricles of the cerebrum through the interventricular foramen to reach the third ventricle in the diencephalon. It then flows through the cerebral aqueduct to the fourth ventricle.

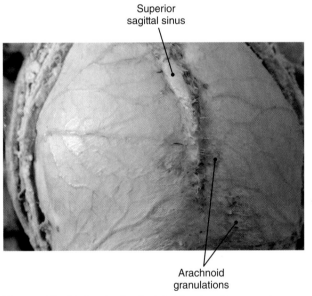

Figure 13–14 Cerebral spinal fluid enters the superior sagittal sinus from the subarachnoid space via the arachnoid granulations.

separated from the pia mater, which is attached to the surface of the spinal cord by the *subarachnoid space* (Figs. 13–15A and B). As in the brain, the subarachnoid space contains CSF.

The spinal cord is enlarged in the cervical and lumbar regions. The **cervical enlargement** contains the added neurons necessary to innervate the upper limb, whereas the **lumbosacral enlargement** contains additional neurons to accommodate the lower extremity (Fig. 13–16A). The spinal cord gradually tapers to

end as the cone-shaped **conus medullaris** (Figs. 13–6A and C). Although the spinal cord terminates, the three meningeal coverings continue inferiorly to attach to the sacrum (Fig. 13–16B). Ventral and dorsal roots of the lower lumbar and sacral spinal segments extend inferiorly from the conus medullaris as a bundle of fibers called the **cauda equina**, or *horse's tail* due to the fibers' resemblance to a horse's tail (Fig. 13–16A and C). The subarachnoid space is enlarged in this area and is known as the **lumbar cistern** (Fig. 13–16C).

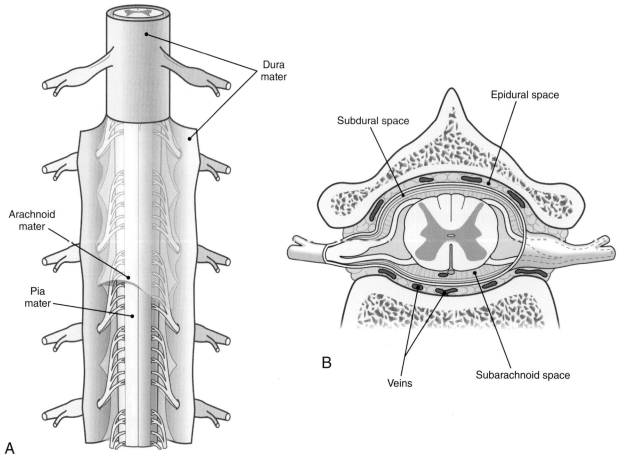

Figure 13–15 (A) The spinal cord is covered by the dura, arachnoid, and pia mater. **(B)** The epidural space separates the dura from the vertebrae and contains veins and fat. The subdural space between the dura and arachnoid mater is very narrow. The subarachnoid space lies between the arachnoid and pia mater.

Clinical Correlation Box 13-6

Lumbar Puncture

Lumbar puncture, also called *spinal tap*, is a procedure to remove a sample of cerebral spinal fluid from the lumbar region of the back. The fluid can be used to diagnose diseases such as meningitis, multiple sclerosis, cancer, and inflammation of the brain or spinal cord. The procedure is based on the anatomy of the spinal cord in this region. Because of differential development, the spinal cord stops at vertebral level L1 to L2; however, the meningeal covers extend to the sacral regions. This leaves an enlarged subarachnoid space known as the *lumbar cistern*. A needle is inserted in between the vertebrae of L3 to L4 or L4 to L5 for collection of the cerebral spinal fluid from the cistern.

Clinical Correlation Box 13-7

Epidural Injections

Injection of drugs in the *epidural space*, which is the space between the dura mater of the spinal cord and the vertebral canal, has become a common procedure for regional nerve blocks and treatment of pain, such as sciatica in the lower extremity. Anesthetics, which block sensation, and analgesics, which block pain, can be injected into the epidural space through a catheter for regional blockage. Drugs are able to diffuse around the dorsal (sensory) roots of the spinal nerve. Likewise, steroids can be injected into the lower back and neck regions to relieve pain caused by inflammation resulting from bulging or degenerating discs (stenosis).

The dorsal surface of the spinal cord is characterized by a shallow midline depression called the **dorsal median sulcus**. The ventral surface displays a much larger midline cleft called the **ventral median fissure** (Fig. 13–17) that contains the blood–vascular supply to the ventral portion of the cord. Thirty-one pairs of **spinal nerves**

(*8 cervical, 12 thoracic, 5 lumbar, 5 sacral, and 1 coccygeal*) are attached to the spinal cord by a series of two pairs of rootlets designated the **dorsal root** and **ventral root** because of their respective attachments to the spinal cord (Fig. 13–17). The ventral root is the motor component of the spinal nerve, whereas the dorsal root is the

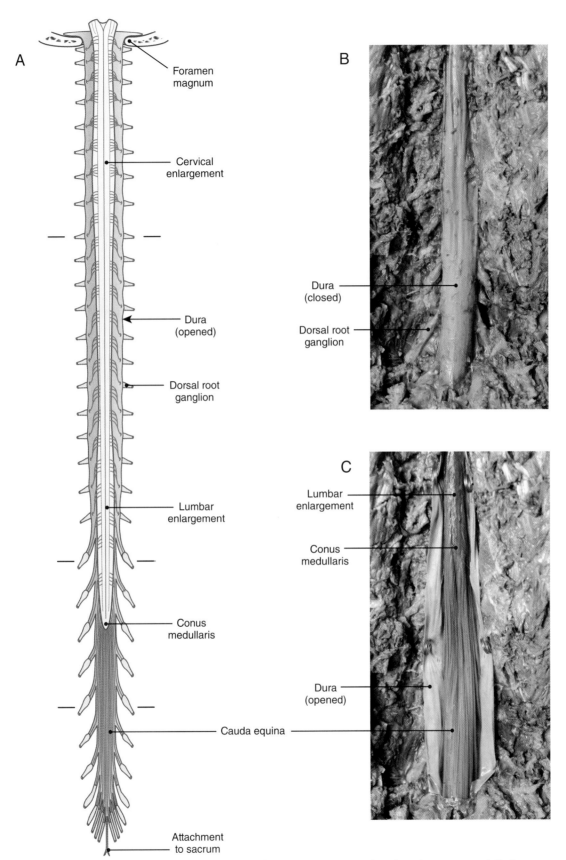

A

Foramen
magnum

Cervical
enlargement

Dura
(opened)

Dorsal root
ganglion

Lumbar
enlargement

Conus
medullaris

Cauda equina

Attachment
to sacrum

B

Dura
(closed)

Dorsal root
ganglion

C

Lumbar
enlargement

Conus
medullaris

Dura
(opened)

Cauda equina

Figure 13–16 (A) The spinal cord begins at the foramen magnum and ends as the conus medullaris at the lower lumbar vertebral level and the dura and arachnoid continue to the sacrum. The cervical and lumbar enlargements indicate the portions of the spinal cord that supply the extremities. **(B)** A view of the lower lumbar region that is enclosed in the dura mater. The dorsal root ganglion represents the area where the ventral and dorsal roots join to form a spinal nerve. **(C)** The ventral and dorsal roots, which form the cauda equina, leave the vertebral canal to form the spinal nerves in the lower lumbar and sacral regions. The nerve roots can be seen through the transparent arachnoid mater within the lumbar cistern.

sensory component of the spinal nerve. The sensory neurons are located in the **dorsal root ganglion** of each dorsal root of a spinal nerve (Fig. 13–17). The ventral and dorsal rootlets leave the vertebral canal through the **intervertebral foramen** to form the spinal nerves (Fig. 13–17). The more relevant spinal nerves to the dental hygienists are the cervical nerves (designated C1 to C8), which supply muscles of the neck and T1 to L2, which contain the sympathetic component of the autonomic nervous system. The sympathetic nervous system will be studied in Chapter 15.

Review Question Box 13-9

1. What is the difference between the epidural and sub-dural spaces?
2. How are the cervical and lumbosacral enlargements similar?
3. What is the relationship between the conus medullaris and the cauda equina?
4. How do the roots of the spinal nerves leave the vertebral canal?

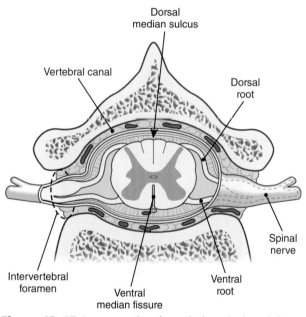

Figure 13–17 A cross section through the spinal cord shows the dorsal median sulcus and the ventral median fissure. The ventral and dorsal roots exit the intervertebral foramen and join to form a spinal nerve. The dorsal root ganglion appears as a swelling on the dorsal root.

SUMMARY

The central nervous system is composed of the brain and spinal cord. Both structures are protected by three layers of connective tissue called the meninges. The outer layer, the dura mater, is very tough. In the skull, the dura is attached directly to the skull. In the spinal cord, the epidural space separates the dura from the vertebral canal. The next layer is the arachnoid mater, which is a delicate membrane. The subarachnoid space, which is filled with cerebral spinal fluid, separates the arachnoid mater from the pia mater. The pia mater is applied directly to the surface of the brain and spinal cord and cannot be separated from the organs.

The brain is composed of the cerebrum, diencephalon, brain stem, and cerebellum. The surface of the cerebrum is characterized by convoluted gyri separated by sulci. Deeper grooves, called fissures, separate the frontal, parietal, temporal, and occipital lobes. The cerebral hemispheres surround the lateral ventricles, which produce and contain cerebral spinal fluid. The precentral gyrus of the frontal lobe is the main motor area. In addition, there are the frontal eye fields, which control eye movement, and Broca's area, which is a motor speech area for forming words. Other areas are associated with personality, intelligence, and problem solving. The postcentral gyrus of the parietal lobes is the main sensory cortex. The temporal lobe is associated with hearing and language, whereas the function of the occipital lobe is related to vision. A fifth lobe, the limbic lobe, lies on the medial surface of the cerebral hemispheres, which are separated by the longitudinal fissure. Its functions are related to emotions.

The diencephalon contains the major sensory relay station, the thalamus. Other structures function in the endocrine system. The third ventricle lies within the diencephalon and is connected to the lateral ventricles by the interventricular foramen of Monroe.

The brain stem is composed of the midbrain, pons, and medulla oblongata. The superior colliculus and inferior colliculus of the midbrain are reflex centers for vision and hearing, respectively. The cerebral aqueduct separates the colliculi from the cerebral peduncles. The pons contains fibers that connect the cerebrum to the cerebellum. The medulla contains cranial nerve nuclei and centers that control respiratory and cardiac rates. The pons and medulla are separated from the cerebellum by the fourth ventricle.

The brain has a dual blood supply: the internal carotid arteries and the vertebral arteries. The vertebral arteries enter the cranial cavity through the foramen magnum and fuse to form the basilar artery, which supplies the cerebellum and brain stem and terminates by forming the two posterior cerebral arteries. The internal carotid artery divides into the anterior cerebral and posterior communicating arteries, which join the posterior cerebral arteries to form the circle of Willis. The middle cerebral artery, a third branch of the internal carotid artery, supplies a major part of the cerebrum including the precentral and postcentral gyri.

Venous blood is collected by the dural sinuses that are formed in folds of the dura. The major folds are the falx cerebri, which separate the cerebral hemispheres, and the tentorium cerebelli, which separate the cerebrum from the cerebellum. The dural sinuses drain into the internal jugular vein.

The brain is bathed by a nutrient fluid called cerebral spinal fluid. The fluid also reduces the weight of the brain in the cranial cavity. The fluid is produced in the ventricles of the brain and circulates in the subarachnoid spaces of the brain and spinal cord. The fluid returns to the venous circulation via the arachnoid granulations in the superior sagittal sinus.

The spinal cord begins at the foramen magnum and ends as the conus medullaris in the upper lumbar region. The dura mater and arachnoid mater extend to the sacral region, forming an enlarged space around the cauda equina called the lumbar cistern. Spinal nerves are attached to the spinal cord by the ventral and dorsal roots. An enlarged swelling, the dorsal root ganglion, contains the sensory neurons of the peripheral nervous system to the trunk. The ventral root contains motor fibers that innervate skeletal muscle.

Learning Activity 13-1

Brain—Lateral View

Match the numbered structures with the correct terms listed below.

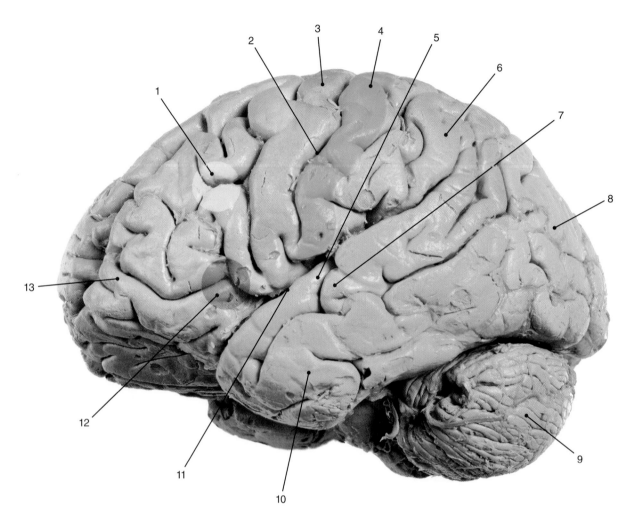

_____ Broca's area

_____ Central sulcus

_____ Cerebellum

_____ Frontal eye field

_____ Frontal lobe

_____ Lateral fissure

_____ Main auditory cortex

_____ Occipital lobe

_____ Parietal lobe

_____ Postcentral gyrus

_____ Precentral gyrus

_____ Temporal lobe

_____ Wernicke's area

Learning Activity 13-2

Brain—Sagittal View

Match the numbered structures with the correct terms listed below.

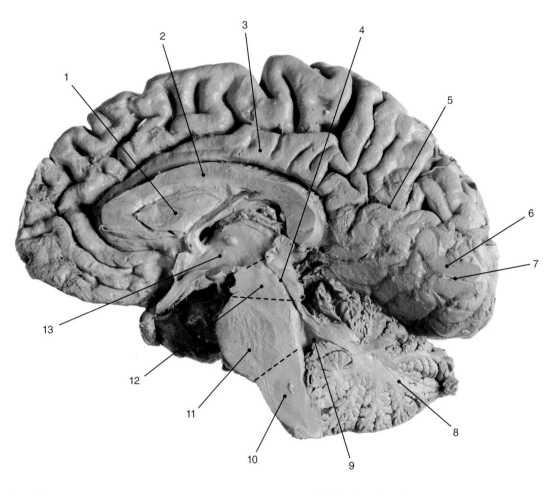

_____ Calcarine fissure

_____ Cerebellum

_____ Cerebral aqueduct

_____ Corpus callosum

_____ Cingulate gyrus/limbic lobe

_____ Diencephalon

_____ Fourth ventricle

_____ Main visual cortex

_____ Medulla

_____ Midbrain

_____ Parieto-occipital fissure

_____ Pons

_____ Septum pellucidum

Learning Activity 13-3

Arterial Supply to the Brain

Match the numbered structures with the correct terms listed below.

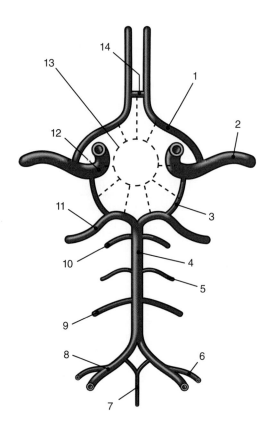

_____ Anterior cerebral artery

_____ Anterior communicating artery

_____ Anterior inferior cerebellar artery

_____ Anterior spinal artery

_____ Basilar artery

_____ Circle of Willis

_____ Internal carotid artery

_____ Middle cerebral artery

_____ Pontine arteries

_____ Posterior cerebral artery

_____ Posterior communicating artery

_____ Posterior inferior cerebellar artery

_____ Superior cerebellar artery

_____ Vertebral artery

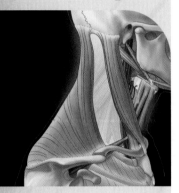

chapter

14

Sensory and Motor Pathways

Objectives

1. Discuss the difference between the following pairs of terms: *effectors* versus *receptors*; *upper motor neurons* versus *lower motor neurons*; *alpha motor neurons* versus *pseudounipolar neurons*; and *spinal nerves* versus *tracts*.
2. On a diagram, label the components of the spinal nerves and the structures they innervate and discuss their functions.
3. Identify and discuss the composition of the three-neuron sensory pathway.
4. Compare the ascending pathways for pain and temperature to conscious touch and proprioception for the body and head.
5. Compare the descending motor pathway for the head and trunk.

Overview

Although the Internet and cell phones have greatly changed our means of communication, the analog telephone (wires) still plays an important role in our communication system. The brain, spinal cord, and peripheral organs communicate by nerve fibers, much like telephone wires. Long-distance telephone calls are channeled through various communication centers across the country to reach their destination. Similarly, the brain and spinal cord are connected by fiber tracts that carry incoming and outgoing information. These fiber tracts determine movement and receive stimuli from peripheral receptors. In this chapter, the major motor and sensory pathways of the trunk and head are discussed.

INTRODUCTION TO SENSORY AND MOTOR PATHWAYS

The initiation of movement and the conscious recognition of sensation require an interaction between the brain, spinal cord, and peripheral structures. Structures that receive motor input—that is, muscles and glands—are called **effectors**, whereas structures that receive sensory stimuli from the environment are called **receptors**. Skeletal muscles are controlled by the **upper motor neurons** in the gray matter of the cerebrum. The axons of these cells, which are called *nerve fibers*, synapse on the **lower motor neurons** in the gray matter of the spinal cord or the brain stem. The motor nerve fibers enter the spinal nerves via the ventral root to reach the skeletal muscle. Receptors are stimulated by temperature, pressure, vibration, pain, as well as other sensations, and the information is carried to the sensory nerves in the spinal cord and brain stem. After multiple synapses with other neurons, the stimulus reaches the cerebrum, where the sensations are perceived at a conscious level (I feel pain; it is cold; the dental drill is vibrating). The sensory nerve fibers are located in the white matter of the brain and spinal cord and are organized into bundles that are called **tracts**. The **pathway** is composed of the neurons and tracts through which a stimulus must travel from the cerebrum to the effector or from the receptor to the cerebrum.

ORGANIZATION OF THE SPINAL CORD

Internally, the spinal cord contains a central column of **gray matter**, which contains the cell bodies of neurons, surrounded peripherally by the **white matter**, which contains nerve fibers (Fig. 14–1). The gray matter has an H-shaped profile in cross section. The "upper arms" of the H are called the **dorsal horns** and comprise the sensory portion of the spinal cord. The "lower arms" are called the **ventral horns** and comprise the motor portion of the spinal cord (Fig. 14–1). The ventral horn contains lower motor neurons, called **alpha motor neurons**, whose axons innervate the skeletal muscle in the trunk and extremities (Fig. 14–2). The white matter is divided into three cordlike segments or **funiculi** (singular: **funiculus**). The **dorsal funiculus** lies between the dorsal horn and dorsal median sulcus, the **lateral funiculus** lies between dorsal and ventral horns, and the **ventral funiculus** is located between the ventral horn and the ventral median fissure (Fig. 14–1). The funiculi contain myelinated nerves that convey messages to and from the spinal cord and higher centers in the brain stem, cerebellum, and cerebrum. The messages are carried in specific bundles of fibers called *tracts*,

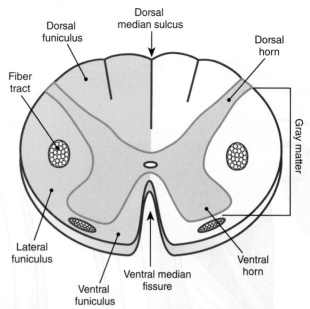

Figure 14–1 This cross section of the thoracic cord illustrates the basic surface and internal features of the spinal cord. The white matter is divided into three funiculi that contain fiber tracts. The gray matter is divided into dorsal and motor horns. The dorsal surface is characterized by a shallow sulcus, whereas the ventral surface is distinguished by a deeper sulcus.

which can be compared to telephone cables, with each cable carrying specific types of information (Fig. 14–1).

The spinal nerves are attached bilaterally to the spinal cord by a series of rootlets designated as either **dorsal root** or **ventral root** because of their respective attachments to the spinal cord (Fig. 14–2). The ventral root is the motor component of the spinal nerve and contains axons of the alpha motor neurons of the ventral horn. The dorsal root is the sensory component of the spinal nerve and contains the processes of the **pseudounipolar** neurons located in a swelling on the dorsal root known as the **dorsal root ganglion** (**DRG**) (Fig. 14–2). The term *ganglion* refers to an aggregation of nerve cell bodies located outside of the brain or spinal cord.

Review Question Box 14-1

1. What is the difference between a receptor and an effector?
2. What is the difference between a ganglion and a nucleus of the central nervous system?
3. Where is the location of the alpha motor neuron and the pseudounipolar neuron?
4. What is a nerve fiber and what is the location in the spinal cord?

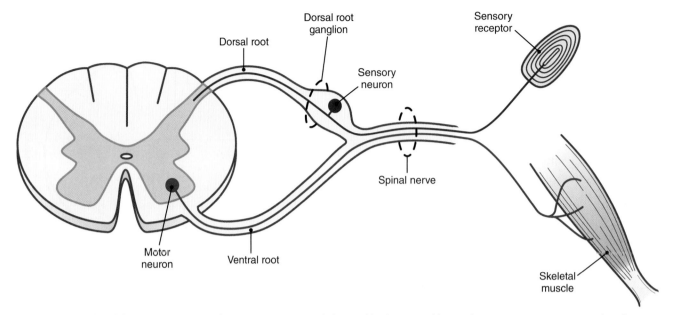

Figure 14–2 The alpha motor neuron, a lower motor neuron, is located in the ventral horn; the sensory neuron, a pseudounipolar neuron, is located in the dorsal root ganglion. Motor fibers enter the spinal nerve via the ventral root and synapse on skeletal muscle. Afferent fibers from sensory receptors enter the spinal cord via the dorsal root of the spinal nerve.

ASCENDING PATHWAYS

The ascending pathways contain **afferent** or **sensory** fibers. Those tracts carrying conscious information (to the sensory areas of the cerebrum) are composed of a three-neuron chain. The nerve cell body of the first neuron is called the **first-order neuron** and is located in the DRG. It carries sensory information from the peripheral receptors to the central nervous system. It synapses with a **second-order neuron** located in either the spinal cord or the brain stem. The axon of this neuron in turn synapses with a **third-order neuron** located in the thalamus. Finally, the axon from the third-order neuron synapses with neurons in the cerebrum (Fig. 14–3).

Trunk

Touch and Proprioception Pathway

The receptors for the sensation of **touch**—which includes the ability to feel pressure, vibration, and two-point discrimination (the ability to distinguish two points of touch to the skin)—are located in the skin. **Proprioception** is the sense of movement in space of the muscles and the body. Proprioceptive receptors are located in the tendons of skeletal muscle and the joints. Sensory fibers from the first-order neuron in the dorsal root ganglion carry sensory input from the trunk and lower extremities. The nerve fibers ascend in the dorsal funiculus, which is composed of two nerve tracts: the fasciculus gracilis and fasciculus cuneatus. The **fasciculus gracilis** carries information regarding touch and proprioception from the lower trunk and lower extremities.

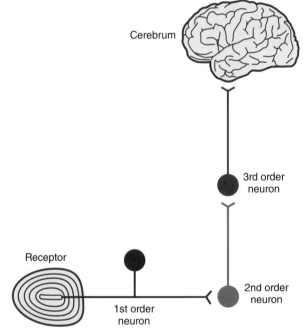

Figure 14–3 Three neurons carry a sensory stimulus to the cerebrum for recognition of a specific modality such as pain or proprioception.

The fasciculus gracilis is formed by nerve fibers entering the spinal cord below T6 and lies medial to the fasciculus cuneatus in the upper thoracic and cervical spinal regions of the spinal cord (Fig. 14–4). The **fasciculus cuneatus** forms above T6 and carries the same information from the upper trunk and upper extremities. These decussate (cross) the midline and synapse with the third-order neurons located in the **contralateral** (opposite side) **thalamus**. The axons of the third-order neuron synapse with neurons in the **postcentral gyrus** (primary sensory area) (Fig. 14–4).

Pain and Temperature Pathways to the Trunk

Pain and temperature receptors of the body are located in the skin. Sensory fibers of the first-order neurons that are located in the DRG carry the stimulus to the spinal cord (Fig. 14–5). Unlike the touch and proprioceptive fibers, the first-order neurons synapse with the second-order neurons that are located in the dorsal horn of the spinal cord (Fig. 14–5). The axons of the second-order neurons decussate the midline and ascend in the **lateral spinothalamic tract** to synapse with third-order neurons in the contralateral thalamus (Fig. 14–5). Fibers from the third-order neurons synapse with sensory neurons in the postcentral gyrus (Fig. 14–5).

Head

Conscious Touch and Proprioception

The senses of touch and proprioception in the head also require three neurons, but take an alternative pathway. The nerve cell bodies for the first-order sensory neurons (pseudounipolar) are located in the **trigeminal ganglion** (Fig. 14–6). Unlike the spinal cord, the trigeminal nerve, a cranial nerve, has more than one sensory nucleus that contains secondary order neurons. Fibers from the first-order neurons

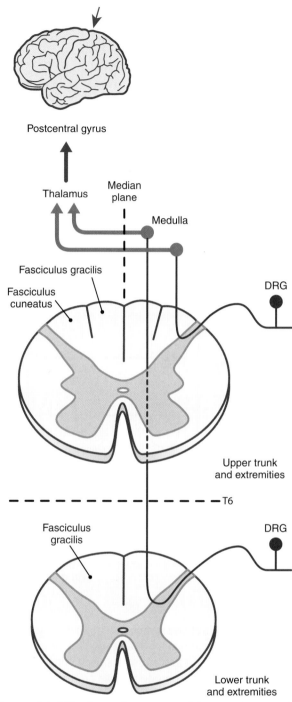

Figure 14–4 The first-order neurons of the conscious touch and proprioceptive pathway for the trunk ascend in either fasciculus gracilis or cuneatus to synapse in nuclei of the medulla. Fibers of the second-order neurons decussate the midline and synapse on the third-order neurons in the thalamus. Fibers of the third-order neurons synapse in the postcentral gyrus.

tracts, which are often called the **dorsal columns**, ascend the **ipsilateral** (same) side of the spinal cord to synapse with the second-order neuron in the nucleus gracilis and nucleus cuneatus, respectively, in the medulla (Fig. 14–4). Axons of the second-order neurons

Clinical Correlation Box 14-1

Lesions of the Dorsal Column

Lesions in the dorsal column can be caused by multiple sclerosis, penetrating injuries such as a knife wound, and compression by tumors. The clinical signs are dependent on the spinal cord level and degree of damage. If the lesion is unilateral and below spinal segment T6 involving only fasciculus gracilis, there would be a loss of touch, vibration, and proprioception of the ipsilateral (same side) lower trunk and lower extremity. A similar lesion above T6 would involve both fasciculi gracilis and cuneatus; thus, there would be a loss of the same modalities on the ipsilateral upper trunk and upper extremity, in addition to the deficit to the lower trunk and extremity. If both dorsal columns are affected, the clinical signs would be the same as described earlier, but deficits would be on both sides of the body.

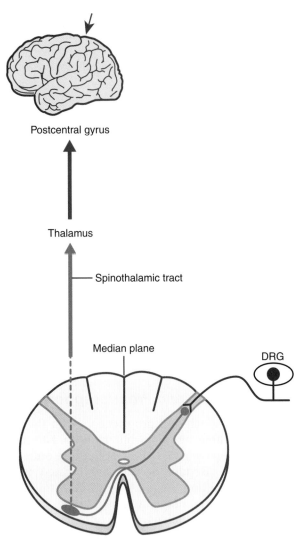

Figure 14–5 The first-order neurons of the pain and temperature pathway for the body are located in the dorsal root ganglion. Their fibers synapse with the second-order neurons of the ipsilateral dorsal horn. The nerve fibers decussate the midline and ascend in the contralateral spinothalamic tract to synapse on the third-order neurons in the thalamus. Fibers from the thalamus synapse in the postcentral gyrus.

Clinical Correlation Box 14-2

Lesions of the Spinothalamic Tract

Lesions in the spinothalamic tract are commonly caused by multiple sclerosis, penetrating injuries, and compression by tumors. Because the spinothalamic tract crosses to the contralateral (opposite side), there would be a loss of pain and temperature sensation on the contralateral side of the body below the injury. For example, an injury to the right spinothalamic tract L1 would cause the loss of pain and temperature sensation below L1 on the left side of the trunk.

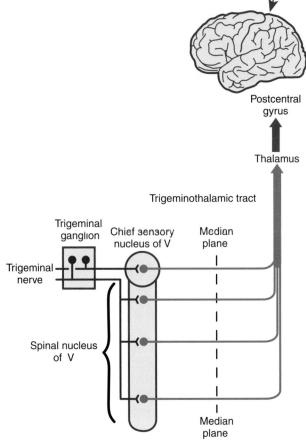

Figure 14–6 The first-order neurons for conscious touch and proprioception, as well as pain and temperature for the head, are located in the trigeminal ganglion and synapse with the second-order neurons. These neurons are located in the chief sensory nucleus for conscious touch and proprioception pathway and in the spinal nucleus of V for the pain and temperature pathway. Fibers of second-order neurons of both pathways cross the midline to synapse in the thalamus. The fibers of the third-order neurons synapse in the postcentral gyrus.

synapse in the **chief sensory nucleus of V** (Fig. 14–6). The term *nucleus* refers to an aggregation of nerve cell bodies located inside the brain or spinal cord. Fibers of the second-order neurons decussate and ascend in the trigeminothalamic tract to synapse with the third-order neurons in the contralateral thalamus (Fig. 14–6). Fibers of the third-order neuron synapse with sensory neurons in the postcentral gyrus (Fig. 14–6).

Pain and Temperature

The first-order neurons for the pain and temperature pathway for the head are also located in the trigeminal nucleus (Fig. 14–6). These fibers synapse with second-order neurons located in the **spinal nucleus of V** (Fig. 14–6). This nucleus begins in the pons and extends inferiorly into the medulla. Fibers from the second-order neurons decussate, ascend in the trigeminothalamic tract, and synapse with third-order neurons located in the contralateral thalamus (Fig. 14–6). The fibers of the third-order neurons ascend and synapse with the sensory neurons in the postcentral gyrus (Fig. 14–6).

Review Question Box 14-2

1. What order neuron crosses in the sensory pathways?
2. What is the location of the first-order neurons for sensory pathways of the head and trunk?
3. Where is the location of the third-order neurons in the sensory pathways of both the trunk and head? Where do their axons terminate?
4. What is the difference between the spinal nucleus of V and the chief sensory nucleus of V?
5. What is the difference between the fasciculus gracilis and fasciculus cuneatus?

DESCENDING PATHWAYS

The descending pathways are **efferent** or **motor** in function. The efferent pathway is composed of two types of neurons: upper motor neurons and lower motor neurons. The nerve fibers of the *upper motor neurons* extend from the brain and synapse on the nerve cell bodies of the *lower motor neurons* in the brain stem or ventral horn of the spinal cord (Fig. 14–7). The lower motor neurons extend their axons into the spinal and cranial nerves to reach skeletal muscle (Fig. 14–7).

Motor Pathways

Trunk

The upper motor neurons are located in the precentral gyrus and other gyri that control skeletal muscle (Fig. 14–8). The axons of the upper motor neurons

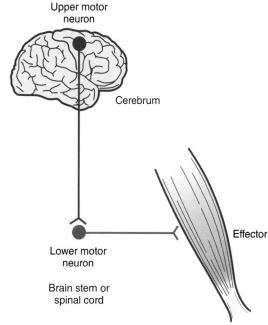

Figure 14–7 The descending motor pathway is formed by two neurons. The upper motor neurons are located in the cerebrum and the lower motor neurons are located in the brain stem and spinal cord. Lower motor neurons directly innervate the effector, which is skeletal muscle.

descend through the midbrain in the cerebral peduncles (Fig. 14–8). At the junction of the medulla and spinal cord, 80% of the fibers cross the midline to form the **lateral corticospinal tract**. The nerve fibers then synapse with the lower motor neurons located in the contralateral ventral horn (Fig. 14–8). The remaining 20% of the fibers descend ipsilaterally as the **ventral corticospinal tract** (Fig. 14–8). The corticospinal tracts control fine motor movement, such as the use of the hands and fingers by a hygienist when scaling teeth.

Clinical Correlation Box 14-3

Trigeminal Neuralgia

Trigeminal neuralgia, also called *tic douloureux*, is a sensory disorder affecting the trigeminal nerve, which innervates the skin of the face, eyelids, and the forehead. The patient feels a very sharp, pulsating pain that can last a few seconds or several minutes. The spasmodic episodes of pain can be stimulated by simply touching the face. The disorder is prevalent in older individuals and generally no specific causes are found. In younger individuals (under 40), the disorder may be caused by multiple sclerosis or pressure placed on the trigeminal nerve by inflammation or tumors.

Clinical Correlation Box 14-4

Lesions of the Lateral Corticospinal Tract

Lesions of the lateral corticospinal tract are injuries to upper motor neurons that can be caused by injury or diseases. Because the fiber tract crosses in the medulla, there is an absence or weakness of voluntary movement on the ipsilateral side below the site of injury. Atrophy of the muscles does not occur, because there is still innervation from the alpha motor neurons (lower motor neurons). The muscle tone is increased, resulting in spasticity. This is caused by the continuation of the stretch reflex, which is normally suppressed by descending tracts.

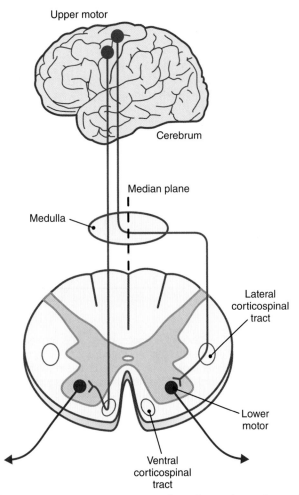

Figure 14–8 Upper motor neurons from the cerebrum descend into the medulla, where 80% of the fibers cross the midline to form the contralateral lateral corticospinal tract. The remaining fibers form the ipsilateral ventral corticospinal tract. The fibers synapse on the lower motor neurons in the ventral horns to innervate the muscles of the trunk.

Clinical Correlation Box 14-5

Poliomyelitis (Polio)

Poliomyelitis (polio) is a virus that attacks the lower motor neurons of the spinal cord and the brain stem. Clinical signs occur on the side of the injury. The muscles innervated by the affected motor neurons are paralyzed or weakened. As a result, there is a reduction in muscle tone. Complete loss of muscle tone is called *flaccid paralysis*, whereas a slight loss is called *flaccid paresis*. The affected muscles undergo atrophy from disuse (*disuse atrophy*).

Head

Similar to the trunk, the upper motor neurons for the head are located in the precentral gyrus. However, the muscles of the head are innervated by lower motor

neurons located in the nuclei of several cranial nerves of the brain stem. Depending on the cranial nerve, the lower motor neurons may receive crossed or uncrossed innervation from upper motor neurons (Fig. 14–9). Disorders are more complex and dependent on the scope of the injury to the brain stem and are beyond the scope of this book. The function of cranial nerve motor neurons will be discussed in Chapter 16.

Review Question Box 14-3

1. Where is the location of the upper motor neurons and lower motor neurons of the trunk and the head?
2. What are the differences between the motor and sensory pathways?

SUMMARY

Three neurons are required for general sensations such as pain, temperature, touch, and proprioception to reach the conscious level (the brain). The route that the neurons take is called a pathway. A sensory stimulus is initiated in receptors that are specific for the various sensory modalities. The stimulus is carried to either the spinal cord or brain stem by the first-order neurons. The nerve cell bodies for these neurons are located in the dorsal root ganglion for the trunk and the trigeminal

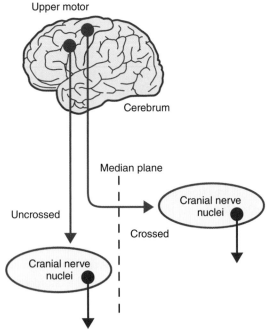

Figure 14–9 The cranial innervation of the lower motor neurons of the head is more complex. The nerve fibers of the upper motor neurons can be either crossed, uncrossed, or both, depending on the cranial nerve.

ganglion for the head. Once entering in the central nervous system, the nerve fibers take alternate courses to synapse on the nerve cell body of the second-order neurons. In the conscious touch and proprioception pathway, fibers that enter below T6 (lower trunk and extremity) ascend in the fasciculus gracilis, whereas fibers that enter above that level (upper trunk and extremity) ascend in the fasciculus cuneatus to synapse with the cell bodies of the second-order neurons in their respective nucleus of the same name in the medulla. The nerve fibers decussate (cross) the midline and ascend to synapse with the nerve cell bodies of the third-order neurons in the thalamus. From there, the fibers synapse in the postcentral gyrus (primary sensory area). For the head, the first-order neurons are located in the trigeminal ganglion and the second-order neurons are located in the chief sensory nucleus of V. The second-order neurons cross to synapse with the third-order neurons in the thalamus, which ascend to the postcentral gyrus.

Second-order neurons for pain temperature of the trunk are located in the ipsilateral dorsal horn, whereas those for the head are located in the spinal nucleus of V. The fibers of the second-order neurons cross to synapse with the third-order neurons in the contralateral thalamus. The fibers of these neurons then synapse in the postcentral gyrus.

The motor pathway consists of two neurons. The upper motor neurons are located in the precentral gyrus (main motor area) and descend to synapse with lower motor neurons in the brain stem and the spinal cord. Eighty percent of the fibers to the spinal cord cross in the medulla and continue as the lateral corticospinal tract; the uncrossed fibers form the ventral corticospinal tract. The innervation of the lower motor neurons of the head is more complex, because some receive crossed, uncrossed, and crossed and uncrossed innervation. The lower motor neurons innervate skeletal muscle (effector).

Injury to the various pathways can cause dysfunction in the sensory and motor pathways.

LEARNING LAB
Exercises for review, practice, and study

Laboratory Activity 14-1

Analyzing the Sensory Pathways

Objective: Learning the sensory pathways for the trunk and head may seem to be a challenging task. However, if you compare the pathways, there are some underlying principles that will make learning the pathways easier. In this exercise, you will analyze the following chart to better understand the pathways.

Principle #1: It takes three neurons to carry information from sensory receptors in the trunk and head to the conscious level in the postcentral gyrus, which is the main sensory area of the cerebrum.

Principle #2: The first neuron is designated as the *first-order* (1°) *neuron*. Its peripheral fibers are attached to the receptor and its central process enters into the spinal cord or brain stem. Its nerve cell body is located in peripheral ganglia.

Principle #3: The second neuron is designated as the *second-order* (2°) *neuron*. Its nerve cell body is located in variable regions, but its axon crosses (X) the midline and ascends to the thalamus.

Principle #4: The nerve cell body of the third neuron, which is designated as the *third-order neuron* (3°), is located in the *thalamus*. Its axon terminates (synapses) on sensory neurons in the *postcentral gyrus*.

Step 1: With these principles in mind, let's analyze the table in Figure 14.10. First, realize the receptors for the conscious touch and proprioception versus the pain and temperature pathway are different. Secondly, the nerve cell bodies of the first-order neurons for both pathways are located in the dorsal root ganglion. However, once the nerve fibers enter the spinal cord, they take two alternate paths.

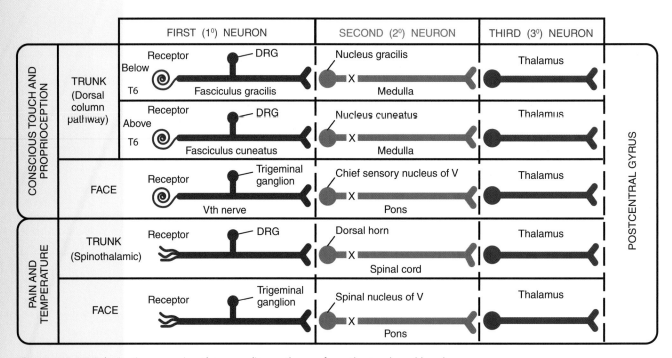

Figure 14–10 Schematic comparing the ascending pathways from the trunk and head.

- For the *conscious touch* and *proprioception* pathway, the axons of the first-order neurons ascend uncrossed in the spinal cord to synapse on the second-order neurons.
  - Sensory fibers for the lower trunk and extremity ascend in the fasciculus gracilis to synapse on the second-order neurons of the nucleus gracilis in the medulla, whereas sensory fibers from the upper trunk and extremity ascend in the fasciculus cuneatus to synapse on the second-order neurons of the nucleus cuneatus.
  - The fibers of the second-order neurons cross the midline and ascend to synapse with the third-order neurons in the thalamus.
  - The nerve fibers of the third-order neuron ascend to synapse in the postcentral gyrus.
- For the *conscious touch* and *proprioception* pathway for the head, the nerve cell bodies of the first-order neurons are located in the trigeminal ganglion, which is analogous to the dorsal root ganglion.
  - Its fibers enter the pons and synapse on the second-order neurons located in the chief sensory nucleus of V.
  - The fibers of the second-order neurons cross the midline and synapse with the third-order neurons in the thalamus.
  - In turn, the fibers of the thalamic neurons (third order) synapse in the postcentral gyrus.

Step 2:   Now let's examine the pain and temperature pathways.

- Note that the nerve cell bodies of the first-order neurons for the trunk are located in the *dorsal root ganglion* and the *trigeminal ganglion* for the head.
- Recognize that the location of the second-order neurons is different for the trunk and the head. In addition, note that the location of the second-order neurons for the pain and temperature pathway is different from the conscious touch and proprioception pathway.
- The nerve cell bodies for the second-order neurons are located in the *dorsal horn* of the spinal cord and the *spinal nucleus of V* for the head.
- Fibers of the second-order neurons cross the midline and synapse on the third-order neurons in the thalamus, which then ascend to synapse in the postcentral gyrus.

For Discussion or Thought:

1. *It is necessary for a specific type of receptor to be stimulated to feel either pain and temperature or conscious touch and proprioception. Additionally, because of the different pathways, injury to one pathway does not necessarily affect the other.*

2. *Structures that are located on the same side (i.e., the right side) are ipsilateral. Nerve fibers cross or decussate the midline to reach the contralateral side (i.e., the left side). How would severing the right half of the spinal cord affect sensory perception on the ipsilateral and contralateral sides of the body?*

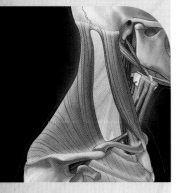

chapter # 15

Autonomic Nervous System

Objectives

1. Describe the structural and functional differences between the somatic nervous system and the autonomic nervous system.
2. Compare the general functional differences between the sympathetic nervous system and the parasympathetic nervous system.
3. Compare the location of the nerve cell bodies of preganglionic neurons and postganglionic neurons of the sympathetic nervous system.
4. Label a diagram of the spinal cord that shows a spinal nerve through the thoracic cord to demonstrate the relationship of the spinal nerves and the sympathetic nervous system.
5. Label and distinguish diagrams of the alternate fiber pathways in the sympathetic nervous system, then discuss the significance of each pathway.

Overview

Movement—that is, contraction of muscle—is part of our everyday life. There is not a time in the day, even while sleeping, in which we are not consciously or unconsciously contracting muscle. Conscious movement, such as walking and talking, involves the voluntary contraction of skeletal muscle by the somatic nervous system. However, breathing, heart rate, digestion, glandular secretion, and perspiration involve the contraction of smooth muscle and cardiac muscles. These activities are considered involuntary and are under the control of the autonomic nervous system. In this chapter, you will study what distinguishes the autonomic nervous system from the somatic nervous system. The division of the autonomic nervous system into the sympathetic and parasympathetic nervous systems will be presented, with emphasis on the sympathetic nervous system. The parasympathetic nervous system will be studied in the next chapter on the cranial nerves.

INTRODUCTION TO THE AUTONOMIC NERVOUS SYSTEM

The **autonomic nervous system** is one of the two efferent (motor) components of the peripheral nervous system; the other is the **somatic nervous system**. The somatic nervous system controls the voluntary movement of skeletal muscles. On the other hand, the autonomic nervous system is involved with the involuntary movement of smooth muscle, glands, and the heart, which are visceral structures. Another major difference is that the somatic nervous system only requires one neuron to carry the stimulus from somatic regions in the spinal cord and brain stem to skeletal muscle (Fig. 15–1A). In contrast, the autonomic nervous system requires two neurons to stimulate the target tissue. The nerve cell bodies of the first neuron are localized in specific areas in the spinal cord and the brain stem. The nerve cell bodies of the second neuron are concentrated in peripheral ganglia that are distant from the spinal cord and brain stem. The first neuron is designated as the **preganglionic neuron**, whereas the neuron whose cell body is located in a ganglion is called the **postganglionic neuron**. The axons arising from the neurons are called **preganglionic fibers** and **postganglionic fibers**, respectively (Fig. 15–1B).

The autonomic nervous system is composed of the **sympathetic nervous system** and the **parasympathetic nervous system**. These two systems generally have opposing functions—that is, the parasympathetic nervous system decreases the heart rate, whereas the sympathetic nervous system increases the heart rate (Table 15–1).

In order for an impulse to travel from one cell to another, neurotransmitters are released into the synaptic space between the cells. In both sympathetic and parasympathetic nervous systems, the neurotransmitter that is released from the fibers of the preganglionic neuron is acetylcholine. The fiber of the postganglionic parasympathetic neuron also secretes acetylcholine, but the fibers of the postganglionic sympathetic neuron secrete adrenaline (epinephrine) into the synaptic space between the neuron and the target tissue—that is, smooth muscle, cardiac muscle, and glands. The dental clinician must consider the patient's medical history before giving injections with epinephrine. Epinephrine added to local anesthetics can cause cardiac arrhythmias in patients with cardiac dysfunction, and thus medically compromise the patient.

Review Question Box 15-1

1. What tissues do the somatic and autonomic nervous systems innervate?
2. Beginning at the spinal cord, how many nerve fibers does it take for the somatic and autonomic nervous systems to reach their target tissues?
3. What is the name of the fibers and location of their nerve cell bodies for the autonomic nervous system?

SYMPATHETIC NERVOUS SYSTEM

The sympathetic nervous system is alternatively called the **thoracolumbar nervous system** because the nerve cell bodies of **preganglionic sympathetic neurons** are located in the **intermediolateral cell column (IMLCC)** between spinal segments **T1 to L2**. Recall that the spinal cord is divided into white matter and gray matter. The gray matter is divided into the dorsal horn (sensory) and the ventral (motor) horn. As the name implies, the IMLCC is a projection of the gray matter that is lateral and between the two horns. The nerve cell bodies of *postganglionic neurons* are located in the **sympathetic ganglion**, which is attached to a **spinal nerve**. The sympathetic ganglia are connected by fibers that form the **sympathetic trunk** (Fig. 15–2). The sympathetic trunk and ganglia extend from the cervical region to the sacrum. At the level of T1 to L2, each sympathetic ganglion is attached to the spinal nerve by a **white communicating ramus** and a **gray communicating ramus** (Fig. 15–2). In other levels of the spinal cord, the sympathetic ganglia are only attached to the spinal nerve by a gray communicating ramus.

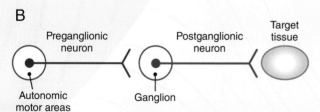

A

Motor neuron

Skeletal muscle

Somatic motor areas

B

Preganglionic neuron

Postganglionic neuron

Target tissue

Autonomic motor areas

Ganglion

Figure 15–1 (A) The innervation of skeletal muscle only requires a single motor neuron whose nerve cell bodies are located in the somatic areas of the spinal cord and brain stem. **(B)** Innervation of smooth muscle, cardiac muscle, and glands require two neurons. The nerve cell body of the preganglionic neuron is located in the autonomic areas of the spinal cord and brain stem, whereas the cell bodies of the postganglionic neurons are located in autonomic ganglia.

TABLE 15–1	Comparison of Effects of the Sympathetic and Parasympathetic Nervous Systems	
Organ	**Effect of Sympathetic Stimulation**	**Effect of Parasympathetic Stimulation**

Eye:
  Pupil
  Ciliary body (muscle)
	Dilation	Constriction

Lacrimal gland	No secretory function	Secretion
Salivary glands	Scanty, thick secretion	Copious, thin secretion
Heart	Increased rate Increased force of contraction	Slowed rate
Bronchioles of the lungs	Dilation	Constriction
Gut	Decreased peristalsis and secretion	Increased peristalsis and secretion
Adrenal medulla	Secretion	None
Skin of the head, the neck, and extremities	Vasoconstriction, sweat secretion, piloerection	None
Blood vessels	Vasoconstriction	None

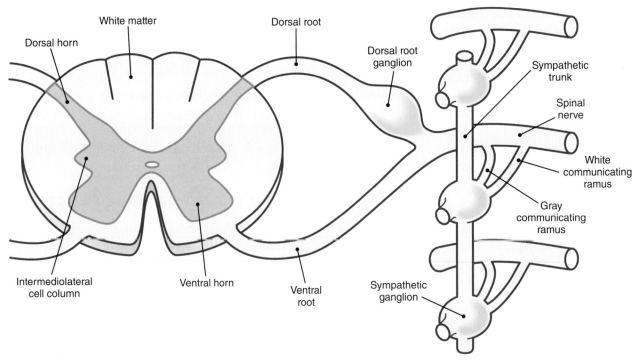

Figure 15–2 A cross section through the spinal cord at the level of the intermediolateral cell column illustrates the relationship of the lateral ganglia of the sympathetic trunk to the spinal nerves. The ganglia are attached by the white and gray communicating rami.

The preganglionic sympathetic fibers (axons) leave the spinal cord through the ventral (motor) root of the spinal cord and enter into the spinal nerve. The fibers then follow the white communicating ramus to reach the ganglion of the sympathetic trunk. The ganglia of the sympathetic chain (chain ganglion) are also called **lateral** or **vertebral ganglia** because of their location next to the vertebral column. Other sympathetic ganglia form plexuses that are located on the surface of the aorta and innervate the viscera of the abdomen. These ganglia are called **collateral ganglia** because they course parallel to the sympathetic trunk, but are located on the surface of the aorta. Alternately, these ganglia are called **prevertebral ganglia** because they are located anterior to the vertebral column (Fig. 15–3).

4. The visceral organs of the neck and thorax are innervated by nerves that branch from the medial aspect of ganglia of the sympathetic trunk.
5. Viscera in the abdomen and pelvis are innervated by collateral ganglia that surround the major branches of the abdominal aorta.
6. To reach the various lateral and collateral ganglia, the preganglionic fibers must ascend or descend in the sympathetic trunk to reach the proper ganglion.

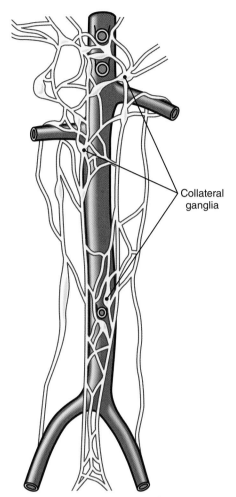

Figure 15–3 The collateral ganglia of the sympathetic nervous system are located along the major branches of the abdominal aorta.

Collateral ganglia

Once the preganglionic nerve fibers reach the lateral ganglion, it can take several alternative pathways. To understand the distribution of the sympathetic fibers, the following principles need to be considered:

1. All preganglionic sympathetic neurons are located in the IMLCC of spinal segments T1 to L2, but the postganglionic neurons are located in either the lateral ganglia of the sympathetic trunk that runs from the cervical region to the sacral region or the collateral ganglia on the abdominal aorta.
2. All preganglionic sympathetic fibers exit the spinal cord through the ventral root and enter into the white communicating ramus to reach the lateral ganglia.
3. Some postganglionic sympathetic fibers exit the lateral ganglia by the gray communicating ramus on the lateral surface of the ganglia and return to the spinal nerve to innervate the smooth muscle of blood vessels in the body wall, and the glands and erector pili (smooth muscle) in the skin.

Review Question Box 15-2

1. What spinal segments contain white communicating rami and why?
2. What is the location of the nerve cell bodies for all preganglionic sympathetic fibers?
3. Where are the locations of the nerve cell bodies for postganglionic sympathetic fibers?

Innervation of the Body Wall at the Same Spinal Segment

The preganglionic sympathetic fibers leave the spinal cord through the ventral roots and enter into the spinal nerve. The nerve fibers then enter the white communicating ramus to synapse with the postganglionic neuron in the sympathetic ganglion (Fig. 15–4). The postganglionic fibers exit the ganglion through the gray communicating ramus and re-enter the spinal nerve and are distributed to the smooth muscle of blood vessels and the erector pili muscle of the skin, as well as glands (Fig. 15–4).

Postganglionic Fibers to the Higher and Lower Spinal Segments

As mentioned earlier, only the thoracic and first two lumbar segments have white communicating rami (Fig. 15–5). Therefore, the lateral ganglia in the cervical region, lower lumbar region, and sacral region do not receive preganglionic sympathetic fibers from their respective segments of the spinal cord. Thus, preganglionic fibers must ascend or descend to reach these ganglia. After leaving the spinal cord, preganglionic fibers enter the *lateral ganglia* via the white communicating ramus, but do not synapse in the ganglion (Fig. 15–5). However, instead of synapsing in the ganglion, the nerve courses either superiorly to the cervical region or inferiorly to the lower lumbar and sacral regions via the fibers of the sympathetic trunk

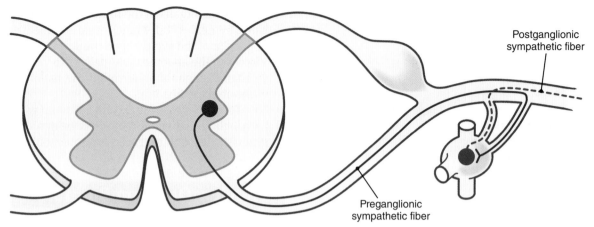

Figure 15–4 In the basic pathway for the sympathetic nervous system, preganglionic fibers leave their preganglionic nerve cell bodies (red), which are located in the intermediolateral cell column, via the ventral roots of the spinal cord. The preganglionic fibers enter the lateral ganglia through the white communicating ramus and synapse with the nerve cell bodies of the postganglionic neurons (blue). The postganglionic nerve fibers exit the gray communicating ramus to join the spinal nerve at the same spinal segment level.

that connect the lateral ganglia (Fig. 15–5). Once the preganglionic nerve fibers reach the appropriate level, the fibers synapse with the postganglionic sympathetic neuron. The postganglionic sympathetic fibers then exit the ganglion through the gray communicating ramus to enter the spinal nerve to be distributed to smooth muscles of blood vessels and structures in the skin (Fig. 15–5).

Review Question Box 15-3

1. How do the postganglionic sympathetic fibers enter into the spinal nerves?
2. Why must preganglionic sympathetic fibers travel up or down to reach cervical, lumbar, and sacral ganglia of the sympathetic trunk?

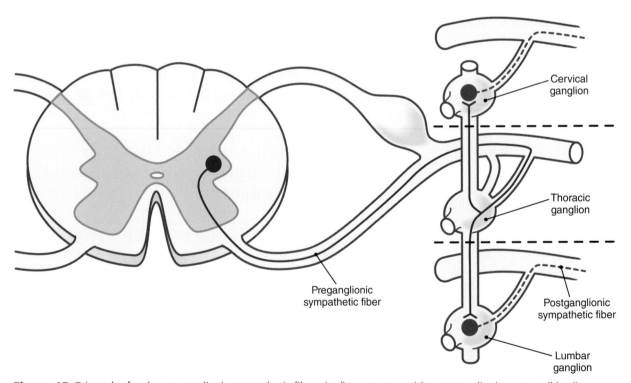

Figure 15–5 In order for the preganglionic sympathetic fibers (red) to synapse with postganglionic nerve cell bodies (blue) in the lateral ganglia of the cervical, lower lumbar, and sacral regions, the fibers must ascend or descend within the sympathetic trunk. Note that cervical and lower lumbar ganglia only have a gray communicating ramus, which contains the postganglionic sympathetic fibers. Only the thoracic ganglia have white communicating rami that contain preganglionic sympathetic fibers.

Innervation of the Thoracic Viscera

The visceral organs of the thorax—the heart, lungs, trachea, and esophagus—are not innervated by spinal nerves. Therefore, the postganglionic sympathetic fibers must take an alternative pathway. The preganglionic sympathetic fibers leave the spinal cord through the ventral root, enter the spinal nerve, and follow the white communicating ramus into the lateral ganglion (Fig. 15–6). The preganglionic sympathetic fibers can synapse with postganglionic neurons at the same segment level or ascend the trunk to synapse in neurons in the cervical ganglia. The postganglionic fibers exit the ganglia through a **visceral nerve** on its medial surface (toward the vertebral column). Visceral nerves from several ganglia form a *plexus* of nerves that innervate the visceral organs.

Innervation of the Viscera of the Abdomen

The visceral organs of the abdomen are separated from the thorax by the diaphragm. The ganglia of the sympathetic trunk do not innervate the visceral organs, but rather are innervated by *collateral ganglia* that are located on the surface of the aorta (Fig. 15–3). Thus, the preganglionic fibers must take an alternate route to reach these ganglia.

After leaving the spinal cord, preganglionic fibers enter the lateral ganglia via the white communicating ramus, but do not synapse in the ganglion (Fig 15–7). Fibers leave the ganglia through **splanchnic** (a term to describe the visceral organs) **nerves** that pass through the diaphragm to synapse on the postganglionic neurons in the collateral ganglia. The postganglionic sympathetic fibers then follow the path of blood vessels to reach the target organs. The splanchnic nerves leave the lateral ganglia on their medial side, similar to the visceral nerves. However, *visceral nerves contain postganglionic fibers*, whereas the fibers in *splanchnic nerves are preganglionic sympathetic fibers*.

Review Question Box 15-4

1. What is the difference between a lateral ganglion and a collateral ganglion?
2. What is the difference between spinal nerves and visceral nerves?

Innervation of the Adrenal Gland

The innervation of the adrenal gland is unusual in that preganglionic sympathetic fibers synapse with cells within the *adrenal medulla* (Fig. 15–8). The adrenal medulla has the same function as the *postganglionic sympathetic neurons*; however, because it is an endocrine

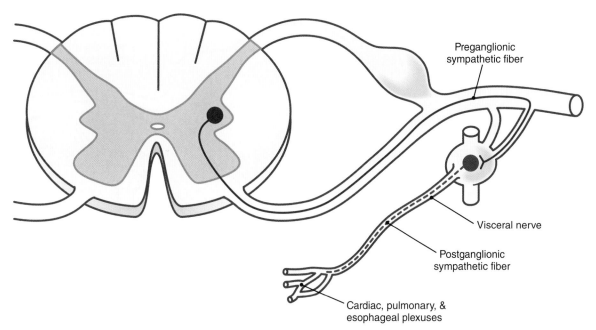

Figure 15–6 Visceral organs of the thorax are innervated by nerve plexuses. Postganglionic sympathetic fibers (blue) contribute to the plexuses by traveling through visceral nerves that exit the medial surface of the lateral ganglia; preganglionic nerve fibers (red) synapse with the postganglionic sympathetic neurons in sympathetic ganglion.

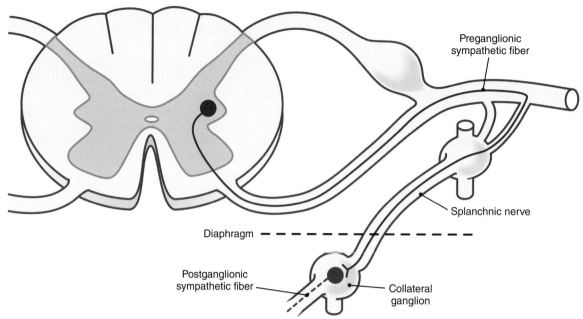

Figure 15–7 The postganglionic sympathetic nerve cell bodies (blue) of the abdominal viscera are located in the collateral ganglia. Preganglionic sympathetic fibers (red) enter through the lateral ganglia of the sympathetic trunk, but do not synapse with neurons of the lateral ganglia. The fibers continue through the splanchnic nerves to synapse with the postganglionic nerve cell bodies in the collateral ganglia.

gland it affects the entire body. Preganglionic fibers enter into the plexus of nerves on the abdominal aorta and follow the blood vessels into the organ. The nerve terminates in the adrenal medulla causing the release of norepinephrine (or adrenaline); hence the "adrenaline rush" during stress, or the so-called "flight or fight" response.

Review Question Box 15-5

1. What is the pathway by which all preganglionic sympathetic fibers enter the ganglia of the sympathetic trunk?
2. Why can the cells of the adrenal medulla be considered analogous to postganglionic sympathetic neurons?

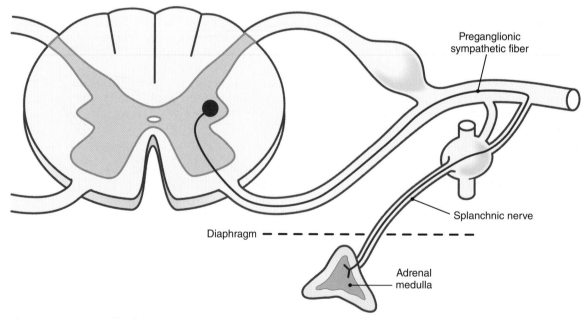

Figure 15–8 The cells of the adrenal medulla are considered to be functionally similar to postganglionic sympathetic neurons. These cells are innervated by preganglionic sympathetic nerve fibers (red) that pass through the splanchnic nerves.

PARASYMPATHETIC NERVOUS SYSTEM

The parasympathetic nervous system is alternatively called the **craniosacral nervous system** because the preganglionic parasympathetic neurons are located in some of the sacral segments of the spinal cord and some of the cranial nerves. The sacral component supplies the pelvic viscera and will not be discussed. The cranial component is of great interest to the dental hygienist, because the cranial nerves control the secretion of the salivary glands, slow the heart rate, as well as change the shape of the lens and constrict the pupil of the eye. The preganglionic parasympathetic fibers arise from neurons located in nuclei of the **oculomotor**, **facial**, **glossopharyngeal**, and **vagus nerves** (Table 15–2). These fibers can take a relatively tortuous pathway to synapse with postganglionic parasympathetic neurons that are located in four ganglia outside of the cranial cavity (Table 15–2). The postganglionic parasympathetic fibers join branches of the trigeminal nerve to reach their target tissues. The details of these pathways will be discussed in Chapter 16.

Review Question Box 15-6

1. Which cranial nerves contain preganglionic parasympathetic neurons?
2. How do the postganglionic parasympathetic fibers reach their target tissues?

SUMMARY

The autonomic nervous system is the portion of the peripheral nervous system that innervates smooth muscle, cardiac muscle, and glands. The autonomic nervous system is subdivided into sympathetic and parasympathetic nervous systems. Even though these systems generally have opposing effects on their target organs, they work together to maintain homeostasis in the body. Unlike the somatic nervous system, which requires only one neuron to innervate skeletal muscle, the autonomic nervous system requires two neurons. The nerve cell bodies of the preganglionic neurons are located in specific areas of the spinal cord and brain stem. Preganglionic sympathetic neurons are located in the intermediolateral cell column of spinal segments T1 to L2, whereas those for the parasympathetic nervous system are located in the sacral region of the spinal cord and the parasympathetic nuclei of the oculomotor, facial, glossopharyngeal, and vagus nerves (cranial nerves). The nerve cell bodies of the postganglionic sympathetic neurons are located in the lateral ganglia of the sympathetic trunk and the collateral ganglia on the surface of the abdominal aorta. The nerve cell bodies of the postganglionic parasympathetic neurons are located in parasympathetic ganglia outside the cranial cavity. Depending on the location of the target organ, the preganglionic and postganglionic sympathetic fibers have alternate pathways. In the basic pathway, preganglionic sympathetic fibers synapse with postganglionic sympathetic neurons in the lateral ganglia at the same spinal cord level. For the cervical, lower lumbar, and sacral regions, the preganglionic sympathetic fibers must ascend or descend in the sympathetic trunk to synapse in lateral ganglia. For the thoracic viscera, the postganglionic sympathetic fibers reach their target organs via visceral nerves, whereas for the abdominal visceral, preganglionic sympathetic fibers pass through the lateral ganglia and exit through splanchnic nerves to synapse with neurons in the collateral ganglia. The parasympathetic nervous system is more complex and will be studied in a later chapter.

TABLE 15–2	Summary of the Location and Distribution of the Parasympathetic Nervous System		
Cranial Nerve	Location of Preganglionic Neurons	Location of Postganglionic Neurons	Distribution of Fibers
III Oculomotor	Nucleus of Edinger–Westphal	Ciliary ganglion	Pupil Ciliary muscle
VII Facial	Superior salivatory nucleus	1. Pterygopalatine ganglion 2. Submandibular ganglion	1. Lacrimal gland Palatine glands 2. Submandibular gland Sublingual gland
IX Glossopharyngeal	Inferior salivatory nucleus	Otic ganglion	Parotid gland
X Vagus	Dorsal motor nucleus	Visceral autonomic ganglia	Heart Lungs GI tract

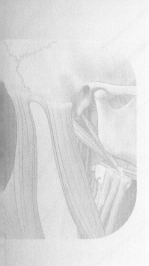

LEARNING LAB

Exercises for review, practice, and study

Laboratory Activity 15-1

Comparing the Functions of the Sympathetic and Parasympathetic Nervous Systems

The sympathetic and parasympathetic nervous systems regulate the contraction of smooth muscle, cardiac muscle, and glandular secretion. Most of the visceral organs are innervated by both systems, generally producing opposite effects. In this way, our bodies are maintained at balance during everyday activities, but can adjust to restful activities such as sleep, and stressful activities such as exercise or even taking an exam. Even though you have not studied the details of autonomic function, you should be able to predict changes in homeostasis (balance) of various activities by consulting Table 15–1 and the information introduced in this chapter.

Scenario 1: You have been jogging with a friend in the hot sun for 30 minutes. During that time, your heart rate increases and you experience a pounding in your heart. In addition, you are breathing deeper and faster and you are perspiring (sweating). Your jogging partner tells you that your pupils look very small. Which of the following is attributed to either the sympathetic or parasympathetic nervous system?

A. Increased heart rate

B. Increased force of contraction

C. Increased breathing rate

D. Increased perspiration

E. Shift of blood supply from the digestive system to the skeletal muscle

F. Decreased pupil size

    The answer to A through E is the sympathetic nervous system. The shift of blood supply from the digestive system to the skeletal system may not be obvious at first. However, the blood supply to the digestive system is reduced by contraction of smooth muscle to bypass the capillary beds and allow a greater nutrient supply to the muscles. As you will study later, the light from the sun caused the pupils to constrict via the parasympathetic nervous system.

Scenario 2: A patient is nervously sitting in the dental chair waiting to undergo an endodontic procedure. She explains that her heart is racing and her chest is pounding. She also complains that her mouth is very dry. What autonomic system is producing the following responses?

A. Increased heart rate and force of contraction

B. Dry mouth from decreased saliva

    The answer to both A and B is the sympathetic nervous system.

Scenario 3: You are having a leisurely meal at your favorite restaurant with a friend. Your heart and breathing rate are normal, but the aroma of the food being prepared in the kitchen makes your mouth water. What is the autonomic response to the following activities?

A. Increased secretion of saliva

B. No increase in heart rate

    The answer to A is the parasympathetic nervous system. For B, the heart rate did not increase because there was not a significant change in either the sympathetic or parasympathetic nervous systems.

For Discussion or Thought:

1. *What conditions changed in the three scenarios that determined whether the parasympathetic or sympathetic component of the autonomic nervous system was dominant?*

Learning Activity 15-1

Sympathetic Nervous System

Match the numbered structures with the correct terms listed below.

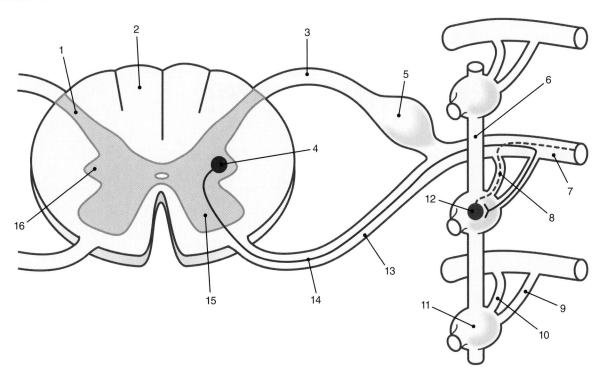

_____ Dorsal horn

_____ Dorsal root

_____ Dorsal root ganglion

_____ Gray communicating ramus

_____ Intermediolateral cell column

_____ Postganglionic sympathetic fiber

_____ Postganglionic sympathetic neuron

_____ Preganglionic sympathetic fiber

_____ Preganglionic sympathetic neuron

_____ Spinal nerve

_____ Sympathetic ganglion

_____ Sympathetic trunk

_____ Ventral horn

_____ Ventral root

_____ White communicating ramus

_____ White matter

16

Cranial Nerves

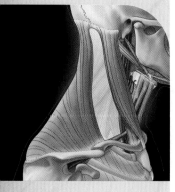

Objectives

1. Define the term *cranial nerves*.
2. Compare the anatomical features of cranial and spinal nerves.
3. Compare the fiber types of the cranial nerves.
4. For each cranial nerve, be able to discuss the (1) location in the central nervous system, (2) passage of fibers out of the cranial cavity, (3) fiber types and their origin, (4) general function of the nerve, (5) target structures, (6) major pathways of nerve fibers, and (7) how they are clinically tested.

Overview

Picture this scene from a television rescue drama. It is a dark, gloomy night. An ambulance arrives at a car accident scene where people surround an accident victim. Eyewitnesses are explaining to the police that an elderly man crossing the street was hit by a pickup truck driven by a young man. The driver was not speeding, but apparently did not see the man as he was turning the corner of an intersection. The truck hit the man in the back, and as he fell, his head struck the curb. The attending paramedics rush to the accident victim and immediately start checking his vital signs. The victim has an irregular heartbeat and is breathing with difficulty. His blood pressure is low, and there are signs of external bleeding. The paramedics start an IV solution and continue their examination. The accident victim is conscious, but does not remember what happened to him. One of the paramedics shines a small light into his eyes, then raises a finger and asks the victim how many fingers he can see. Next the paramedic asks the victim to follow his finger as he moves it from left to right and up and down. The paramedic checks the victim's facial features, and everything appears normal. Although the victim is dazed from the accident, he does not feel dizzy and has no signs of nausea. His back is bruised and sore, but he is able to shrug his shoulders.

On request, the victim can stick out his tongue without deviation to one side. The victim is rushed to the hospital for further examination. After 2 days of observation in the intensive care unit, the elderly man is released from the hospital with a badly bruised back, no broken bones, and normal vital signs.

The paramedic in this scenario was testing the accident victim's cranial nerve functions to determine possible neurological damage to his head caused by the trauma. Although hygienists may check their patients' blood pressure and pulse, testing the functions of all the cranial nerves is not normally necessary. However, you may treat medically compromised patients, and a medical emergency could occur with a patient in your care. In this chapter, you will study the 12 cranial nerves and their functions, and learn what the testing of cranial nerves indicates.

INTRODUCTION TO CRANIAL NERVES

There are 12 pairs of cranial nerves that arise from the brain and spinal cord and exit through foramina in the cranial cavity to innervate structures in the head and neck. Although each nerve is named, the nerves are also designated by Roman numerals numbered sequentially from an anterior to posterior direction.

COMPARISON OF CRANIAL NERVES AND SPINAL NERVES

To understand cranial nerves, it is best to compare them to spinal nerves. Spinal nerves are formed by the dorsal and ventral roots, which are attached to the spinal cord. Three fiber types are found in spinal nerves: *efferent fibers to skeletal muscle, afferent fibers* (Chapter 14), and *autonomic fibers to smooth muscle, cardiac muscle, and glands* (Chapter 15). The efferent fibers arise from the motor neurons within the ventral horn of the gray matter. The afferent fibers arise from the sensory neurons in the dorsal root ganglia and enter the spinal cord through the dorsal root (see Fig. 14–2). The preganglionic fibers originate from the neurons located in the intermediolateral cell column (Chapter 15) in the thoracolumbar region for the sympathetic nervous system and from the sacral region for the parasympathetic nervous system. The preganglionic sympathetic fibers gain access to the ganglia of the sympathetic trunk through the white communicating ramus, and the fibers of the postganglionic sympathetic neurons leave through the gray communicating ramus (see Fig. 15–2). The sacral autonomic fibers take an alternate pathway to innervate the pelvic organs and will not be discussed in this book.

Unlike spinal nerves, the cranial nerves do not contain the same fiber types. Some cranial nerves are either motor or sensory in function (Table 16–1). Thus, most

TABLE 16–1	Comparison of Spinal Nerves to Cranial Nerves
Spinal Nerves	**Cranial Nerves**
Have separate motor and sensory roots	Most do not have separate motor and sensory roots
Have sensory ganglia	Some have none, whereas others may have two
Contain preganglionic sympathetic fibers	No preganglionic sympathetic fibers
Have white and gray communicating rami	No communicating rami

cranial nerves do not have separate motor and cranial roots. Not all cranial nerves have sensory ganglia, while others may have two. Cranial nerves do not contain preganglionic sympathetic fibers, but some may have preganglionic parasympathetic fibers (Table 16–1). Unlike spinal nerves, cranial nerves do not have white and gray communicating rami (Table 16–1).

General Versus Special Sensation

Afferent modalities (sensory information) from peripheral receptors are categorized as either **general** or **special sensation**. Pain, temperature, touch, and pressure are examples of general sensation. These sensations arise from receptors that are spread throughout the entire body. General sensation is associated with both cranial and spinal nerves. However, only the receptors for cranial nerves perceive the special sensations of taste, smell, vision, hearing, and equilibrium. The receptors for these senses are localized in small distinct areas such as the retina, olfactory area of the nasal cavity, the internal ear, and taste buds.

Review Question Box 16-1

1. What fiber type is found in spinal nerves, but is not in cranial nerves?
2. What fiber type is found cranial nerves, but is not in spinal nerves?

CRANIAL NERVES

The cranial nerves are numbered from anterior to posterior according to where they exit through openings in the floor of the cranial cavity and their attachments to the central nervous system (Fig. 16–1; Table 16–2).

Cranial Nerve I

The **olfactory nerve** (**I**), unlike most cranial nerves, is attached to the cerebrum (Table 16–2) and contains fibers that only carry the special sensation of *smell* (Table 16–3). Structures generally identified as the olfactory nerve on the ventral surface of the brain (Fig. 16–1)

are actually extensions of the cerebrum and not a peripheral nerve. Recall that peripheral nerves extend from the central nervous system to either effectors (muscle) or, in this case, to receptors. The first-order neurons (Chapter 14) are located within a specialized area (olfactory epithelium) of the nasal mucosa that covers the roof of the nasal cavity and extends onto the surface of the upper portions of the superior nasal conchae and the nasal septum (Fig. 16–2). The connective tissue under the olfactory epithelium contains olfactory glands that secrete a serous fluid that moistens the epithelium. The peripheral processes of the neurons project beyond the surface of the epithelium and function as sensory receptors, which are stimulated by chemicals. Therefore, aromatic molecules must dissolve in the nasal secretions to stimulate the receptors. The central processes of the first-order neuron form several nerve filaments that pass through the opening of the cribriform plate of the ethmoid bone. The nerves synapse on second-order neurons (Chapter 14) within the **olfactory bulbs** (Fig. 16–2), which lie on the cranial surface of the cribriform plate on either side of the crista galli. The sensory information is relayed to the olfactory areas of the

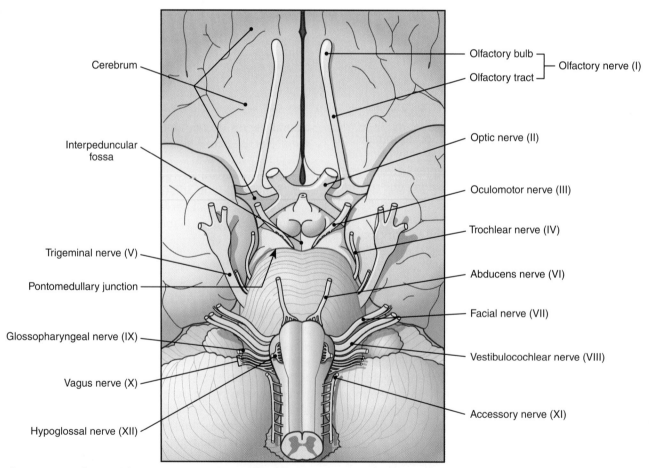

Figure 16–1 The cranial nerves are viewed ventrally with their respective attachments to the cerebrum, diencephalon, medulla, and spinal cord. The olfactory (I) nerve is represented by the olfactory tract and bulb. Note that the attachment of the trochlear (IV) nerve is out of view because it arises off the dorsal surface of the midbrain.

TABLE 16–2	Cranial Nerve Attachments to the CNS and Exit Points From the Cranial Cavity		
	Cranial Nerve	**Attachment to the CNS**	**Exit Point**
I	Olfactory	Cerebrum	Cribriform plate
II	Optic	Diencephalon	Optic canal
III	Oculomotor	Midbrain	Superior orbital fissure
IV	Trochlear	Midbrain below the inferior colliculus	Superior orbital fissure
V	Trigeminal	Pons	Ophthalmic division—superior orbital fissure Maxillary division—foramen rotundum Mandibular division—foramen ovale
VI	Abducens	Pontomedullary junction	Superior orbital fissure
VII	Facial	Pontomedullary junction	Internal acoustic meatus
VIII	Vestibulocochlear	Pontomedullary junction	Internal acoustic meatus
IX	Glossopharyngeal	Medulla	Jugular foramen
X	Vagus	Medulla	Jugular foramen
XI	Accessory	Cervical spinal cord	Jugular foramen
XII	Hypoglossal	Medulla	Hypoglossal canal

cerebrum by the **olfactory tract** (Fig. 16–1). The olfactory areas are connected to centers that control salivation as when smelling something pleasant, or nausea when smelling an unpleasant odor.

Cranial Nerve II

The **optic nerve** (**II**) carries special sensory information concerning *vision* from the retina (Table 16–3). The retina is formed by a complex layering of neurons and

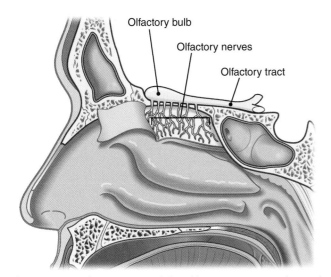

Figure 16–2 The receptors of the olfactory nerves are located in the epithelium in the superior region of the nasal cavity, as viewed by this sagittal section. The nerves pass through the cribriform plate to synapse in the olfactory bulbs. Nerve fibers continue through the olfactory tract to reach the cerebrum.

Olfactory bulb

Olfactory nerves

Olfactory tract

Clinical Correlation Box 16-1

Shearing of the olfactory nerves can occur from a horizontal fracture of the cribriform plate caused by trauma to the head while diving into water or a car accident. This can cause the loss of smell on the ipsilateral (same) side of the fracture. Additionally, cerebral spinal fluid, which supplies nutrition and protects the brain and spinal cord, can leak from the subarachnoid space and enter into the nasal cavity. Conversely, air and the contents of the nasal cavity (including infectious microorganisms) can enter into the cranial cavity.

nerve fibers. Photoreceptors—the rods and cones—are located in the deepest layer of the **retina** (Fig. 16–3). The cones perceive color and function better in bright light. The rods are more sensitive than the cones and can function in low light, but cannot perceive color. Photoreceptors transfer information to the ganglion cell layer at the surface of the retina. Axons from these cells form the optic nerve and enter into the cranial cavity through the optic canal (Table 16–2). The axons of the nasal half of the retina cross in the **optic chiasm** to reach the contralateral cerebral cortex. The axons continue through as the **optic tract** carrying information to relay to areas in the **thalamus** before reaching the visual area in the occipital lobe (Fig. 16–4). Some axons pass to the superior colliculus for visual reflexes (see the next section).

TABLE 16–3	Summary of Cranial Nerve Functions and Fiber Types	
Nerve	**Fibers***	**General Functions (Not inclusive)**
Olfactory	S	Smell
Optic	S	Vision
Oculomotor	M, P	Eye movement, pupillary constriction, and rounding of the lens
Trochlear	M	Eye movement
Trigeminal	M, S	Motor to the muscles of mastication; general sensation to the face, mouth, teeth, and anterior two-thirds of the tongue
Abducens	M	Eye movement
Facial	M, S, P	Motor to the muscles of facial expression; taste to the anterior two-thirds of the tongue and soft palate; motor to the submandibular and sublingual salivary glands
Vestibulocochlear	S	Hearing, equilibrium, and balance
Glossopharyngeal	M, S, P	Motor to a muscle of the pharynx; general sensation to the pharyngeal wall; general sensation and taste to the posterior one-third of the tongue; motor to the parotid gland
Vagus	M, S, P	Motor to the muscles of the larynx, pharynx, and palate; visceral sensation; motor to the organs of the thorax and abdomen
Accessory	M	Motor to the trapezius and sternocleidomastoid muscles
Hypoglossal	M	Motor to the muscles of the tongue

*S = sensory; M = motor; P = parasympathetic

Box 16-1 Visual Pathways

The nose divides our view into left and right visual fields and blocks light reflecting off an object from directly entering the eyes from all directions. Functionally, each retina is divided into nasal and temporal hemiretinas (half retinas). In Figure 16–4, light emitted from the object in the right visual field (red) strikes the temporal hemiretina of the left eye and the nasal hemiretina of the right eye. Photoreceptors in the retina transfer the information to the brain through the optic nerves. The nasal fibers cross at the optic chiasm and join the temporal fibers of the left retina to form the left optic tract. The optic tract carries the information from the opposite visual field, in this case the right, to the thalamus or the superior colliculus. Fibers from the thalamus synapse in the primary visual cortex of the occipital lobe. Alternatively, some fibers synapse with neurons in the superior colliculus. Nerve fibers leave the superior colliculus and synapse with preganglionic parasympathetic neurons in the nucleus of Edinger–Westphal of the oculomotor nerve, which then synapse in the ciliary ganglion. Postganglionic parasympathetic fibers cause the pupil to constrict, thus protecting the retina from bright light.

Review Question Box 16-2

1. Why is the olfactory tract and bulb called the *olfactory nerve*, but the optic tract is not called the optic nerve?
2. What fiber type is found in both olfactory and optic nerves?

Cranial Nerve III

The **oculomotor nerve (III)** exits the brain stem anterior to the pons and can be seen in the depression between the cerebral peduncles known as the **interpeduncular fossa** (Fig. 16–1). The nerve exits the cranial cavity through the superior orbital fissure to reach the orbit (Table 16–2). The nerve contains motor fibers, which supply skeletal muscle, and parasympathetic fibers, which supply smooth muscle. The *motor fibers*, which supply skeletal muscle, arise from a cluster of nuclei called the *oculomotor complex*. These fibers supply the levator muscle of the upper eyelid, and four of the six extrinsic (meaning "outside of") muscles that control the movement of the eyeball. The **superior rectus muscle** (Fig. 16–5) elevates and adducts the eye toward the nose, the **inferior rectus muscle** (Fig. 16–5) depresses (lowers) and adducts the eye toward the temporal region, the **medial rectus muscle** (Fig. 16–5) adducts the eye, and

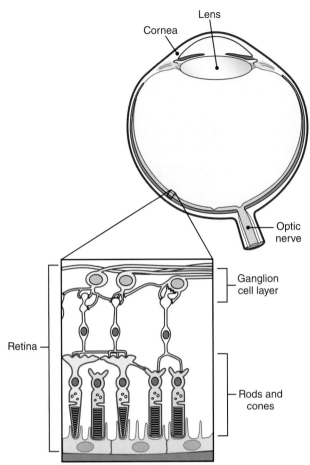

Figure 16–3 The rods and cones are photoreceptors located in the deep layers of the retina. The optic nerve is formed from axons arising from neurons in the ganglion cell layer.

the **superior oblique muscle** (Fig. 16–5) lowers and abducts the eye (Table 16–4). The oculomotor nerve contains *preganglionic parasympathetic fibers* that arise from neurons in the nucleus of Edinger–Westphal and synapse on postganglionic parasympathetic neurons in the **ciliary ganglion** (Fig. 16–4). The postganglionic parasympathetic fibers innervate the smooth muscle of the eye, which constrict the pupil in response to light and round the lens to accommodate near vision (Fig. 16–4 and Table 16–3).

Cranial Nerve IV

The **trochlear nerve** (**IV**) is the only cranial nerve that arises from the dorsal surface of the midbrain just caudal to the inferior colliculus. It courses through the superior orbital fissure to enter the orbit (Table 16–2). The nerve contains motor fibers that only innervate the *superior oblique muscle* (Table 16–3), which depresses and abducts the eye (Fig. 16–5 and Table 16–4). Injury to this nerve is not common. When it does occur, the individual will tilt his or her head toward the affected side to realign the eye to read or look downward.

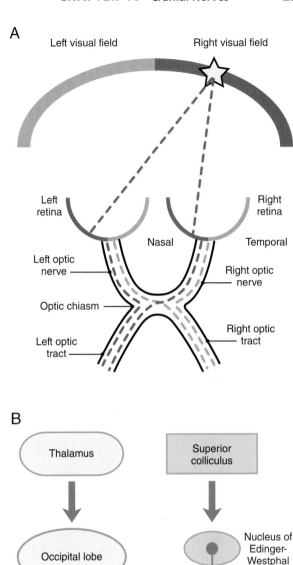

Figure 16–4 (A) The retina is divided functionally into temporal (lateral) and nasal (medial) hemiretinas (half of a retina). Light reflecting off an object from the right visual field strikes the photoreceptors in the temporal hemiretina on the left side and the nasal hemiretina on the right side. Visual information is carried by the optic nerves toward the brain. The right nasal fibers cross in the optic chiasm to join the temporal fibers of the left eye to form the optic tract. **(B)** The fibers have two alternate pathways. The fibers can synapse in the thalamus and the information can be relayed to the occipital lobe. Alternatively, the fibers can synapse in the superior colliculus, which can initiate the papillary reflex.

Because of the proximity of the pituitary gland to the optic chiasm, a tumor of the gland can affect vision. The growth of the tumor can place pressure on the nasal crossing fibers in the chiasm. Therefore, there is a loss of vision in the nasal hemiretinas of both eyes, which affects peripheral vision.

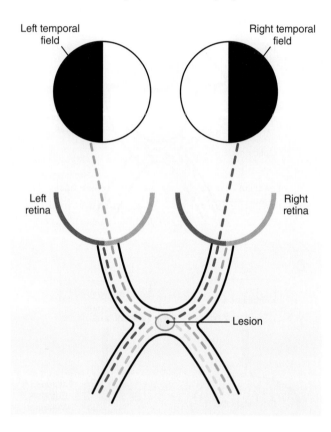

Cranial Nerve V

The **trigeminal nerve** (**V**) is the largest and most complex of the cranial nerves. It is attached by motor and sensory roots to the lateral aspect of the pons (Fig. 16-1 and Table 16-3). The trigeminal nerve is the major sensory nerve of the head and oral cavity and its motor components innervate the muscles of mastication (Table 16-3). Thus, the trigeminal nerve is clinically important to the dental hygienist. Nerve cell bodies of the sensory neurons are located in the trigeminal ganglion. The peripheral fibers form three distinct bundles, which are called *divisions*, as they exit the ganglion (Fig. 16-6). The **ophthalmic division**, which is also designated as V_1, exits the cranial cavity via the superior orbital fissure (Fig. 16-6) to supply sensory fibers to the orbit and the anterior portion of the scalp (Tables 16-2 and 16-3). The maxillary division, V_2, leaves through the foramen rotundum (Fig. 16-6) to supply sensory fibers to the nasal

Box 16-2 Pupillary Reflex

When bright light enters the eyes, the pupil will automatically constrict to protect the retina. The **pupillary light reflex**, as this automatic response is called, is initiated by the optic nerve. Not all visual information reaches the visual cortex. Fibers of the ganglion cells (first-order neurons) can bypass the thalamus and synapse within the *superior colliculus*, which is a relay nucleus in the midbrain (Fig. 16-4). Axons from this nucleus synapse on preganglionic parasympathetic neurons located in the *nucleus of Edinger–Westphal*, which is part of a complex of nuclei that form the oculomotor nerve. The postganglionic parasympathetic neurons, whose fibers actually innervate the constrictor muscle of the pupil, are located in the *ciliary ganglion* (Fig. 16-4).

The pupillary reflex is frequently used to test the function of the oculomotor nerve of an individual who sustains a concussion from a blow to the head or a stroke.

and oral cavities, maxillary teeth, and surrounding soft tissues, as well as the skin over the zygoma (Tables 16-2 and 16-3). The **mandibular division**, or V_3, has both sensory and motor fibers that leave the cranial cavity through the foramen ovale (Fig. 16-6). The sensory fibers supply the mandibular teeth and surrounding soft tissue, the tongue, the floor of the mouth, and the skin of the chin and the cheek wall (Tables 16-2 and 16-3). In addition, the fibers of postganglionic parasympathetic neurons join branches of the trigeminal nerve to reach their target. This nerve will be discussed in further detail in Chapter 17.

Cranial Nerve VI

The **abducens nerve** (**VI**) is a small nerve that arises at the junction of the pons and medulla oblongata (Fig. 16-1) and enters the orbit through the superior orbital fissure (Table 16-2). The nerve serves as the motor supply to the **lateral rectus muscle**, which abducts the eye in a lateral direction (Fig. 16-5; Tables 16-3 and 16-4). A person with a lesion of the abducens nerve will not be able to move the affected eye laterally, which will cause double vision or **diplopia**.

1. What fiber type is common to the oculomotor, trochlear, and abducens nerves?
2. What cranial nerve that innervates the eye contains preganglionic parasympathetic fibers?

TABLE 16–4	Summary of the Innervation and Function of the Extrinsic Eye Muscles		
Muscle	**Cranial Nerve**	**Eye Movement**	**Position of the Eyes**
Superior rectus	III	Elevates and adducts	
Inferior oblique	III	Elevates and abducts	
Medial rectus	III	Adducts	
Lateral rectus	VI	Abducts	
Inferior rectus	III	Depresses and adducts	
Superior oblique	IV	Depresses and abducts	

Right   Nose   Left

Superior rectus   Inferior oblique

Medial rectus   Lateral rectus

Superior oblique   Inferior rectus

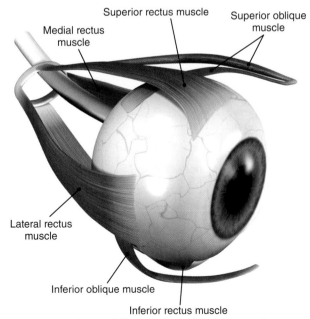

Figure 16–5 The medial rectus, lateral rectus, superior rectus, and inferior rectus muscles are attached radially along the anterior aspect of the eye. The superior and inferior oblique muscles insert posteriorly.

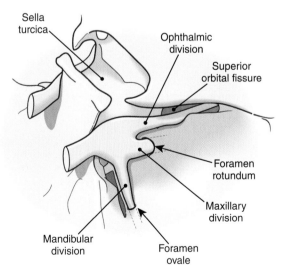

Figure 16–6 The sensory neurons of the trigeminal nerve are located in the trigeminal ganglion. Their fibers are divided into three divisions, which exit the cranial cavity separately to reach their target areas. The ophthalmic division (V_1) exits the superior orbital fissure, the maxillary division (V_2) leaves through the foramen rotundum, and the mandibular division (V_3) passes through the foramen ovale.

Cranial Nerve VII

The functions of the **facial nerve** (**VII**) are clinically relevant to the dental hygienist. The facial nerve supplies *efferent fibers* to the muscles of facial expression, the posterior belly of the digastric muscle, and the stylohyoid muscles; preganglionic parasympathetic fibers, which control the *secretion* of the lacrimal, submandibular, sublingual, palatine, and nasal glands; and *afferent fibers* for *taste* to the anterior two-thirds of the tongue, with the exception of the vallate papillae (Table 16–3). The facial nerve also supplies afferent fibers that carry pain and temperature sensations to parts of the outer ear, soft palate, and pharynx. However, these are of lesser clinical importance and will not be detailed (Table 16–3).

The *facial nerve* is attached to the brain stem by two roots at the pontomedullary junction (Fig. 16–1; Table 16–2). The larger motor root contains fibers that innervate skeletal muscles. The smaller root contains afferent fibers and preganglionic parasympathetic fibers (Fig. 16–1). The neurons of the motor root are located in the facial nucleus, whereas the preganglionic parasympathetic neurons are located within the *superior salivatory nucleus*. The two roots enter the **internal acoustic meatus** and join to form the facial nerve (Fig. 16–8). Although the nerve exits the cranial cavity through the internal acoustic meatus (Table 16–2), the nerve must also pass through the petrous portion of the temporal bone to reach the **stylomastoid foramen**, where motor fibers exit the skull to innervate the muscles of the face (Figures 16–7 and 16–8). Immediately after exiting the foramen, the facial nerve sends branches to the ear, and more relevant to the dental hygienist, sends branches to the stylohyoid muscle and to the posterior belly of the digastric muscle. The trunk of the facial nerve enters into the substance of the parotid gland where it divides into five principal branches that are named according to the region they innervate as **temporal**, **zygomatic**, **buccal**, **marginal mandibular**, and **cervical nerves** (Fig. 16–7).

The nerve cell bodies of the special sensory neurons are located in the **geniculate ganglion**, which is embedded inside the petrous portion of the temporal bone (Fig. 16–8). The sensory fibers enter the **chorda tympani nerve**, which branches off the main trunk of the facial nerve just before the facial nerve exits the skull through stylomastoid foramen (Fig. 16–8). The nerve then joins the **lingual nerve**, a branch of the *mandibular division* of the trigeminal nerve, to access the anterior two-thirds of the tongue (Fig. 16–8). It is important to understand that the sensation of taste is the function of the fibers of the chorda tympani branch of the facial nerve and that pain and temperature sensations are carried by the trigeminal fibers in the lingual nerve.

The *preganglionic parasympathetic neurons* are located in the superior salivatory nucleus of the facial nerve.

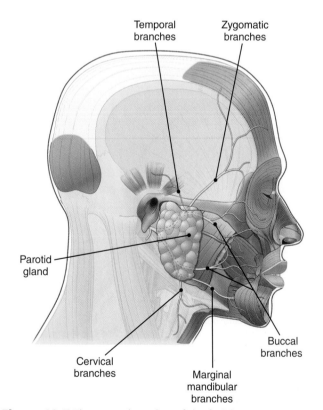

Temporal branches · Zygomatic branches · Parotid gland · Cervical branches · Marginal mandibular branches · Buccal branches

Figure 16–7 The motor branches of the facial nerve must pass through the parotid gland to innervate the muscles of facial expression.

Box 16-3 Motor Branches of the Facial Nerve

The *temporal branch* (Fig. 16–7) crosses over the zygomatic arch to supply efferent fibers to the muscles of the temporal region, which include the frontalis, procerus, and corrugator supercilii muscles, and the superior portion of the orbicularis oculi muscle.

The *zygomatic branch* (Fig. 16–7) passes over the zygomatic process to reach the corner of the eye. This nerve supplies the inferior portion of the orbicularis oculi muscle and all the elevators of the lip.

The *buccal branch* (Fig. 16–7) courses inferior to the zygomatic process to reach the corner of the mouth. This nerve also supplies the elevators of the upper lip, plus the muscles of the nose, the buccinator, and the orbicularis oris muscles.

The *marginal mandibular branch* (Fig. 16–7) courses along the margin of the mandible to innervate the depressors of the lower lip and mentalis muscle.

The *cervical branch* (Fig. 16–7), which is the most inferior of the five branches, innervates the platysma muscle of the neck.

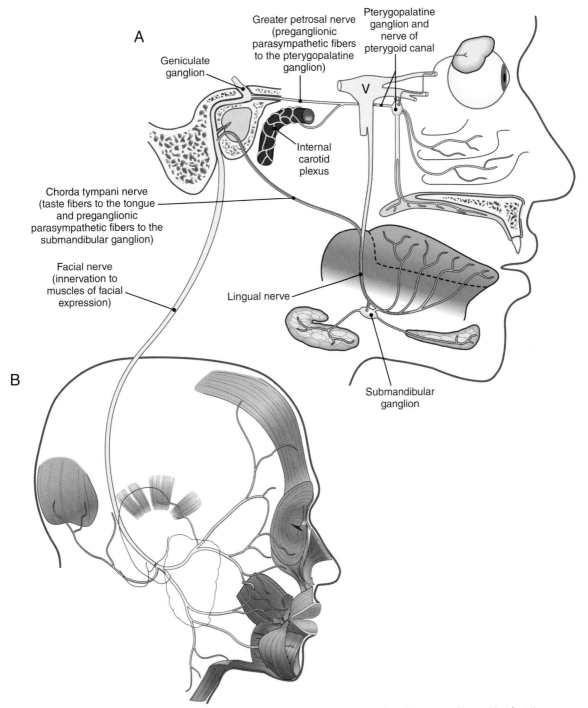

Figure 16–8 This schematic of the facial nerve illustrates the alternate paths of its nerve fibers. The facial nerve exits the cranial cavity through the internal acoustic meatus. **(A)** Preganglionic parasympathetic fibers take two alternate pathways. In one pathway, the preganglionic fibers from the greater petrosal nerve join the postganglionic sympathetic fibers of the internal carotid plexus to form the nerve of the pterygoid canal. The parasympathetic fibers synapse in the pterygopalatine ganglion, where the postganglionic parasympathetic fibers are distributed to the palate, nasal cavity, and maxillary sinus. In the other pathway, preganglionic parasympathetic fibers enter the chorda tympani nerve, which joins the lingual nerve of the mandibular division of the trigeminal nerve. The fibers synapse in the submandibular ganglion, where postganglionic parasympathetic fibers leave to innervate the submandibular and sublingual glands. The nerve cell bodies of the taste fibers are located in the geniculate ganglion. The peripheral fibers course the chorda tympani and lingual nerves to innervate the taste buds of the anterior two-thirds of the tongue. **(B)** Motor fibers to skeletal muscle pass through the geniculate ganglion without synapsing and exit through the stylomastoid foramen to reach the facial muscles and to the posterior belly of the digastric and stylohyoid muscles.

Preganglionic parasympathetic fibers join the motor root of VII as it enters the internal acoustic meatus. The fibers travel through the geniculate ganglion, but do not synapse. The fibers then diverge into two separate pathways. One group of fibers enters the chorda tympani nerve along with the taste fibers (Fig. 16–8) to join the lingual nerve. The preganglionic fibers synapse on postganglionic parasympathetic neurons located in the **submandibular ganglion**, which is attached to the lingual nerve (Fig. 16–8). Postganglionic parasympathetic fibers from the submandibular ganglion control the enzymatic secretion of the submandibular and sublingual glands.

The other preganglionic parasympathetic fibers leave the geniculate ganglion as the greater petrosal nerve. The greater petrosal nerve (Fig. 16–8) exits through a small opening in the petrous bone to surface on the floor of the cranial cavity. The nerve courses anteriorly to reach the pterygoid canal, where it joins the postganglionic sympathetic fibers of the deep petrosal nerve to form the nerve of the pterygoid canal (Fig. 16–8). The nerve cell bodies of the postganglionic sympathetic nerve fibers are located in the superior cervical ganglion and travel along the **internal carotid artery** as the **internal carotid plexus** to reach their target tissues. The nerve passes through the canal to enter the pterygopalatine fossa. The preganglionic parasympathetic fibers synapse with the *postganglionic parasympathetic neurons* within the **pterygopalatine ganglion** (Fig. 16–8). Postganglionic parasympathetic fibers ride "piggyback" on branches of the trigeminal nerve to innervate glands of the nasal cavity, intrinsic salivary glands of the palate, glands of the maxillary sinus, and the lacrimal gland. Specific branches of the trigeminal nerve will be studied in detail in Chapter 17.

Review Question Box 16-4

1. In which ganglia do the preganglionic parasympathetic fibers of the facial nerve synapse?
2. What fiber types arise from neurons in the geniculate ganglion?
3. The secretions of which glands are controlled by the facial nerve?
4. What fiber types are found in the chorda tympani nerve?
5. What fiber types are found in the nerve to the pterygoid canal and what is the location of their nerve cell bodies?

Cranial Nerve VIII

The **vestibulocochlear nerve (VIII)**, which is attached to the pontomedullary junction lateral to the facial nerve (Fig. 16–1), is a sensory nerve. The special sensory nerve fibers exit through internal acoustic meatus to innervate the inner ear (Tables 16–2 and 16–3). The nerve has two components, the **vestibular** and **cochlear nerves**. The cell bodies of the first-order neurons of the vestibular nerve are located in the **vestibular ganglion** (Fig. 16–9). Receptors in the vestibular apparatus detect motion, which are projected to higher brain centers. Vestibular input controls *posture* and *equilibrium*. In addition, vestibular input influences the movements of the eyes that stabilize the eyes during head movements, thus preventing the movement of images of an object on the retina (fixed gaze). The nerve cell bodies of the *cochlear nerve* are located in the **spiral ganglion** within the cochlea (Fig. 16–9). The receptors are localized within the membranous canal inside the bony spirals of the cochlea. After multiple synapses, *auditory* information reaches the temporal lobe. Auditory information reaches other centers, which initiate turning the eyes, head, and body toward a loud sound.

Review Question Box 16-5

1. What ganglia contain the nerve cell bodies of neurons of the vestibular and cochlear nerves?
2. How are the nerve fibers of the vestibulocochlear nerve classified?

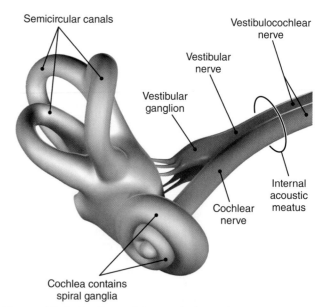

Figure 16–9 The fibers of the vestibulocochlear (VIII) nerve pass through the internal acoustic meatus to innervate structures of the inner ear. The nerve cell bodies of the special sensory neurons of the cochlear nerve are located in the spiral ganglion in the bone of the central portion of the cochlea. The nerve cell bodies for the vestibular nerve are located in the semicircular canals.

Cranial Nerve IX

The **glossopharyngeal nerve (IX)**, which contains both sensory and motor fibers, is attached to the medulla of the brain stem caudal to the vestibulocochlear nerve (Fig. 16–1 and Table 16–2). The glossopharyngeal nerve has four general functions of importance to the dental hygienist: *secretion* (parasympathetic control) of the parotid gland, **taste** (special sensory) to the posterior one-third of the tongue; *general sensation* to the posterior one-third of the tongue, pharynx, the tonsillar regions, and the carotid sinus; and *motor innervation* to a muscle (Table 16–3), which aids in swallowing.

Immediately after the glossopharyngeal nerve exits the cranial cavity through the **jugular foramen**, two small swellings appear on the nerve. The swellings, the superior and inferior ganglia of IX, contain the cell bodies of the first-order sensory neurons (Fig. 16–10). The nerve follows the course of the stylopharyngeus muscle to reach its targets (Fig. 16–10). The first of the afferent branches, the *pharyngeal nerve* (Fig. 16–10), joins the pharyngeal plexus of nerves on the posterior surface of the pharynx and supplies pain and temperature fibers to the pharyngeal wall. After entering the pharynx, the nerve gives off *tonsillar* and *lingual* branches (Fig. 16–10). These branches supply pain and temperature fibers to the mucosa of their respective areas. In addition, the lingual branch contains taste fibers

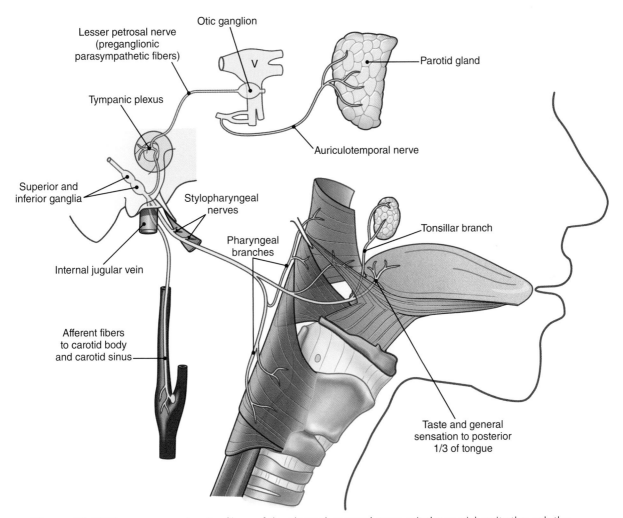

Figure 16–10 The sensory and motor fibers of the glossopharyngeal nerve exit the cranial cavity through the jugular foramen. The nerve cell bodies of the sensory neurons are located in the superior and inferior ganglia. Some sensory fibers extend to the carotid sinus, whereas others remain in the glossopharyngeal nerve as it courses along the stylopharyngeus muscle and supply pain and temperature fibers to the mucosa of the pharynx. The motor fibers leave the nerve to innervate the stylopharyngeus muscle. Sensory fibers continue to the tonsil and tongue. The tonsillar and lingual branches contain general sensory fibers, whereas the lingual branch also contains taste fibers. The preganglionic parasympathetic nerve fibers leave the inferior ganglion as the tympanic nerve that joins the tympanic plexus and leaves as the lesser petrosal nerve. The fibers synapse in the otic ganglion. The postganglionic nerve fibers join the auriculotemporal nerve of the mandibular division of the trigeminal nerve to innervate the parotid gland.

that innervate taste buds of the posterior one-third of the tongue and the circumvallate papillae.

The efferent fibers of the glossopharyngeal nerve arise from motor neurons located in the nucleus ambiguus in the medulla of the brain stem. The glossopharyngeal nerve only innervates one muscle, the **stylopharyngeus muscle** (Fig. 16–10), one of the longitudinal muscles of the pharynx. Contraction of this muscle aids in swallowing (deglutition).

The secretion of the parotid gland is controlled by preganglionic parasympathetic fibers arising from neurons located in the *inferior salivatory nucleus* of the glossopharyngeal nerve. The preganglionic parasympathetic fibers branch off the inferior ganglion as the *tympanic nerve*. The nerve enters the tympanic cavity and joins the tympanic plexus located in the middle ear (Fig. 16–10). The nerve leaves the plexus as the *lesser petrosal nerve* (Fig. 16–10). This small nerve exits the middle ear by passing through a small opening in the petrous portion of the temporal bone. The nerve travels anteriorly and leaves the cranial cavity through the foramen ovale. The nerve fibers synapse with the postganglionic parasympathetic neurons in the **otic ganglion**, which is attached to the mandibular division of the trigeminal nerve (Fig. 16–10). Postganglionic parasympathetic fibers join the *auriculotemporal branch* of the mandibular nerve to reach the parotid gland (Fig. 16–10).

Cranial Nerve X

The **vagus nerve** (**X**) (*vagus* literally means "wandering") is the major source of fibers of the parasympathetic nervous system. In addition, the vagus nerve contains efferent fibers to skeletal muscle and taste fibers on the palate and epiglottis (Table 16–3).

The *preganglionic parasympathetic fibers* originate from neurons in the dorsal motor nucleus of X. Vagal fibers leave the brain stem caudal to the glossopharyngeal nerve (Fig. 16–1) and exit the skull through the jugular foramen (Table 16–2). Along its long journey to its termination in the abdomen, its fibers innervate the viscera in the thorax and abdomen (Fig. 16–11).

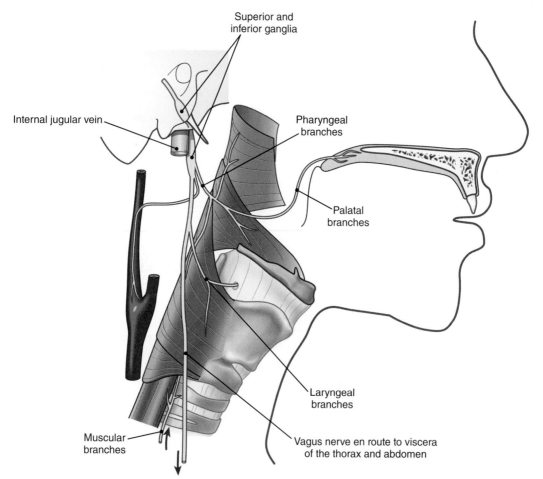

Figure 16–11 Preganglionic parasympathetic fibers of the vagus nerve take a wandering path through the neck to visceral structures of the thorax and abdomen. Motor fibers to skeletal muscle innervate the muscles of the pharynx, larynx, and palate. Sensory neurons are located in the superior and inferior ganglia. The fibers carry general sensation from the larynx and the special sensation of taste from the palate and epiglottis.

Like the glossopharyngeal nerve, the *motor fibers* of the vagus nerve originate from neurons in the nucleus ambiguus. The motor fibers innervate the muscles of the pharynx, larynx, and palate (Fig. 16–11). The *sensory neurons* of the vagus nerve are located in the superior and inferior ganglia of X, which are two small swellings on the vagus nerve as it exits the jugular foramen (Fig. 16–11). Pain and temperature fibers supply the larynx, whereas taste fibers supply taste buds on the palate and epiglottis (Fig. 16–11). The vagus nerve also supplies sensory fibers to the carotid sinus of the internal carotid artery for cardiovascular reflexes and the carotid body, which is located between the bifurcation of the common carotid artery. Fibers to the carotid body are concerned with respiratory reflexes related to the oxygen concentration in the peripheral blood.

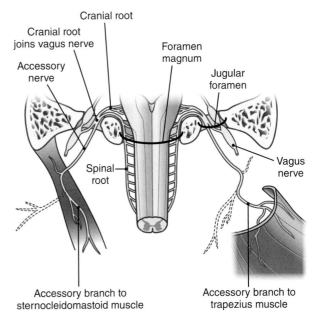

Figure 16–12 The traditional cranial component of the accessory nerve has motor neurons within the nucleus ambiguus, along with the motor neurons of the glossopharyngeal (IX) and vagus (X) nerves. The fibers of the spinal component arise from the spinal cord and ascend to enter the cranial cavity via the foramen magnum. Within the cranial cavity, the cranial and spinal components join to exit the jugular foramen with the vagus nerve. As the nerves exit, the cranial component rejoins the vagus nerve to supply skeletal muscle. Most anatomists now consider the cranial component to be fibers of the vagus nerve.

Review Question Box 16-6

1. What nerve fibers directly innervate the parotid gland and what is the location of their nerve cell bodies?
2. What is the location of the nerve cell bodies of the sensory fibers of the glossopharyngeal and vagus nerves?
3. What is the relationship of the glossopharyngeal nerve and the vagus nerve in the innervation of the pharynx?
4. Why is the vagus nerve called the "wandering" nerve?

Cranial Nerve XI

Traditionally, the **accessory nerve** arises from both the medulla and spinal cord (Fig. 16–1 and Table 16–2). Its *cranial component* (Fig. 16–12) is formed by nerve fibers from neurons in the nucleus ambiguus. These fibers join the vagus nerve to supply the muscles of the larynx and pharynx. Although still controversial, many anatomists consider the cranial component to be a part of the vagus nerve. The nerve fibers of the *spinal component* (Fig. 16–12) originate in neurons in the accessory nucleus in the upper cervical segment of the spinal cord. These fibers are distinct from the ventral roots of the spinal nerve. Rootlets from the accessory nucleus join and ascend the spinal cord to form the accessory nerve. The nerve enters the posterior cranial cavity through the **foramen magnum**, and then exits the **jugular foramen** (Fig. 16–12) to innervate the **trapezius** and **sternocleidomastoid muscles** (Table 16–3).

Cranial Nerve XII

The **hypoglossal nerve** arises as a series of rootlets from the medulla and exits the cranial cavity through the hypoglossal canal (Fig. 16–1 and Table 16–2). The nerve enters the oral cavity by passing between the mylohyoid

and hyoglossus muscles. Its *motor fibers* innervate the extrinsic and intrinsic muscles of the tongue (Table 16–3). Note that the palatoglossus muscle is a muscle of the palate and is innervated by the vagus nerve, not the hypoglossal nerve.

Review Question Box 16-7

1. Which cranial nerves contain only special sensory fibers?
2. Which cranial nerve contains only motor fibers to skeletal muscle?
3. Which cranial nerves contain preganglionic parasympathetic fibers?

SUMMARY

The cranial nerves are components of the peripheral nervous system that innervate the structures of the head and neck, with the exception of the vagus nerve, which also innervates the viscera of the thorax and abdomen. Most of the cranial nerves originate in nuclei located on the brain or brain stem, with the exception of the accessory nerve, which originates from the cervical spinal cord. Unlike a spinal nerve, which contains motor, sensory, and autonomic fibers, each cranial nerve has its own specific fiber types. Only four cranial nerves contain preganglionic parasympathetic fibers and none contain sympathetic fibers. In addition to general sensory fibers, such as temperature, pain, and touch, some cranial nerves contain special sensory fibers for smell, taste, vision, hearing, and equilibrium.

- The *olfactory nerve (I)* contains special sensory fibers for smell.
- The *optic nerve (II)* contains fibers for the special sensation of vision.
- The *oculomotor nerve (III)* has motor fibers to skeletal muscle that elevates the upper eyelid, and most of the muscles that move the eye. In addition, this nerve contains parasympathetic fibers that innervate smooth muscles that round the lens and constrict the pupil.
- The *trochlear nerve (IV)* has motor fibers to only one skeletal muscle, the superior oblique muscle of the eye.
- The *trigeminal nerve (V)* is the main general sensory nerve of the head. All three divisions—ophthalmic, maxillary, and mandibular—contain sensory fibers, whereas the mandibular division also contains motor fibers, in particular, the muscles of mastication (and others).
- The *abducens nerve (VI)* supplies motor fibers to only the superior oblique muscle.
- The *facial nerve (VII)* is a complex nerve. It supplies motor fibers to the muscles of facial expression, the stylohyoid muscle, and the posterior belly of the digastric muscle. The nerve supplies preganglionic parasympathetic fibers that regulate the secretion of the lacrimal, submandibular, and sublingual glands. It supplies taste fibers to the anterior two-thirds of the tongue.
- The *vestibulocochlear nerve (VIII)* has two components that supply special sensation. The vestibular nerve contains fibers for equilibrium, whereas the cochlear nerve contains fibers for hearing.
- The *glossopharyngeal nerve (IX)* contains several fiber types. This nerve has motor fibers to one muscle of the pharynx, the stylopharyngeus muscle. The nerve also has preganglionic parasympathetic fibers, which supply the parotid gland. This nerve contains general sensation fibers to the pharynx and posterior one-third of the tongue, and special sensory fibers for taste on the posterior one-third of the tongue.
- The *vagus nerve (X)* is also a complex nerve. It supplies motor fibers to the pharynx, larynx, and soft palate. Its preganglionic parasympathetic fibers supply the viscera of the thorax and abdomen. This nerve supplies general sensory fibers to the mucosa of the pharynx and larynx and taste fibers to the palate and epiglottis.
- The *accessory nerve (XI)* supplies motor fibers to the trapezius and sternocleidomastoid muscles.
- The *hypoglossal nerve (XII)* contains motor fibers that innervate the intrinsic and extrinsic muscles of the tongue.

LEARNING LAB

Exercises for review, practice, and study

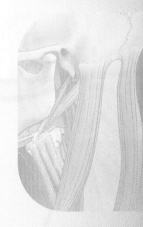

Laboratory Activity 16-1

Testing Cranial Nerve Function

Objective: Dental professionals do not routinely test cranial nerve function. However, if an emergency should occur with a medically compromised patient or someone faints getting out of the chair and hits his or her head, some very simple tests can help to assess the severity of the incident.

Step 1: *Olfactory nerve*—Pass a small packet of ammonia quickly in front of the patient's nose. The patient should respond to the offensive odor.

Step 2: *Optic nerve*—Test for blurred vision by sticking up two fingers and asking how many fingers.

Step 3: *Oculomotor nerve*—Test the patient's pupillary reflex by shining a light in the eyes. The pupils should reflexively close.

Step 4: *The oculomotor, trochlear,* and *abducens* nerves can be tested by asking the patient to follow an object (finger) in an H-shape pattern. By testing eye movements, it is possible to test for the individual nerves.

- Moving the object toward the nose tests the medial rectus muscle, which is innervated by III.
- While the object is positioned toward the nose, move the object in the superior direction. This tests the inferior oblique muscle, which is also innervated by III.
- Moving the object inferiorly tests the superior oblique muscle, which is innervated by IV.
- Moving the object lateral toward the temple tests the lateral rectus muscle, which is innervated by VI.
- Moving the object upward tests the superior rectus muscle and moving it downward tests the inferior rectus muscle. Both are innervated by III.

Step 5: *Trigeminal nerve*—The patient should be able to open and close the mouth.

Step 6: *Facial nerve*—The patient should be able to smile and to wrinkle the forehead.

Step 7: *Vestibulocochlear nerve*—The patient should not be dizzy and is able to hear.

Step 8: *Glossopharyngeal nerve*—The patient should be able to feel pain, temperature, and taste on the posterior one-third of the tongue.

Step 9: *Vagus nerve*—Ask the patient if he or she feels nauseated or is vomiting. Positive responses indicate involvement with the vagus nerve.

Step 10: *Accessory nerve*—The patient should be able to shrug the shoulders.

Step 11: *Hypoglossal nerve*—Have the patient stick out his or her tongue. The tongue should not deviate to the left or right.

For Discussion or Thought:

1. Why is it important to test for cranial nerve function?

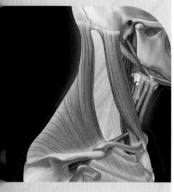

17

Trigeminal Nerve

Objectives

1. Identify the fiber types that arise from the trigeminal nerve and indicate the location of their nerve cell bodies.
2. Identify the branches of the three divisions of the trigeminal nerve on diagrams and be able to discuss their distribution to their target organs.
3. Discuss the relationship of the postganglionic parasympathetic neuron and its fibers to the branches of the trigeminal nerve.

Overview

Small communities, towns, cities, and countries are connected by a series of roadways and major highways. Similarly, structures of the head are joined by the extensive branching of the trigeminal nerve. Nerve fibers that do not originate from the trigeminal nerve can also serve as feeder roads to the larger trigeminal highway system. In this chapter, you will study the trigeminal nerve and how other cranial nerve and autonomic nerve fibers travel on its branches to reach their target organs.

INTRODUCTION TO THE TRIGEMINAL NERVE

The **trigeminal nerve (V)** has several functions that are important to the dental profession. First, it is the major general sensory nerve to many of the mucous membranes of the head, to the teeth and surrounding tissues, and to the face (with the exception of the skin over the angle of the mandible, which is innervated by the cervical plexus). Second, it supplies motor fibers, as well as proprioceptive

(sense of position and movement) fibers, to the muscles of mastication. Third, its branches serve as a distribution highway for parasympathetic fibers and fibers from other cranial nerves to search their target organs.

The nerve cell bodies of the motor neurons are located within the motor nucleus of V. On the other hand, the cell bodies of the first-order neurons that carry the general sensations of pain, temperature, and touch are located in the **trigeminal ganglion**. The trigeminal ganglion is considered analogous to the dorsal root ganglia of the spinal cord.

The trigeminal nerve is divided into three divisions: the **ophthalmic division**, which is also designated as **V₁**; the **maxillary division** or **V₂**; and the **mandibular division** or **V₃**. Each of these divisions carries afferent fibers that pass through the trigeminal ganglion (Fig. 17–1) before entering the pons. Motor fibers exit the pons and join the mandibular division to be distributed to skeletal muscles (Table 17–1).

There are four small parasympathetic ganglia that contain the nerve cell bodies of postganglionic parasympathetic neurons that are associated with branches of the trigeminal nerve. These ganglia do not receive preganglionic fibers from the trigeminal complex, but their postganglionic fibers are distributed by branches of the trigeminal nerve. These are the ciliary, pterygopalatine, otic, and submandibular ganglia. The **ciliary ganglion** is associated with the *ophthalmic division*, the **pterygopalatine ganglion** with the *maxillary division*, and the **otic** and **submandibular ganglia** with the *mandibular division*.

OPHTHALMIC DIVISION (V₁)

The first division of the trigeminal nerve, which is called the *ophthalmic nerve* (*V₁*), enters the orbit through the **superior orbital fissure** (see Fig. 16–6). The ophthalmic nerve divides into three major branches: the lacrimal, frontal, and nasociliary nerves (Table 17–2). The **lacrimal nerve** is a small branch that passes laterally through the orbit to innervate the lacrimal gland and the adjacent skin and conjunctiva (Fig. 17–2). The **frontal nerve** is the large middle branch, which courses superiorly in the orbit and terminates on the surface of the face and scalp as the supraorbital and supratrochlear nerves. The **supraorbital nerve** (Fig. 17–2) reaches the outer surface of the skull by passing through the supraorbital foramen or notch (see Fig. 2–9). This nerve supplies the skin of the upper eyelid, the forehead, the anterior scalp, and the mucous membrane of the frontal sinus. The **supratrochlear nerve** (Fig. 17–2) is more medially placed and supplies the skin of the upper eyelid and the skin of the lower and medial part of the forehead. The third and most medial branch, the **nasociliary nerve** (Fig. 17–2), is the most complex because of its numerous branches. A small branch of the nasociliary nerve communicates with the ciliary ganglion. This branch is called the **long root** or *sensory root* **of the ciliary ganglion** (Fig. 17–2) because it contains afferent fibers. These nerve fibers pass through the ganglion without synapsing and exit the **short ciliary nerves** to supply afferent fibers to the cornea, iris, and ciliary body (Fig. 17–2). The *ciliary ganglion* contains *postganglionic parasympathetic neurons*. Recall that the *preganglionic parasympathetic fibers, which* arise from the *oculomotor*

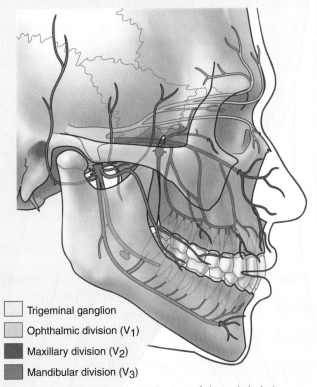

- ☐ Trigeminal ganglion
- ☐ Ophthalmic division (V₁)
- ■ Maxillary division (V₂)
- ■ Mandibular division (V₃)

Figure 17–1 The general distribution of the ophthalmic, maxillary, and mandibular divisions of the trigeminal nerve is indicated. The sensory components of the nerves arise from the trigeminal ganglion.

TABLE 17–1	Summary of the Trigeminal Nerve
Divisions	**Fiber Types**
Ophthalmic division (nerve) V₁	Sensory only
Maxillary division (nerve) V₂	Sensory only
Mandibular division (nerve) V₃	Sensory and motor

TABLE 17–2	Summary of the Ophthalmic Nerve
Major Branches	**Target Organs**
Lacrimal	Lacrimal gland
	Conjunctiva and adjacent skin
Frontal	
Supratrochlear	Skin of upper eyelids and medial forehead
Supraorbital	Skin of the upper eyelids, the forehead, the anterior scalp, and the frontal sinus
Nasociliary	
Long ciliary	Eyeball
Infratrochlear	Medial eyelids and side of nose
Anterior and posterior ethmoidal	Frontal, ethmoid, and sphenoid sinuses
Anterior ethmoidal	Skin of the surface of the noses

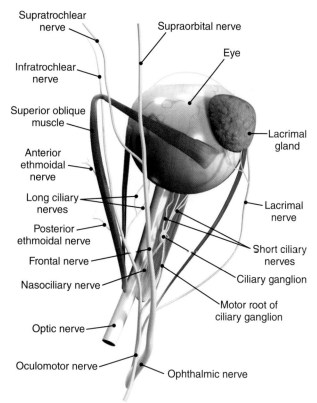

Figure 17–2 The ophthalmic nerve has three major branches that supply the orbit and the skin of the forehead. The lacrimal nerve innervates the lacrimal glands and continues on the surface of the eyelid. The frontal nerve passes through the orbit and terminates on the surface as the supraorbital and supratrochlear nerves. The nasociliary nerve gives off the sensory root of the ciliary ganglion, the long ciliary nerves, the anterior and posterior ethmoidal branches, and terminates on the surface as the infratrochlear nerve. Note that the supratrochlear nerve passes superior to the bend in the superior oblique muscle, whereas the infratrochlear nerve lies inferior to the muscle.

nerve, synapse with the neurons in the ganglia (Chapter 16). These postganglionic parasympathetic fibers exit through the short ciliary nerves to innervate the sphincter pupillae and the ciliary muscles (contraction causes the rounding of the lens). In addition, the short ciliary nerves contain *postganglionic sympathetic* fibers from the *superior cervical ganglion* that innervate the dilator pupillae muscle. The next two or three branches, the **long ciliary nerves**, pierce the posterior surface of the sclera of the eyeball to supply afferent fibers to the iris and cornea.

There are three terminal branches of the nasociliary nerve. The **infratrochlear nerve** supplies afferent fibers to the skin on the medial parts of the eyelids and the side of the nose (Fig. 17–2). The **anterior** and **posterior ethmoidal nerves** supply afferent fibers to the frontal, ethmoid, and sphenoid paranasal sinuses (Fig. 17–2). In addition, *external nasal branches* of the anterior ethmoidal nerve supply the skin on the surface of the nose.

1. What are the three major branches of the ophthalmic nerve?
2. Do sensory nerve fibers synapse in the ciliary ganglion?
3. What type of nerves is found in the ciliary ganglion?
4. What fiber types are found in the short ciliary nerve and where are the locations of their nerve cell bodies?

MAXILLARY DIVISION (V₂)

The *maxillary division or V₂* (Fig. 17–1) is generally called the *maxillary nerve.* It is extremely important to the dental clinician and hygienist because it supplies sensory innervation to the maxillary teeth and surrounding soft tissue, the palate, and the skin and upper lip of the maxilla. The dental clinician anesthetizes branches of the maxillary nerve during cavity preparations, extractions, and other invasive procedures of the maxillary teeth. Understanding the pathway of this nerve will help explain the tingling sensations and numbness in certain areas of the face that are associated with the anesthesia of the maxillary teeth. The clinician uses these "side effects" as signs to assess the effectiveness of the anesthetic before beginning a clinical procedure, thus preventing unnecessary pain to the patient. Intraoral injections will be covered in more detail in Chapter 18.

The maxillary division leaves the cranial cavity through the **foramen rotundum** and enters into the **pterygopalatine fossa**, a space in the shape of an inverted four-sided pyramid located posterior to the maxilla and anterior to the pterygoid process of the sphenoid bone (Fig. 17–3A). The roof of the fossa, which forms the base of the triangle, is the greater wing of the sphenoid bone. The anterior wall is the maxilla, the medial wall is the palatine bone, and the posterior wall is the pterygoid process of the sphenoid bone. The lateral wall is not formed by bone, but is a narrow slit, the **pterygomaxillary fissure**, between the maxilla and the pterygoid process (Figs. 17–3A and B). The fossa is connected to the nasal cavity by the **sphenopalatine foramen**, to the orbit by the **inferior orbital fissure**, to the infratemporal fossa by the pterygomaxillary fissure, and to the hard palate by the **greater palatine canal** (Fig. 17–3B).

Within the fossa, the maxillary nerve gives off small branches, which connect to the **pterygopalatine ganglion** (Fig. 17–4). This ganglion contains postganglionic parasympathetic neurons, which cause the secretion of tears from the lacrimal glands and the secretion of glands in the mucosae of the nasal cavity, palate, nasopharynx, and the paranasal sinuses. The branches of this ganglion will be studied in more detail in the next section.

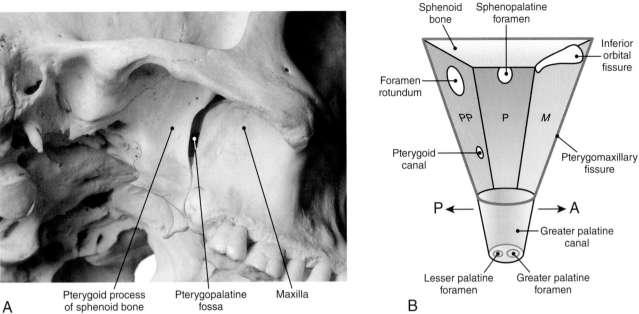

A

B

Figure 17–3 (A) The pterygopalatine fossa is a narrow space between the maxillary bone and the pterygoid process of the sphenoid bone. The pterygomaxillary fissure, which is outlined in red, is the lateral entranceway into the fossa. **(B)** The fossa is described as an inverted four-sided pyramid. The base or roof of the fossa is formed by the sphenoid bone (yellow dashes). The anterior side of the space is bordered by the maxillary bone (M), the medial side by the palatine bone (P), the posterior side by the pterygoid process (PP), and lateral side is the pterygomaxillary fissure (outlined in red). Structures within the fossa communicate with the orbit through the inferior orbital fissure, the nasal cavity through the sphenopalatine foramen, the palate via the greater and lesser palatine foramina of the greater palatine canal, and the infratemporal fossa through the pterygomaxillary fissure. Nerves enter the fossa through the foramen rotundum and pterygoid canal.

Figure 17–4 In this sagittal section through the lateral wall of the nasal cavity, the greater palatine canal has been opened and the sphenopalatine foramen widened to expose the pterygopalatine ganglion and its branches. The ganglion is attached to the maxillary nerve by the small pterygopalatine nerves. The nerve of the pterygoid canal contains preganglionic parasympathetic fibers that synapse in the ganglion and postganglionic parasympathetic fibers, which are distributed through some of its branches. The branches include the nasopalatine, pharyngeal, and greater and lesser palatine nerves.

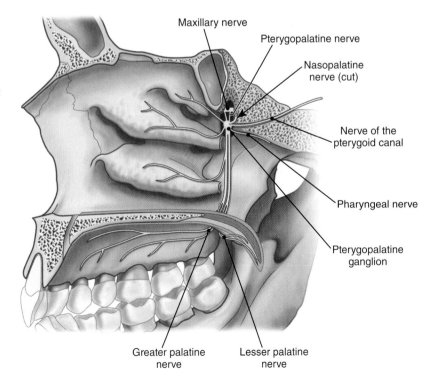

Major Branches of the Maxillary Nerve

Pterygopalatine Ganglion Branches (Table 17–3)

Within the pterygopalatine fossa, the **pterygopalatine nerves** attach the pterygopalatine ganglion to the maxillary nerve (Fig. 17–4). The afferent nerve fibers pass through the ganglion without synapsing to be distributed to their target tissues. Several branches arise from the ganglion. Two of the branches, the greater palatine and lesser palatine nerves, descend within the *greater palatine canal* to reach the palate via the **greater** and **lesser palatine foramina**, respectively (Fig. 17–3B). The **greater palatine nerve** travels anteriorly and terminates near the first premolar tooth and supplies the mucosa of the hard palate adjacent to the molar and premolar teeth (Fig. 17–4). The **lesser palatine nerve** courses posteriorly to supply the mucosa of the soft palate (Fig. 17–4). A pharyngeal branch supplies the mucosa of the nasopharynx. Another branch, the **nasopalatine nerve**, supplies the mucosa of the nasal cavity and courses through the incisive foramen to innervate the mucosa of the primary palate and the palatal gingiva of the maxillary incisors and canine teeth (Fig. 17–5).

Zygomatic Nerve (Table 17–3)

The **zygomatic nerve**, which contains sensory and autonomic fibers, branches off the maxillary nerve in the pterygopalatine fossa and enters the orbit (Figs. 17–6 and 17–7). Postganglionic parasympathetic fibers that arise from the pterygopalatine ganglion innervate the lacrimal gland. These fibers follow a circuitous route. The fibers leave the zygomatic nerve and enter a communicating branch that joins the lacrimal nerve of V_1 to reach the lacrimal gland (Figs. 17–6 and 17–7). The sensory fibers exit the lateral wall of the orbit as the zygomaticofacial and zygomaticotemporal

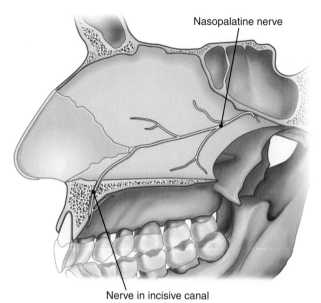
Nasopalatine nerve

Nerve in incisive canal

Figure 17–5 The mucosa of the nasal septum has been stripped in this sagittal view of the nasal cavity. Branches of the nasopalatine nerve supply the mucosa of the nasal septum before entering the incisive canal. Terminal branches of the nerve innervate the palatal mucosa and gingivae of the anterior teeth.

nerves. The **zygomaticofacial nerve** supplies the skin over the zygomatic arch, whereas the **zygomaticotemporal nerve** supplies the skin of the temporal region (Fig. 17–7).

Posterior Superior Alveolar Nerve (Table 17–3)

The **posterior superior alveolar nerve** branches from the maxillary nerve as it exits the pterygopalatine fossa through the pterygomaxillary fissure to reach the infratemporal fossa (Fig. 17–6). The nerve courses inferiorly on the posterior surface of the maxilla and enters into the bone via the posterior superior alveolar foramen. Within the maxilla, this nerve communicates with the middle superior alveolar and anterior superior alveolar

TABLE 17–3	Summary of the Maxillary Nerve
Branches	**Target Organs**
Greater palatine nerve	Hard palate and gingiva of the maxillary molar and premolar teeth
Lesser palatine nerve	Soft palate and uvula
Nasopalatine nerve	Nasal septum and gingiva of the maxillary incisors and the canine teeth
Zygomatic nerve	Skin over the cheek and portions of the temporal region
Posterior superior alveolar nerve	Maxillary molar teeth except the mesiobuccal root of the first molar and surrounding gingiva
Infraorbital nerve	
Palpebral, nasal, and labial nerves	Lower eyelid, lip, nose, and cheek
Middle superior alveolar nerve	Premolar and mesiobuccal root of the first molar
Anterior superior alveolar nerve	Maxillary incisor teeth

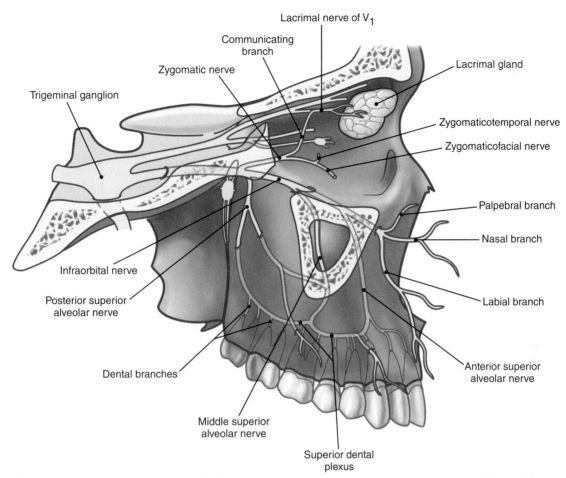

Figure 17–6 The posterior superior, middle superior, and anterior superior alveolar branches of the maxillary nerve form the superior dental plexus, which supply dental branches to the maxillary teeth. The zygomatic branch enters the orbit and sends off a communicating branch to the lacrimal nerve of V_1. The maxillary nerve becomes the infraorbital nerve as it passes through the orbit and exits to terminate as the palpebral, the nasal, and the labial nerves.

nerves to form the **superior dental plexus** (Fig. 17–6) (see the next section). This plexus supplies the lining mucosa of the maxillary sinus, the maxillary gingiva, and the maxillary teeth. The fibers of the posterior superior alveolar nerve supply all the maxillary molar teeth, with the possible exception of the mesiobuccal root of the first molar tooth (see Chapter 18).

Infraorbital Nerve (Table 17–3)

The **infraorbital nerve** gives off two important branches that supply the maxillary teeth, the anterior and middle superior alveolar nerves. The **anterior superior alveolar nerve** (Fig. 17–6) supplies the incisors, canines, and surrounding gingiva, as well as the maxillary sinus. The **middle superior alveolar nerve** (Fig. 17–6) is present about 30% of the time. The nerve supplies the two premolars and the mesiobuccal root of the first molar. The infraorbital nerve terminates as several small cutaneous branches, which supply the external nose, lower eyelid, and upper lip (Fig. 17–6).

> ### Review Question Box 17-2
>
> 1. What are the boundaries of the pterygopalatine fossa?
> 2. What nerves branch from the pterygopalatine ganglion?
> 3. What cranial nerve is the source of the preganglionic parasympathetic fibers that synapse in the pterygopalatine ganglion?
> 4. What branch of the maxillary nerve contains autonomic fibers that innervate the lacrimal gland?
> 5. What is the one fiber type that is found in all branches of the maxillary nerve and where is the location of the nerve cell bodies?

MANDIBULAR DIVISION (V₃)

The *mandibular division* (V_3), or mandibular nerve, is the largest division of the trigeminal nerve. It is also extremely important to the dental clinician and hygienist

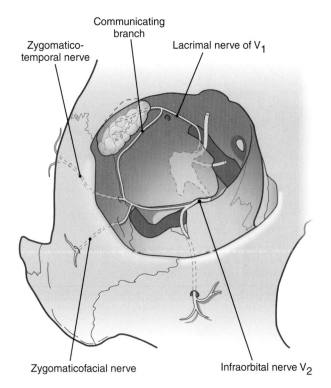

Zygomatico-
temporal nerve

Communicating
branch

Lacrimal nerve of V₁

Zygomaticofacial nerve

Infraorbital nerve V₂

Figure 17–7 The anterior view of the orbit with the eyeball removed reveals branches of the zygomatic nerve and the maxillary nerve. The zygomatic nerve divides into the zygomaticofacial and zygomaticotemporal nerves, which supply the skin of the zygoma and temporal region. Before the zygomaticotemporal nerve exits the orbit, it sends a communicating branch to the lacrimal nerve of V₁, which contains postganglionic parasympathetic fibers to the lacrimal gland.

because the nerve contains motor fibers to the muscles of mastication (and others) and general sensory fibers that supply the lower lip, the lower jaw, the mucous membranes of the cheek and floor of the mouth, the anterior two-thirds of the tongue, the mandibular teeth and gingiva, the temporomandibular joint, the parotid gland, and the skin anterior to the ear and temporal region (Table 17–4). In addition, two parasympathetic

ganglia—the otic and submandibular ganglia—are attached to its branches.

Upon exiting the skull through the foramen ovale, the nerve divides into an anterior division and a posterior division. The *anterior division* is primarily motor and supplies the following muscles that you have already studied: the muscles of mastication (temporalis, medial and lateral pterygoid, masseter), mylohyoid muscle, anterior belly of the digastric muscle, and tensor veli palatini muscles. One sensory branch, the **long buccal nerve** (Fig. 17–8), arises from the anterior division and supplies the skin of the cheek wall and the buccal mucosa and gingiva of the mandibular molars.

The *posterior division*, which is mostly sensory, has three nerve branches: the auriculotemporal, lingual, and inferior alveolar nerves. The **auriculotemporal nerve** branches from the posterior division just inferior to the foramen ovale (Fig. 17–8). The nerve encircles the middle meningeal artery (Fig. 17–9) as it passes lateral to innervate the parotid gland, the temporomandibular joint, and the skin anterior to the ear. In addition, the nerve receives *postganglionic parasympathetic fibers* from the **otic ganglion**, which lies next to the mandibular nerve (Fig. 17–9). Recall from Chapter 16 that the *preganglionic parasympathetic fibers* are derived from the *glossopharyngeal nerve (IX)*. These fibers synapse in the otic ganglion, and the postganglionic parasympathetic fibers join the auriculotemporal nerve to stimulate the secretion of the parotid gland.

The **inferior alveolar nerve** (Figs. 17–8 and 17–9) branches from the mandibular nerve near the origin of the lingual nerve. The first branch of the inferior alveolar nerve is the **mylohyoid nerve** (Figs. 17–9 and 17–10). This nerve contains motor fibers that supply the mylohyoid muscle and the anterior belly of the digastric. After branching of the mylohyoid nerve, the inferior alveolar nerve enters into the mandible through the **mandibular foramen**. While passing

TABLE 17–4	Summary of the Mandibular Nerve
Branches	**Target Organs**
Motor branches	Motor to the muscles of mastication
Long buccal nerve	Sensory to the skin of the cheek wall and buccal mucosa Gingiva of the mandibular molars
Auriculotemporal nerve	Sensory to the ear, temporal skin, parotid gland, and temporomandibular joint
Inferior alveolar nerve Incisive nerve Mental nerve Nerve to the mylohyoid muscle	Sensory to all the mandibular teeth and their buccal gingivae Sensory to the mandibular incisors and canines Sensory to the mucosa and skin of lower lip and chin Motor to the mylohyoid and anterior belly of the digastric muscles
Lingual nerve	Sensory to: Anterior two-thirds of the tongue Mucosa of the floor of the mouth Lingual mandibular gingiva Submandibular and sublingual glands

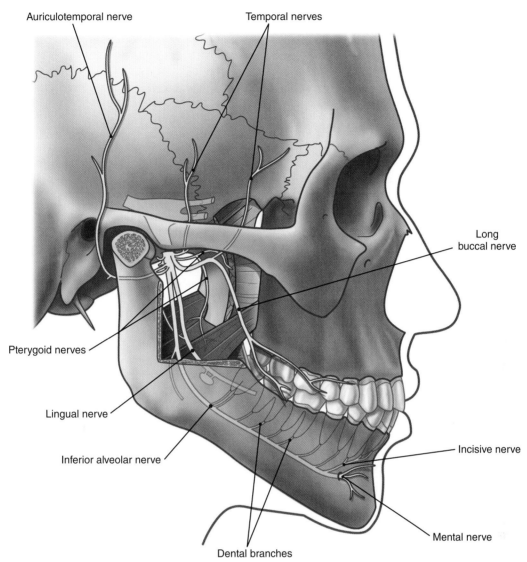

Figure 17–8 This overview of the mandibular nerve shows the branches of its anterior and posterior divisions. The anterior division innervates the muscles of mastication—that is, the temporal and pterygoid nerves, and its long buccal branch contains sensory fibers to the skin and mucosa of the cheek wall. The posterior division has three branches: the auriculotemporal nerve, the inferior alveolar nerve, and the lingual nerve. The inferior alveolar nerve enters the mandibular canal and extends dental branches to the mandibular teeth. In the premolar region, the nerve divides into a mental branch, which supplies the skin of the cheek and lip and the incisive nerve, which supplies the anterior teeth.

through the bone, the nerve supplies *dental branches*, which supply the molar and premolar teeth and the adjacent buccal gingiva. The inferior alveolar nerve ends in two terminal branches. One branch, the **mental nerve** (Fig. 17–8), exits the mandible through the **mental foramen** to supply the mucosa and skin of the lower lip and chin. The second terminal branch, the **incisive nerve** (Fig. 17–8), remains in the mandible. The incisive nerve supplies the canine and incisor teeth and the adjacent labial gingiva.

The **lingual nerve** (Fig. 17–10) innervates the anterior two-thirds of the tongue, the floor of the mouth, and the lingual mandibular gingiva. It contains three fiber types: *general sensory*, *special sensation* (*taste*),

and *preganglionic parasympathetic fibers*. The taste fibers and preganglionic fibers are derived from the **facial nerve (VII)** and reach the lingual nerve by the **chorda tympani nerve** (Figs. 17–9 and 17–10) (Chapter 16). Fibers of general sensation (pain, temperature, and touch) arise from the trigeminal ganglion. Understanding the motor and sensory innervations of the tongue can be very important in distinguishing nerve damage to the facial nerve or to the mandibular division of the trigeminal nerve. The preganglionic fibers synapse in the **submandibular ganglion**, which is attached to the lingual nerve (Fig. 17–10). The postganglionic efferent fibers leave the ganglion to supply the submandibular and sublingual salivary glands.

Review Question Box 17-3

1. What is the only sensory nerve of the anterior division of the mandibular nerve and what does it supply?
2. What fiber types are found in the lingual nerve and where is the location of the nerve cell bodies for each fiber type?
3. What fiber types are found in the auriculotemporal nerve and where is the location of the nerve cell bodies for each fiber type?
4. What do the fibers arising from the submandibular ganglion innervate?
5. What fiber types are found in the inferior alveolar nerve and where is the location of the nerve cell bodies for each fiber type?
6. What is the incisive nerve?

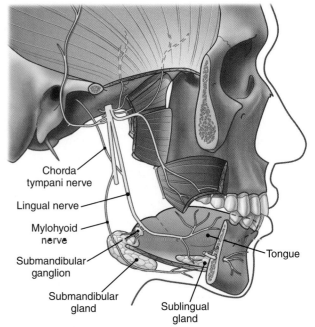

Figure 17–10 In this lateral view, the zygomatic arch has been removed to reveal branches of the mandibular nerve in the infratemporal fossa. The lingual nerve courses in an anteroinferior direction to supply general sensation to the anterior two-thirds of the tongue, the floor of the mouth, and the gingiva of the mandibular teeth. The chorda tympani branch of the facial nerve, which carries taste fibers to the anterior two-thirds of the tongue and preganglionic parasympathetic fibers destined for the submandibular ganglion, joins the lingual nerve. The submandibular ganglion is attached to the lingual nerve and its postganglionic parasympathetic fibers innervate the submandibular and sublingual glands.

SUMMARY

The trigeminal nerve is the major source of general sensory fibers to the face, teeth, and mucous membranes of the oral cavity, nasal cavity, and paranasal sinuses. Its motor fibers supply the muscles of mastication, the anterior belly of the digastric muscle, the mylohyoid muscle, and the tensor veli palatini muscle. Postganglionic parasympathetic fibers arising from autonomic ganglia use branches of the three divisions of the trigeminal nerve as highways to reach their target organs.

The nerve cell bodies of the sensory neurons are located in the trigeminal ganglion and are distributed by the ophthalmic, maxillary, and mandibular nerves, which are the three divisions of the trigeminal nerve. The ophthalmic nerve (V_1) enters the orbit and divides into three major branches. The lacrimal nerve supplies sensory fibers to the lacrimal gland, the skin of the upper eyelid, and the conjunctiva. The frontal nerve passes superiorly in the orbit and divides into two terminal branches, the supraorbital and supratrochlear nerves,

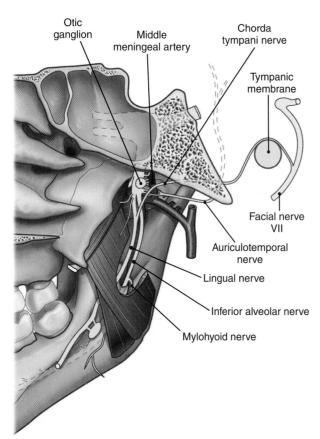

Figure 17–9 In this sagittal section along the medial surface of the mandible, a portion of the medial pterygoid muscle has been removed to expose branches of the mandibular nerve. The mylohyoid nerve branches from the inferior alveolar nerve before it enters the mandibular foramen. The chorda tympani branch of the facial nerve joins the lingual nerve from a posterior direction. The otic ganglion sends fibers to the auriculotemporal nerve for distribution to the parotid gland.

which supply the upper eyelid and the skin of the forehead and anterior scalp. The sensory branches of the nasociliary nerve, which form the sensory root of the ciliary ganglion, pass through the ganglion and travel in the short ciliary nerves to reach the anterior structures of the eyeball. Postganglionic parasympathetic fibers from the ciliary ganglion also use the short ciliary nerves to supply the ciliary body that rounds the lens and the constrictor muscles of the pupil. Postganglionic sympathetic fibers from the superior cervical ganglion also pass through the ciliary ganglion and short ciliary nerves to innervate the dilator muscle of the pupil. The long ciliary branches send sensory branches to the posterior region of the eyeball, whereas the posterior and anterior ethmoid branches supply sensory innervation to the frontal, ethmoid, and sphenoid sinuses. The infratrochlear nerve innervates the skin of the medial eyelid and nose. An external nasal branch also supplies the skin of the nose.

The maxillary nerve (V_2) enters the pterygopalatine fossa and gives off branches that attach the pterygopalatine ganglion to the maxillary nerve. Branches from the ganglion contain both postganglionic parasympathetic fibers arising from the pterygopalatine ganglion and sensory fibers from the trigeminal ganglion. The greater and lesser palatine nerves supply the glands and mucosa of the hard and soft palate. The nasopalatine nerve innervates the glands and mucosa of the nasal cavities and supplies sensory fibers to the mucosa and gingiva of the anterior palate adjacent to the incisor and canine teeth. The zygomatic nerve contains postganglionic parasympathetic fibers that supply the lacrimal gland and sensory fibers to the skin of the face via the zygomaticofacial and zygomaticotemporal nerves. Before entering the orbit, the maxillary nerve gives off the posterior superior alveolar nerve, which supplies the molar teeth, with the possible exception of the mesiobuccal root of the first molar. After entering the orbit, the maxillary nerve becomes the infraorbital nerve. The middle superior alveolar (present 30% of the time) and anterior superior alveolar nerves branch off the infraorbital nerve in the orbit. The infraorbital nerve then exits the skull to supply the lower eyelid, lateral surface of the nose, and the upper lip.

The mandibular nerve (V_3) divides into anterior and posterior divisions. The anterior division innervates the muscles of mastication and its long buccal branch supplies sensory fibers to the cheek wall in the vicinity of the molar teeth. There are three branches of the posterior division. The auriculotemporal nerve contains sensory fibers that innervate the parotid gland, temporomandibular joint, and the skin anterior to the ear. It also contains postganglionic parasympathetic nerve fibers from the otic ganglion that innervate the parotid gland. The lingual nerve supplies general sensory fibers to the anterior two-thirds of the tongue, the floor of the mouth, and the lingual mandibular gingiva. Taste fibers to the anterior two-thirds of the tongue originate from the facial nerve and course through the chorda tympani nerve to join the lingual nerve. In addition, preganglionic parasympathetic fibers from the facial nerve travel through the chorda tympani and lingual nerves to reach the submandibular ganglion, whose postganglionic fibers innervate the submandibular and sublingual glands. The inferior alveolar branch gives off the nerve to the mylohyoid muscle before it enters the mandibular foramen to supply the mandibular teeth. Within the mandibular canal, the inferior alveolar nerve branches into its two terminal branches. The mental nerve exits the canal to supply the mucosa and skin of the lower lip and chin. The incisive nerve supplies the incisive and canine teeth.

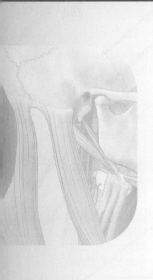

LEARNING LAB
Exercises for review, practice, and study

Laboratory Activity 17-1

Cutaneous Innervation of the Face

Objective: In this exercise, you will study the distribution pattern of the sensory nerves to the face.

- A *dermatome* is a predictable area of skin innervated by a nerve. With the exception of the face and portions of the scalp, the dermatome is innervated by spinal nerves.
- Let's use the innervation of the skin of the fingers of the hand by the ulnar nerve as an example. This nerve lies in a groove on the back of the elbow. If you hit this area, you will feel a sharp pain. A layperson would say that he or she hit the "funny bone." If this area becomes depressed—that is, resting your weight on your elbow too long—you will develop numbness in your fingers and when the pressure is released there is a tingling sensation. Actually, these sensations involve the fifth digit (little finger) and the lateral half of the fourth digit (the ring finger). These cutaneous areas are innervated specifically by the eighth cervical nerve.
- Clinicians can use dermatome patterns to determine injury to specific spinal cord segments.
- Similarly, with the exception of a small area of skin over the angle of the mandible, the skin of the face is supplied by the three divisions of the trigeminal nerve. The skin of the angle of the mandible is innervated by cervical spinal nerves. Within each of these three regions, predictable areas of skin are innervated by specific branches of each division.

Test yourself by completing the exercise on the next page.

Match the numbered structures with the correct terms listed below.

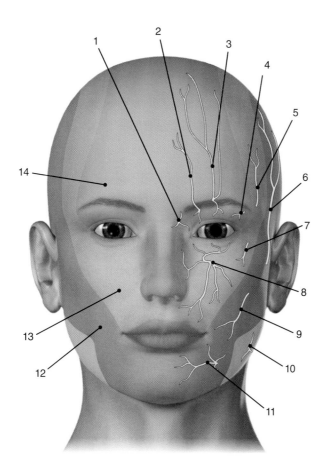

_____ Auriculotemporal nerve   _____ Maxillary division

_____ Cervical nerves   _____ Mental nerve

_____ Infraorbital nerve   _____ Ophthalmic division

_____ Infratrochlear nerve   _____ Supraorbital nerve

_____ Lacrimal nerve   _____ Supratrochlear nerve

_____ Long buccal nerve   _____ Zygomaticofacial nerve

_____ Mandibular division   _____ Zygomaticotemporal nerve

For Discussion or Thought:

1. *Pain management by intraoral injections of anesthetics for dental procedures not only affects the teeth, but also the surrounding soft tissue and skin. Dental clinicians routinely test the profoundness of the anesthesia by testing the effects on the skin and soft tissues.*

2. *It also explains the pattern of pain that results from herpes zoster (shingles), which affects the ophthalmic division. Herpes varicella virus, or chickenpox, generally infects children. After the initial infection, the virus becomes dormant and resides in the ganglia of nerves. As we grow older or the immune system becomes weakened, the virus becomes active again and spreads along the path of the nerves. The skin innervated by the nerves becomes red, develops a blistering rash, is itchy, and can become extremely painful. Knowing the dermatome pattern allows the clinician to assess which specific nerve or nerves are affected.*

Learning Activity 17-1

Branches of the Ophthalmic Division and Related Structures

Match the numbered structures with the correct terms listed to the right.

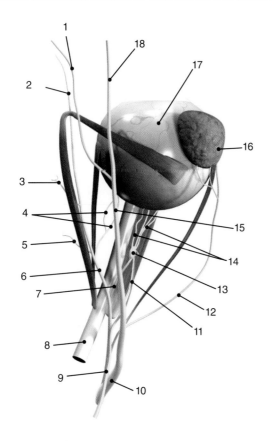

_____ Anterior ethmoidal nerve

_____ Ciliary ganglion

_____ Eyeball

_____ Frontal nerve

_____ Infratrochlear nerve

_____ Lacrimal gland

_____ Lacrimal nerve

_____ Long ciliary nerves

_____ Motor root of the ciliary ganglion

_____ Nasociliary nerve

_____ Oculomotor nerve

_____ Ophthalmic nerve

_____ Optic nerve

_____ Posterior ethmoidal nerve

_____ Sensory root of the ciliary ganglion

_____ Short ciliary nerve

_____ Supraorbital nerve

_____ Supratrochlear nerve

Learning Activity 17-2

Branches of the Maxillary Division and Related Structures

Match the numbered structures with the correct terms listed below.

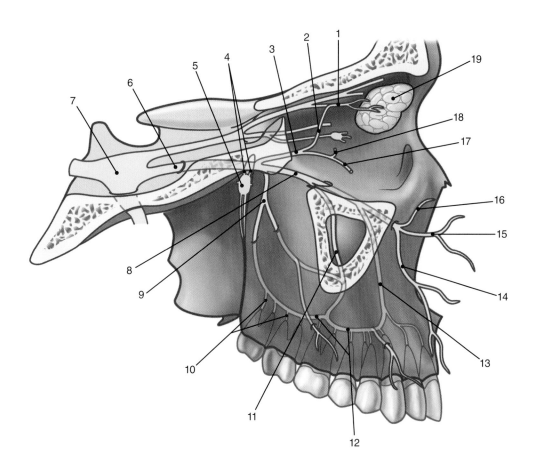

_____ Anterior superior alveolar nerve

_____ Communicating branch

_____ Dental branches

_____ Infraorbital nerve

_____ Labial nerve

_____ Lacrimal gland

_____ Lacrimal nerve of V_1

_____ Maxillary nerve

_____ Middle superior alveolar nerve

_____ Nasal nerve

_____ Palpebral nerve

_____ Posterior superior alveolar nerve

_____ Pterygopalatine branches

_____ Pterygopalatine ganglion

_____ Superior dental plexus

_____ Trigeminal ganglion

_____ Zygomatic nerve

_____ Zygomaticofacial nerve

_____ Zygomaticotemporal nerve

Learning Activity 17-3

Branches of the Mandibular Division and Related Structures

Match the numbered structures with the correct terms listed below.

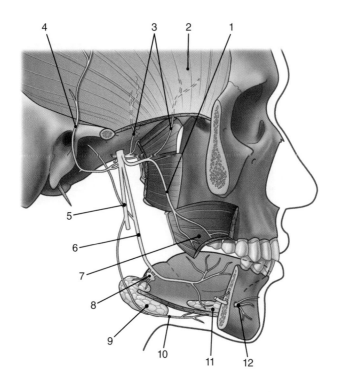

_____ Auriculotemporal nerve

_____ Buccinator muscle

_____ Deep temporal nerves

_____ Inferior alveolar nerve

_____ Lingual nerve

_____ Long buccal nerve

_____ Mental nerve

_____ Mylohyoid nerve

_____ Sublingual gland

_____ Submandibular ganglion

_____ Submandibular gland

_____ Temporalis muscle

chapter 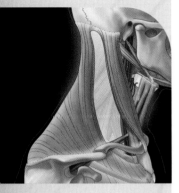

18

Anatomy of Intraoral Injections

Objectives

1. Explain the difference between supraperiosteal (infiltration) anesthesia and nerve blocks.
2. Identify the regional pattern of sensation for branches of the trigeminal nerve that innervate the teeth and surrounding soft tissues.
3. Locate the general injection sites for branches of the trigeminal nerve and be able to state what nerves must be anesthetized for the roots and soft tissue surrounding individual teeth.

Overview

A mother brings her 10-year-old son who has a sore mouth to your dental office. He fell off his bicycle while riding on the sidewalk in front of a neighbor's house. His mouth is swollen and his right central incisor tooth is chipped and needs to be crowned. The child has never had a dental procedure that requires an intraoral injection. After dispensing the anesthetic, the tooth becomes insensitive to pain, but the child complains to the dentist and to his mother that his lower eyelid, the side of his nose, and his upper lip are numb on the right side of his face. Should his mother be concerned? In this chapter, you will learn the answer to this question, and similar questions for other intraoral injections that are required for routine dental procedures.

INTRODUCTION TO THE ANATOMY OF INTRAORAL INJECTIONS

The prevention of pain by local anesthesia is the corner-stone of all dental practices. Understanding the innervation of each root of individual teeth and its surrounding soft tissues is absolutely essential in administering anesthetics. This also requires a thorough understanding of the pathways and distributions of the branches of the mandibular and maxillary divisions of the trigeminal nerve as well as the structures that are in the vicinity of the injection site that could be affected by the errant placement of a hypodermic needle. There are several techniques that can be used, depending on the requirements of a clinical procedure or the degree of infection that may be present. In this chapter, the anatomical basis for these procedures is presented, as well as precautions that need to be considered when administering local anesthesia.

REVIEW OF THE MAXILLARY NERVE AND ASSOCIATED STRUCTURES

The *sensory fibers* of the maxillary nerve arise from neurons in the *trigeminal ganglion*. The maxillary nerve exits the skull through the foramen rotundum to enter the **pterygopalatine fossa**. The fossa, which contains the **pterygopalatine ganglion**, is a pyramid-shaped space between the pterygoid process of the sphenoid bone and the maxillary bone (Fig. 18–1A). The fossa lies lateral to the nasal cavity, posterior to the orbit, and medial to the infratemporal fossa.

The *pterygopalatine ganglion* contains postganglionic parasympathetic neurons and is attached to the maxillary nerve by two small pterygopalatine branches. Sensory fibers from the maxillary nerve pass through the ganglion and are distributed to target tissues by branches of the ganglion. The **lesser palatine** and **greater palatine nerves** (Fig. 18–1B) descend in the greater palatine canal to surface onto the hard palate through their respective lesser and greater palatine foramina. The lesser palatine nerve is inconsequential to dental procedures because it innervates the soft palate. On the other hand, the greater palatine nerve innervates the mucosa of the hard palate and the palatal gingiva of the molars and premolar teeth (Table 18–1). The **nasopalatine nerve** branches from the ganglion and passes through the sphenopalatine foramen to reach the nasal cavity (Fig. 18–1B). The *septal branch* of this nerve is important to the dental clinician because it passes through the **incisive canal** of the anterior portion of the hard palate (Fig. 18–1B) to supply the mucosa of the primary palate and the palatal gingiva of the anterior teeth (Table 18–1). Terminal branches of the nasopalatine nerve cross the midline to the contralateral side and must be considered in cases of incomplete anesthesia of the central incisors.

The maxillary nerve courses laterally to exit the fossa by passing through the pterygomaxillary fissure and gives off the **posterior superior alveolar nerve**. Branches of the nerve enter the posterior surface of the maxillary bone through the **posterior superior alveolar foramina** and course through the wall of the maxillary sinus to innervate the mucosa of the sinus, and the roots and buccal gingiva of the molars (Fig. 18–1A), with the possible exception of the *mesiobuccal root* of the first molar (Fig. 18–2 and Table 18–1). The maxillary nerve enters the orbit through the inferior orbital fissure and becomes the **infraorbital nerve**. About 30% of the time, a **middle superior alveolar nerve** branches from the infraorbital nerve as it passes along the floor of the orbit (Fig. 18–1A). The nerve, when present, passes through the lateral wall of the maxillary sinus to innervate the mucosa of the maxillary sinus, the mesiobuccal root and gingiva of the first molar, and the

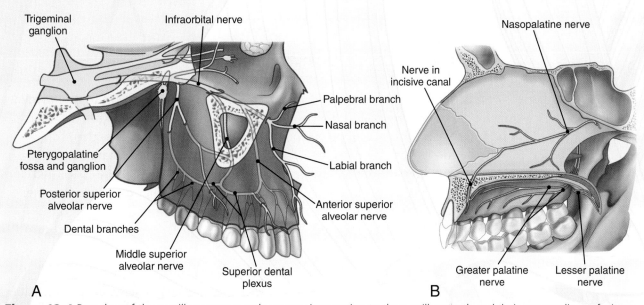

Figure 18–1 Branches of the maxillary nerve supply sensory innervation to the maxillary teeth and their surrounding soft tissue, as well as the mucosa of the hard palate. The posterior superior, the middle superior, and the anterior superior alveolar nerves form the superior dental plexus, which supplies the teeth **(A)**, whereas the greater palatine nerve and nasopalatine nerve innervate the mucosa of the hard palate **(B)**.

TABLE 18–1	Nerve or Trunk Blocks for the Maxillary Nerve		
Nerve	**Injection Site**	**Teeth**	**Palatal Tissue**
Posterior superior alveolar nerve	Mucobuccal fold at the level of the second molar	All roots of the first, second, and third molars, except the mesiobuccal root of the first molar, and their facial gingiva	Not applicable
Middle superior alveolar nerve	Mucobuccal fold above the second premolar	Mesiobuccal root of the first molar, premolars, and their facial gingiva	Not applicable
Anterior superior alveolar nerve	Mucobuccal fold above the lateral incisor	Canines, incisors, their labial gingiva, and upper lip	Not applicable
Infraorbital nerve	Mucobuccal fold of the first premolar directed toward the infraorbital foramen	Canine, incisors, and labial gingiva, the lower eyelid, the side of the nose and the upper lip	Not applicable
Greater palatine nerve	Junction between the hard palate and the lateral edge of the alveolar bone distal to the second molar	Not applicable	Hard palate and palatal gingiva of the molars and premolars
Nasopalatine nerve	Incisive papilla	Not applicable	Anterior hard palate Palatal alveolar periosteum of the anterior teeth Palatal mucosa Palatal gingiva

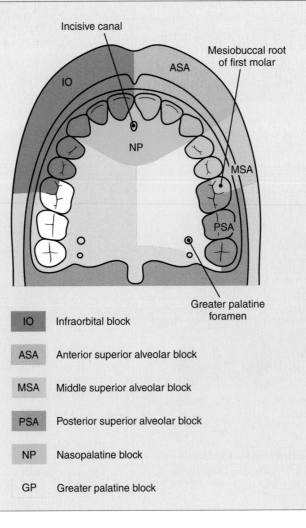

Incisive canal

Mesiobuccal root of first molar

ASA

IO

NP

MSA

PSA

Greater palatine foramen

IO	Infraorbital block
ASA	Anterior superior alveolar block
MSA	Middle superior alveolar block
PSA	Posterior superior alveolar block
NP	Nasopalatine block
GP	Greater palatine block

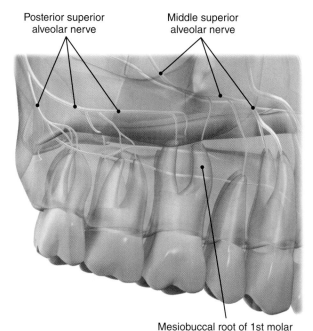

Posterior superior   Middle superior
alveolar nerve   alveolar nerve

Mesiobuccal root of 1st molar

Figure 18–2 The posterior superior alveolar nerve supplies the roots of all the maxillary molar teeth, with the possible exception of the mesiobuccal root of the first molar, which is supplied along with the premolars by the middle superior alveolar nerve. Even though the middle superior alveolar nerve is present only 30% the time, for practical purposes it should be treated as being present.

roots and buccal gingiva of the premolars (Table 18–1). The infraorbital nerve enters a canal of bone along the orbital rim that opens onto the surface of the skull as the infraorbital foramen. As the nerve passes through the canal, it gives off the **anterior superior alveolar nerve**, which travels through the anterior wall of the maxilla (Fig. 18–1A). The nerve supplies the mucosa of the maxillary sinus and the roots and buccal gingiva of the anterior teeth and the premolars if the middle superior alveolar nerve is not present (Table 18–1). Terminal branches of the anterior superior alveolar nerve cross the midline to the contralateral side and must be considered in cases of incomplete anesthesia of the central incisors. The infraorbital nerve terminates as the *nasal, superior labial,* and *inferior palpebral nerves* (Fig. 18–1A). These terminal branches can be used to test the effectiveness of an infraorbital nerve block.

Review Question Box 18-1

1. What branches of the maxillary nerve innervate the mucosa of the palate and palatal gingiva, but not the maxillary teeth?

2. What branches of the infraorbital nerve innervate the teeth?

3. How do the nerve branches that innervate the maxillary second and third molars enter the maxilla?

REVIEW OF THE MANDIBULAR NERVE AND THE INFRATEMPORAL FOSSA

The afferent fibers of the mandibular division of the trigeminal nerve arise from neurons in the trigeminal ganglion, which is located in the middle cranial fossa (Fig. 18–3A). The mandibular nerve exits the fossa through the foramen ovale to enter into the infratemporal fossa and immediately divides into anterior and posterior divisions (Fig. 18–3A). The anterior division is mostly efferent and supplies motor fibers to the muscles of mastication. However, one branch, the **long buccal nerve**, is sensory and is very important to the dental clinician when administrating anesthetics to the mandibular molar teeth (Figs. 18–3A and B). The long buccal nerve innervates the buccal mucosa and the buccal (facial) gingiva of the mandibular molars (Table 18–2). On the other hand, most of the posterior division is sensory. Several of its branches are of clinical interest. The inferior alveolar nerve and the lingual nerve enter the infratemporal fossa by passing in between the lateral and medial pterygoid muscles (Fig. 18–3B).

The mylohyoid nerve, which innervates the mylohyoid muscle and the anterior belly of the digastric muscle, branches from the **inferior alveolar nerve** before it enters the mandibular foramen on the medial surface of the mandible (Figs. 18–3A and B). Although this nerve is considered a motor nerve, studies indicate that the nerve also has sensory fibers, which must be considered when there is incomplete anesthesia of the incisor teeth. After entering the mandibular foramen, the inferior alveolar nerve courses anteriorly through the mandibular canal. Along its pathway, the nerve extends dental branches to the roots of all the mandibular teeth and associated buccal gingiva of all mandibular teeth except for the molars (Fig. 18–3A and Table 18–2). Upon reaching the second premolar tooth, the inferior alveolar nerve divides into its two terminal branches. The **mental nerve** exits the canal and reaches the surface via the mental foramen (Fig. 18–3A). The nerve supplies the skin of the chin and lower lip (Table 18–2). Insensitivity of the lip and chin is one way to test the completeness of an inferior alveolar nerve block. The **incisive nerve** continues anteriorly to supply the roots of the anterior teeth and facial gingiva (Fig. 18–3A and Table 18–2). Terminal branches of the incisive nerve cross the midline to the contralateral side. These crossing fibers must be considered in cases of incomplete anesthesia of the central incisors.

The **lingual nerve** courses on the surface of the medial pterygoid muscle anterior and parallel to the inferior alveolar nerve (Fig. 18–3B). The nerve turns anteriorly to enter into the floor of the mouth. The lingual nerve supplies pain and temperature fibers to the anterior two-thirds of the tongue, the floor of the mouth, and the lingual gingiva of the mandibular teeth

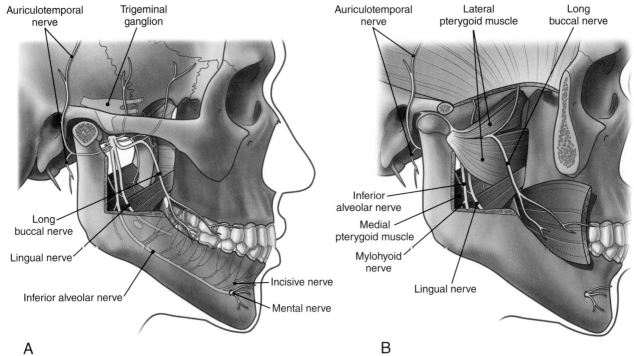

A

B

Figure 18–3 The sensory fibers of the mandibular division arise from the trigeminal ganglion. Upon exiting the cranial cavity, the mandibular nerve divides into anterior and posterior divisions, which is indicated by the dashed line **(A)**. The long buccal nerve enters the infratemporal fossa between the two heads of the lateral pterygoid muscle **(B)** and courses anteriorly to innervate the cheek wall **(A)** and **(B)**. The inferior alveolar and lingual nerves enter the infratemporal fossa between the medial and lateral pterygoid muscles **(B)**. The inferior alveolar nerve courses through the mandibular canal to supply the mandibular teeth. The nerve terminates as the mental nerve and the incisive nerve **(A)**. The nerve to the mylohyoid muscle branches from the inferior alveolar nerve **(B)**. The lingual nerve lies on the surface of the medial pterygoid muscle as it travels anteriorly to reach the tongue **(B)**. The auriculotemporal nerve passes deep to the mandibular condyle **(B)** to reach the skin anterior to the ear **(A)**.

(Table 18–2). Numbness of the lip and tongue is a test for a successful mandibular nerve block.

The **auriculotemporal nerve** branches immediately off the posterior division as the mandibular nerve exits the skull through the foramen ovale. The auriculotemporal nerve courses along the roof of the infratemporal fossa and passes deep to the mandibular condyle to reach the skin anterior to the ear (Figs. 18–3A and B). The nerve is important to the dental clinician because it supplies afferent fibers to the temporomandibular joint, but it is not necessary to anesthetize the nerve for routine dental procedures.

Review Question Box 18-2

1. What sensory branches of the mandibular nerve are located in the infratemporal fossa?
2. What branch of the mandibular nerve supplies the cheek wall and lingual mucosa of the mandibular molar teeth?
3. What sensory branch of the mandibular nerve is not anesthetized during most dental procedures?

SUPRAPERIOSTEAL ANESTHESIA VERSUS NERVE BLOCKS

The administration of local anesthetics to the maxillary and mandibular teeth differs because of the variance in thickness of the cortical plates of the mandibular and maxillary arches. The **supraperiosteal injection** is used for the maxillary teeth to anesthetize the terminal nerve branches in the area of treatment. The needle of an aspirating syringe is placed into the **mucobuccal fold (vestibular fornix)** above the roots of each tooth. Because the cortical bone is thin and porous along the maxillary arch, the anesthetic can infiltrate through the bone to reach the nerves. For this reason, this technique is also called **infiltration anesthesia**. Additional injections are administered for the palatal gingiva, the periodontal ligament, and the interdental gingiva for dental procedures that require anesthesia to soft tissues.

The cortical plates of the mandible are too thick for an anesthetic to penetrate by diffusion. Therefore, the larger trunks of the nerve are anesthetized, which means there is also a larger area of anesthesia. Techniques to anesthetize nerve trunks are known as **nerve blocks**. Nerve blocks are also administered in the maxillary arch

TABLE 18–2	Nerve or Trunk Blocks for the Mandibular Nerve		
Nerve	**Injection Site**	**Teeth**	**Soft Tissue**
Inferior alveolar nerve	Mucosa lateral to the pterygo-mandibular fold	Mandibular teeth	Buccal gingiva of the mandibular teeth
Lingual nerve	Mucosa lateral to the pterygo-mandibular fold	Not applicable	Lingual gingiva of all teeth, the floor of the mouth, and the tongue
Long buccal nerve	Medial to the border of the ramus of the mandible at the occlusal plane of the maxillary molars	Not applicable	Buccal gingiva and mucosa of the mandibular molars
Mental nerve	Between the roots of the first and second premolar	Not applicable	Skin of chin and the lower lip; the mucosa of the lower lip
Incisive nerve	Between the roots of the first and second premolar	Incisors, canines, and premolars	Mucosa of the lower lip; roots and gingiva of the incisor, canine, and premolar teeth

Mental foramen

B	Buccal block
IA	Inferior alveolar block
IN	Incisive block
L	Lingual block

when full anesthesia is not achieved, such as in the area of an infection or to prevent discomfort to a patient who would require multiple injections for procedures on more than one tooth.

Review Question Box 18-3

1. Why are infiltration injections not suitable for dental procedures of the mandible?
2. Why would it be necessary to administer nerve blocks for dental procedures on the maxillary teeth?

NERVE BLOCKS TO BRANCHES OF THE MAXILLARY NERVE

Operative procedures on maxillary teeth that do not violate the surrounding gingiva generally only require infiltration anesthesia along the roots of the teeth. However, there are occasions when infiltration anesthesia may not be the best choice. For example, inflamed or chronically infected tissues are more difficult to anesthetize, because diffusion of the anesthetic is impeded. Multiple injections of several teeth in the same arch could cause discomfort for the patient after the anesthesia wears away. Procedures, such as

Box 18-1 Aspirating Syringe

An *aspirating syringe* is a type of hypodermic syringe used in dental procedures. The syringe is designed to allow a clinician to retract on the plunger for the testing of the presence of blood in the syringe before delivering the anesthesia. The hypodermic needle is beveled to allow easy penetration into the tissue. If the bevel of the needle is placed on the surface of the bone, it will prevent the gouging of the needle tip into the tissue.

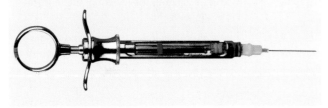

extractions and crown preparations, require additional injections. Nerve blocks would be a better approach in these circumstances.

Posterior Superior Alveolar Nerve Block

The *posterior superior alveolar nerve block* is used to anesthetize the maxillary molar teeth, with the possible *exception of the mesiobuccal root* (middle superior alveolar nerve when present) of the first molar and their buccal gingiva (Table 18–1). The needle is placed into the mucobuccal fold at the level of the zygomatic arch above the second maxillary molar tooth and directed posterior toward the posterior superior alveolar foramina, where the anesthetic is deposited (Fig. 18–4 and Table 18–1).

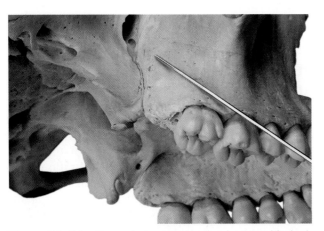

Figure 18–4 For the posterior superior alveolar nerve block, the needle is inserted above the second maxillary molar and directed in the vicinity of the posterior superior alveolar foramina.

Precautions

The needle must pass through the *buccinator muscle* to reach the foramina. Although unlikely to happen, if the needle is directed too far laterally, the needle could penetrate the cheek wall. One of the primary concerns with any injection is the penetration or tearing of blood vessels. The *posterior superior alveolar branches of the maxillary artery* and the *pterygoid plexus* are in the same area (Figs. 18–5A and B). *Aspiration*, which is checking for the presence of blood in the syringe by retracting the plunger, is the best preventive technique. Slight penetration does not damage a vessel, but tearing a vessel could cause a *hematoma*, which is a swelling of blood. The hematoma will eventually disappear, but would certainly alarm the patient. Another concern for all injections is *tearing the periosteum* with the needle, which can be painful when the anesthesia wears away. To reduce this possibility, the beveled side of the needle is placed on the surface of the bone, which allows the needle to glide over the periosteum.

Middle Superior Alveolar Nerve Block

Although the *middle superior alveolar nerve* is not always present, it is necessary to give the injection for procedures of the maxillary premolar and mesiobuccal root of the first molar (Table 18–1) as a precaution. The needle is inserted in the mucobuccal fold above the second premolar tooth and advanced vertically approximately 6 to 12 mm to reach its target area (Fig. 18–6 and Table 18–1).

Precautions

The tissue above the mucobuccal fold and between the facial muscles and the periosteum is sparse. Injecting too large of a volume of anesthetic too quickly would be initially painful to the patient. Although the blood vessels are small in this area, aspirate for blood.

Anterior Superior Alveolar Nerve Block

Blockage of the *anterior superior alveolar nerve* will anesthetize the maxillary central incisors, the lateral incisors, the canine teeth (and the premolars if the middle superior alveolar nerve is not present) and their labial gingiva, and the upper lip. The needle is placed in the mucobuccal fold above the lateral incisor and directed toward the apex of the canine tooth (Fig. 18–7 and Table 18–1).

Precautions

As for the premolars, the tissue surrounding the teeth is sparse. Thus, injecting too large a volume of anesthetic too quickly would be initially painful to the patient.

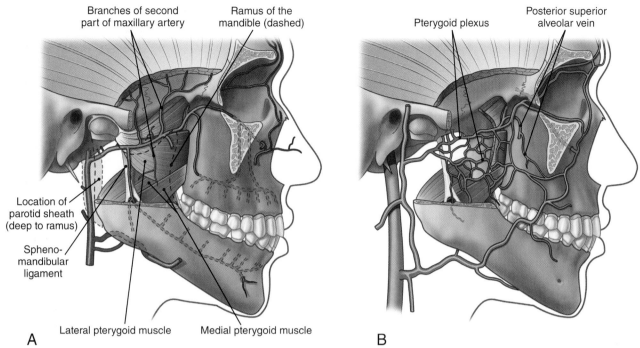

Branches of second
part of maxillary artery

Ramus of the
mandible (dashed)

Pterygoid plexus

Posterior superior
alveolar vein

Location of
parotid sheath
(deep to ramus)

Spheno-
mandibular
ligament

Lateral pterygoid muscle

Medial pterygoid muscle

A

B

Figure 18–5 The posterior superior alveolar artery and the posterior superior alveolar vein of the pterygoid plexus are endangered while attempting the posterior superior alveolar nerve block **(A)** and **(B)**. The medial and lateral pterygoid muscles, the parotid sheath, and the ramus of the mandible border the pterygomandibular space **(A)**. Branches of the second part of the maxillary artery **(A)** and the pterygoid plexus **(B)** are vulnerable to penetration by a needle. The sphenomandibular ligament can potentially block the diffusion of an anesthetic **(A)**.

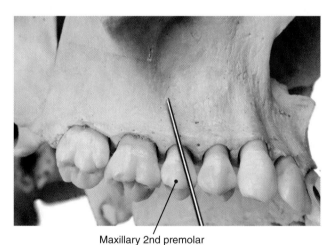

Maxillary 2nd premolar

Figure 18–6 For the middle superior alveolar nerve block, the hypodermic needle is inserted into the mucobuccal fold above the second maxillary premolar tooth.

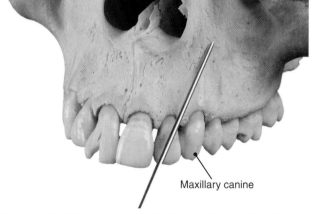

Maxillary canine

Figure 18–7 The mucobuccal fold above the maxillary lateral incisor is the insertion point of the needle for the anterior superior alveolar nerve block.

As for all injections, aspirate for blood. There is also *crossover of nerve fibers* to the central incisors from the opposite side, and additional injection may be required.

Greater Palatine Nerve Block

The *greater palatine nerve block* is useful for anesthesia to the palatal gingiva of one or more maxillary molar or premolar teeth. The insertion point of the needle is at the level of the distal border of the maxillary second molar tooth (Fig. 18–8 and Table 18–1). The target area is the soft tissue at the junction of the lateral edge of the palate and the alveolar process just anterior to the greater palatine foramen (Fig. 18–8). It is not necessary to place the needle into the foramen, because the nerve courses anteriorly from the foramen to supply the mucosa of the palate and the palatal gingiva.

Greater palatine foramen

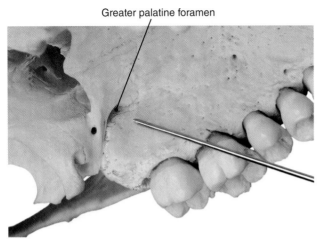

Figure 18–8 The greater palatine nerve is blocked by dispensing an anesthetic just anterior to the greater palatine foramen. The needle is placed between the junction of the palate and the alveolar process just distal to the maxillary second molar tooth.

Incisive canal

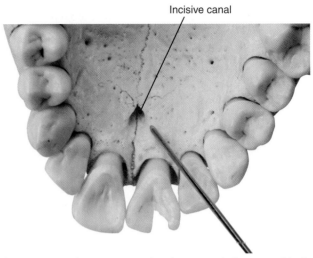

Figure 18–9 The target area for the nasopalatine nerve block is the lateral border of the incisive canal, which is deep to the incisive papilla.

Precautions

As with other areas of the maxilla, the tissue is sparse, and it is necessary to use caution with volume and pressure. The intent of the technique is not to place the needle into the greater palatine foramen because of the risk of breaking a needle tip in the foramen or shearing the blood vessels that pass through the foramen.

Nasopalatine Nerve Block

The *nasopalatine nerve* is blocked for procedures that would violate the mucosa of the primary palate and the palatal gingiva of the anterior teeth—that is, the canine and incisor teeth (Table 18–1). The needle point is directed into the lateral side of the incisive papilla in the vicinity of the opening of the incisive canal (Fig. 18–9 and Table 18–1). This area is extremely sensitive, and application of a topical anesthetic will reduce discomfort to the patient.

Precautions

Placement of the needle into the foramen should be avoided to prevent shearing of blood vessels or damaging the nasopalatine nerve. There is also *crossover of nerve fibers* to the central incisors from the opposite side, and additional injection may be required.

Infraorbital Nerve Block

Administering an anesthetic to the *infraorbital nerve* is an alternate method of blocking sensation from the anterior teeth and their labial gingiva, and the upper lip (Table 18–1). The needle is placed in the mucobuccal fold above the first premolar tooth and directed toward the infraorbital foramen (Fig. 18–10 and Table 18–1). The foramen is located underneath a ridge of the orbital

rim just medial to the lowest point of the orbit. The placement of the needle is just inferior to the foramen (Fig. 18–10). The anesthetic diffuses into the infraorbital canal, where the anterior superior alveolar nerve branches from the infraorbital nerve. This procedure also numbs the lower eyelid, the lateral portion of the nose, and the upper lip. Although these secondary side effects are useful to determine the effectiveness of the anesthetic, many patients find the loss of sensation to these areas annoying.

Precautions

As with the previous procedures, there is a risk of tearing branches of the infraorbital vein and artery, which can be avoided by aspiration. There is also the potential of

Infraorbital foramen

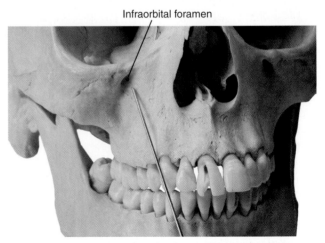

Figure 18–10 For the infraorbital nerve block procedure, the needle is inserted into the mucobuccal fold above the first maxillary premolar tooth and directed toward, but not into, the infraorbital foramen.

breaking a needle in the foramen, but the greater risk is penetrating the thin bone of the floor of the orbit and injecting the anesthetic into the area. This would not only cause loss of sensation, but the patient would not be able to move the eye, depending on the affected nerve branches. These effects are usually transient, but are also very frightening to the patient.

Review Question Box 18-4

1. What measure can be used to prevent pressure on nerves and blood vessels while administrating infiltration injections to the roots of the maxillary teeth?
2. What is the hazard of placing a needle into the infraorbital foramen?
3. Why can a central incisor still be sensitive to pain after a successful ipsilateral anterior superior alveolar nerve block?
4. Why can the mesiobuccal root of the first molar still be sensitive to pain after a posterior superior alveolar nerve block?

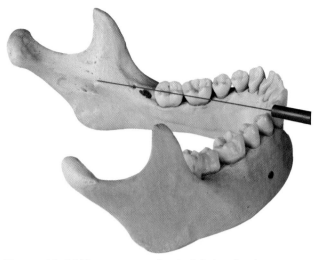

Figure 18–11 The target area for the inferior alveolar nerve block is just superior to the lingula of the mandible. The target area is approached from the first premolar tooth on the opposite side of the mouth. The needle is directed along the occlusion plane and penetrates the soft tissue between the pterygomandibular raphe and the ramus of the mandible.

NERVE BLOCKS TO BRANCHES OF THE MANDIBULAR NERVE

Unlike the maxilla, the bones surrounding the mandibular teeth are too dense for the anesthetic to penetrate by diffusion for infiltration techniques to be effective. Therefore, the inferior alveolar nerve must be blocked for dental procedures that involve the mandibular teeth. However, as for the maxillary teeth, other nerve blocks are required to block sensations from soft tissue.

Inferior Alveolar Nerve Block

The *inferior alveolar nerve block* will prevent sensation from the mandibular teeth, the buccal gingiva, and the mucosa associated with the premolar, the canine, and the incisor teeth, as well as the lower lip. The needle of the syringe is angled toward the mandible from the position of the second premolar tooth on the opposite side of the injection site in the occlusal plane (Fig. 18–11 and Table 18–2). The needle is inserted lateral to the **pterygomandibular raphe**, in a depression called the **pterygotemporal depression**, between the raphe and the ramus of the mandible. As the needle is inserted, it passes through the *buccinator muscle* and is advanced approximately 2.5 cm until it comes in contact with the bone just above the mandibular foramen.

Precautions

While injecting local anesthesia for the nerves located in the infratemporal fossa, other structures that are in harm's way must be considered. The *inferior alveolar*

nerve lies in a subdivision of the infratemporal fossa that dental clinicians call the *pterygomandibular space*. The space is bordered medially by the *medial pterygoid muscle*; laterally by the ramus of the mandible; superiorly by the lateral pterygoid muscle; and posteriorly by the connective tissue sheath of the parotid gland. Because there is no structural anterior boundary, it serves as the entranceway for the hypodermic needle to reach its target in the pterygomandibular space (Fig. 18–5A). This area contains branches of the *second part of the maxillary artery* (Fig 18.5A), the numerous anastomosing branches of the *pterygoid plexus* (Fig. 18–5B), and the *sphenomandibular ligament* (Fig 18.5A).

As with all injections, the syringe should be aspirated for blood. Puncturing an artery can cause the rapid formation of a hematoma and secondary effects of the anesthesia in the circulating blood. Injecting into a vein will also cause a hematoma, but a slower rate because the blood pressure is less in a vein than in an artery. Traumatic injury to the maxillary artery would not only result in a hematoma in the fossa, but could also result in *trismus*, which is the inability to open the mouth. In addition, injecting the needle into the lateral pterygoid muscle could cause tissue damage, which could produce a hematoma and result in trismus. If the needle is directed too far posteriorly, the needle could penetrate the parotid gland. Recall that the nerves that innervate the muscles of facial expression pass through the parotid gland to reach these muscles. Anesthesia to nerves supplying these muscles would cause *temporary facial paralysis*, which would be alarming to the patient. Upon entering the mandibular foramen, the inferior alveolar nerve lies in between the ramus of the mandible and the *sphenomandibular ligament* (Fig. 18–5B). Realize that if the anesthetic is deposited inferior to the attachment of the ligament to the lingula of the mandible, the connective tissue of the ligament could prevent its diffusion to the nerve, which would retard, reduce, or prevent complete anesthesia.

Lingual Nerve Block

In dental procedures that involve the lingual gingiva of the mandibular teeth, a *lingual nerve block* is required (Table 18–2). This procedure causes numbness and blocks sensation from the same side of the floor of the mouth and the anterior two-thirds of the tongue. The injection procedure is the same for the inferior alveolar nerve block, and is often accomplished at the same time to prevent discomfort to the patient. Once the needle touches bone, the needle is retracted approximately 1 cm and the anesthetic is deposited.

Precautions

The concerns are similar to the inferior alveolar nerve block, although the sphenomandibular ligament is inconsequential because the lingual nerve lies on the surface of the medial pterygoid muscle.

Long Buccal Nerve

The *long buccal nerve* supplies the buccal gingiva and the buccal mucosa in the vicinity of the mandibular molar teeth (Table 18–2). This procedure is accomplished by placing the needle in the buccal mucosa distal to the position of the third molar. The needle should strike the bone at the junction of the ramus and the body of the mandible (Fig. 18–12), and the anesthetic is then deposited.

Precautions

The *buccal artery* follows the path of the long buccal nerve. Although it is small, the syringe should be aspirated for blood as in all intraoral injection procedures.

Mental Nerve Block

The *mental nerve* supplies sensory fibers to the skin of the chin and lower lip (Table 18–2). The procedure is generally used to suture lacerations of the lower lip. The needle of the syringe is inserted into the buccal mucosa between the roots of the first and second premolar teeth in the mucobuccal fold. The needle should touch bone slightly posterior to the mental foramen (Fig. 18–13). Placing the needle in the mental foramen is not necessary, because the anesthetic is deposited on the nerve as the nerve exits the foramen to reach the surface.

Precautions

Placing the needle into the mental foramen should be avoided because of the danger of damaging the mental nerve as it passes through the foramen. This could be painful to the patient and could cause permanent damage to the nerve.

Incisive Nerve Block

An *incisive nerve block* can be used to partially block the mandible when access to the mandibular foramen is compromised by infection. The dental procedure affects the premolar, canine, and incisive teeth and labial gingiva (Table 18–2). Although the incisive nerve directly innervates the canine and incisive teeth, the anesthetic

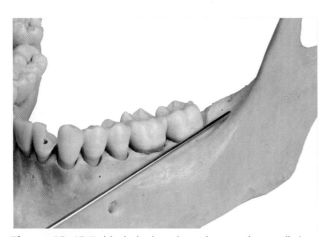

Figure 18–12 To block the long buccal nerve, the needle is inserted in the mucosa medial to the border of the ramus of the mandible at the occlusal plane of the maxillary molars. The needle should come in contact with the junction of the body and the ramus of the mandible.

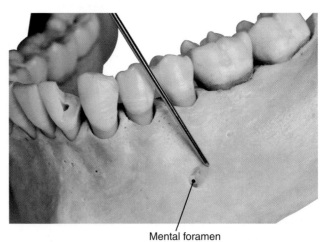

Mental foramen

Figure 18–13 The mental nerve is blocked as it exits the mental foramen. The needle penetrates the mucobuccal fold between the first and second premolar teeth. The needle should be placed posterior to, but not inserted into, the mental foramen.

will diffuse posteriorly in the mandibular canal to reach the dental branches of the premolars. The needle of the syringe is inserted to the buccal mucosa between the two premolars at the level of mucobuccal fold. The needle is glided along the bone and is gently inserted into the mental foramen and the anesthetic is deposited into the mandibular canal (Fig. 18–14).

Precautions

There is a high risk of damaging the mental nerve when placing the needle into the mental foramen. Shearing of mental nerve fibers passing to the surface could permanently damage the nerve and would be uncomfortable, or could cause persistent pain and tingling sensations.

In addition, the incisive nerve has fibers that cross from the contralateral side. A second injection medial to the root of the central incisor may also be required.

Review Question Box 18-5

1. What measures can be used to prevent damage to blood vessels and the periosteum during the inferior alveolar nerve block?

2. How does the location of the sphenomandibular ligament affect the diffusion of anesthetics during an inferior alveolar nerve block?

3. What is the effect of injecting an anesthetic into the parotid gland?

4. What is the pterygomandibular space and what is its significance to intraoral injections of the mandible?

5. What is the difference between a mental nerve block and an incisive nerve block?

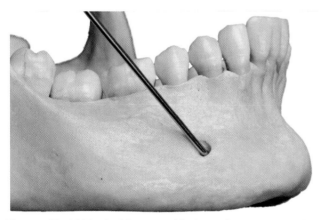

Figure 18–14 The incisive nerve block requires a more posterior approach to insert the needle into the mental foramen.

SUMMARY

The management of pain during dental procedures is essential in any dental practice and requires a thorough understanding of the innervation of the teeth and surrounding soft tissues by branches of the maxillary and mandibular nerves. Local anesthesia can be achieved by infiltration anesthesia or nerve blocks. Infiltration of anesthetics through the thin, porous supporting bone of the maxillary teeth to reach the nerve endings is adequate for maxillary teeth. However, nerve blocks are required for the mandibular teeth or when inflammation around the maxillary teeth does not allow diffusion of the anesthetic. Also, a nerve block may be preferential for procedures involving multiple maxillary teeth. There are certain general precautions that should be followed. First, in areas where there is little tissue space, a small volume of anesthetic should be slowly dispensed to reduce pressure on nerves and blood vessels. Second, the syringe should always be aspirated to ensure that a blood vessel has not been punctured or damaged. Third, the bevel of the needle should be directed to the surface of the bone to avoid tearing the periosteum. Fourth, injecting directly into a foramen should be avoided unless required by the procedure.

The maxillary teeth are innervated by a plexus of nerves formed by the posterior superior, the middle superior, and the anterior superior alveolar nerves. The posterior superior alveolar nerve innervates the molar teeth and buccal gingiva, with the possible exception of the mesiobuccal root of the first molar tooth. The middle superior alveolar nerve supplies the mesiobuccal root of the first molar and premolar teeth, whereas the anterior superior alveolar nerve innervates the anterior teeth. In procedures involving the palatal gingiva of the molar and premolar teeth, such as a tooth extraction, the greater palatine nerve must be blocked. For similar procedures for the anterior teeth, the nasopalatine nerve must be blocked.

The mandibular teeth are innervated by the inferior alveolar nerve. The lingual nerve must also be blocked for procedures involving the lingual gingiva of all the teeth and the long buccal nerve must be anesthetized for the gingiva and mucosa of the mandibular molar teeth. The inferior alveolar and lingual nerves are located in the pterygomandibular space. The inferior alveolar nerve lies between the ramus of the mandible and the sphenomandibular ligament as it enters the mandibular canal. Depositing an anesthetic medial and inferior to the sphenomandibular ligament results in incomplete anesthesia to the nerve because the connective tissue limits the diffusion of the anesthetic to the nerve. The clinician must also realize that branches of the maxillary artery, the pterygoid plexus of veins, the pterygoid muscles, and the parotid gland can be damaged by an incorrectly placed needle.

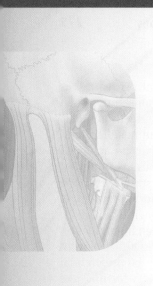

LEARNING LAB

Exercises for review, practice, and study

Learning Activity 18-1

What Went Wrong?

Scenario 1: You are participating in a simulated private practice rotation with a senior dental student to role play as part of a dental health team. The first appointment of the day is a 35-year-old male who has been scheduled for a routine crown preparation on his left mandibular first molar. According to his medical records, he has no apparent allergies to any medications. You check his pulse and blood pressure, and his vital signs are normal. The attending dentist asks your group what nerves must be anesthetized for this procedure?

1. What is your answer?

You correctly answer the *left inferior alveolar*, *lingual*, and *long buccal nerves*. The dental student uses a single injection for both the inferior alveolar nerve and the lingual nerve, and a second injection for the long buccal nerve.

Within minutes, the patient is blinking more frequently on the right side of the face than on the left. The team suspects that the patient is having a reaction to the anesthetic and is concerned that the patient will go into shock. You recheck his vital signs, and his vital signs are normal. Further examination indicates that the patient cannot move his muscles on the left side of his face. The team is now concerned he has suffered a stroke and calls emergency medical services. The paramedics confirm the patient did not have a systemic reaction to the anesthetic and did not have a stroke.

2. What went wrong?

Although the patient claims to have no allergies to medication, you must consider the potential for an allergic or systemic reaction. In this case, the patient has normal vital signs, but the facial paralysis could indicate a stroke. Again, that was not the case. His facial paralysis on the same side of the injection indicates an alternate explanation. The inferior alveolar nerve and the lingual nerve are located in the pterygomandibular fossa, which is bordered posteriorly by the parotid gland. If the anesthetic is deposited into the parotid gland, the facial nerve could be affected and cause facial paralysis on the side of the injection.

Within a couple of hours, the patient slowly gains controls of his facial muscles, thus confirming the anesthetic was inadvertently injected into the parotid gland.

Learning Activity 18-2

Your First Intraoral Nerve Block

Scenario: You are being trained by a clinician in the dental clinic to administer intraoral injections. You have been assigned a patient who needs a crown on his maxillary first molar tooth. Before you begin, you must determine which nerves need to be anesthetized, explain your choices, and be able to discuss the injection site and any precautions for the injections.

1. Which nerves must be blocked and why?

a. Posterior superior alveolar nerve: Because soft tissue will be traumatized during the preparation of the tooth for a crown, infiltration anesthesia would not achieve the pain insensitivity required. The posterior superior alveolar nerve supplies the roots of the first molar and the facial (buccal) gingiva, with the possible exception of the mesiobuccal root.

b. Middle superior alveolar nerve: Even though the nerve is present only 30% of the time, it supplies the mesiobuccal root of the first maxillary molar tooth and should be treated as if it is always present.

c. Greater palatine nerve: The palatal gingiva of all the maxillary teeth is innervated by the greater palatine nerve, and thus must be anesthetized for the procedure.

2. What precautionary measures should be considered prior to all injections?

a. The length and bore of the hypodermic needle is important. Using the improper length needle can increase risk to surrounding tissues and decrease the accuracy of the placement of the needle at target. Smaller diameter needles will make the penetration of the needle less painful.

b. The bevel of the needle should always be placed on the surface of the bone to prevent the tearing of the periosteum.

c. Avoid placing the needle into a foramen unless it is required by the procedure. This will help prevent tearing of nerves and vessels passing through the openings.

d. Aspirate the syringe for blood. If there is blood in the syringe, redirect the needle and aspirate again until the syringe is clear.

e. In areas where there is little tissue space between the teeth, bone, and mucosa, use a small volume of anesthetic and deposit it slowly to prevent placing pressure on the tissues.

3. What is the injection site and what is in harm's way of the target?

a. The branches of the *posterior superior alveolar* nerve enter the maxilla by the foramina on the posterior surface of the maxillary tuberosity. The hypodermic needle is inserted into the mucobuccal fold above the second maxillary molar and is directed posteromedially along the surface of the bone for approximately 2.5 cm. The anesthetic is deposited after aspiration of the syringe. Care must be taken not tear the branches of the posterior superior alveolar artery and vein, which accompany the nerve along its path, or tear the periosteum.

b. The *middle superior alveolar nerve* passes through the bone of the lateral surface of the maxillary sinus in the vicinity of the secondary maxillary premolar tooth. The needle is inserted into the mucobuccal fold, and although the blood vessels are very small, the syringe is aspirated for blood before dispensing the anesthetic. The tissue space is very small; therefore, a small volume of anesthetic should be slowly released. Turning the bevel of the needle to face the bone will decrease the risk of tearing the periosteum.

c. The *greater palatine nerve* enters the mucosa of the hard palate by passing through the greater palatine foramen located slightly distal to the maxillary second molar. The needle is inserted into the mucosa just posterior to the second molar at the junction between the hard palate and alveolar process. Placing the needle into the foramen should be avoided to prevent tearing of the greater palatine artery and vein that accompany the nerve or breaking the needle in the greater palatine canal. The narrow tissue space between the mucosa and bone of the hard palate requires the slow release of a small volume of anesthetic.

You have answered the preliminary questions, and now, anatomically speaking, it is time to inject.

For Discussion or Thought:

1. How do you decide which nerves must be blocked for a particular procedure?

2. What hazards should be considered when administrating an intraoral injection?

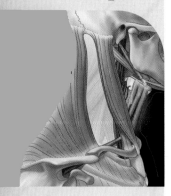

chapter

19

Orofacial Reflexes

Objectives

1. Distinguish between the terms *reflex* and *reflex arc*; name the components of a reflex arc.
2. Distinguish between interneurons and reflex centers.
3. Compare the pathways for the cornea, the blink-to-light, and the tear reflexes.
4. Compare the pathways for the cough and gag reflexes.

Overview

What generally happens when you accidentally touch something hot, such as a stove, with your hand? You instinctively remove your hand to prevent burning yourself. After a short delay, you tell yourself that you moved your hand because the stove was hot. This instinctive response is an example of a reflex. In this chapter, you will study reflexes that are associated with the face and oral cavity that can affect your patient's comfort during oral examinations.

INTRODUCTION TO OROFACIAL REFLEXES

A **reflex** is a predictable, involuntary response to an outside stimulus. Many responses are protective to prevent injury to the body or a fixed pattern such as breathing or swallowing. In the example in the Overview, the command to move the hand does not arise from the brain, but from motor neurons in the spinal cord. You remove your hand first, and then consciously say to yourself, "I removed my hand because it was hot." To recognize

the stimulus as temperature, the information must reach the brain by an alternate pathway—the spinothalamic tract. Voluntary commands to move the hand arise from the cerebrum and are transferred to the motor neurons in the spinal cord by the corticospinal tract.

A **reflex arc** refers to the pathway or structures through which a stimulus must travel to invoke a response. The reflex arc is composed of a **sensory limb** and a **motor limb**. The *sensory limb* is formed by a **receptor** that receives the stimulus and a **sensory neuron** that carries the impulse via spinal or cranial nerves to the central nervous system. The *motor limb*, which begins at a **motor neuron**, transmits the impulse via spinal or cranial nerves to an **effector**, which can be a muscle or a gland. A reflex can be **monosynaptic**, in which the central process of the sensory neuron synapses directly on the motor neuron (Fig. 19–1) or **polysynaptic**, in which the sensory neuron synapses on one or more **interneurons** (Fig. 19–2). Interneurons are neurons that transfer the sensory impulse to the motor neuron. Reflexes involving the visceral organs (visceral reflexes) are complex and frequently require a **reflex center**, which is composed of multiple neurons to coordinate multiple activities. Respiratory rate, blood pressure, and heart rate are examples of visceral reflexes that have respiratory and cardiovascular centers in the medulla of the brain stem. Sensory neurons synapse with the neurons in the reflex center. Then, nerve fibers from the reflex center synapse on motor neurons of the brain stem and spinal cord.

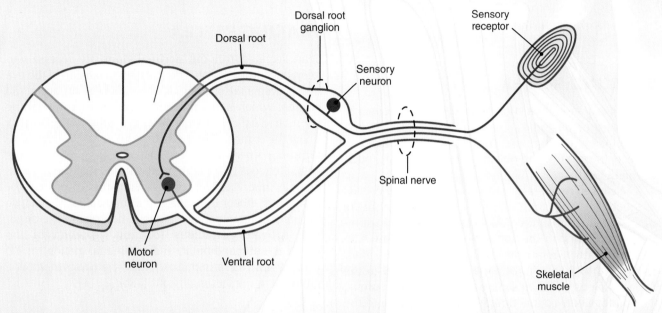

Figure 19–1 The reflex arc has an afferent limb, which is composed of a receptor and a sensory nerve, and an efferent limb formed by a motor neuron and skeletal muscle. In a monosynaptic reflex, the afferent nerve synapses directly on the motor neuron.

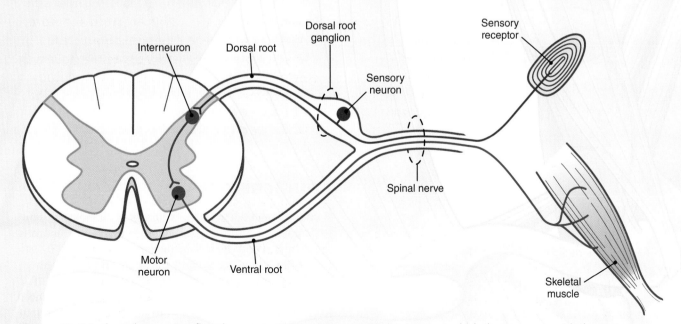

Figure 19–2 In the polysynaptic reflex, the sensory nerve synapses on an interneuron, which then synapses with the motor neuron, which causes the muscle to contract.

Although it is not necessary for a dental hygienist to know the details of the polysynaptic reflex arc, the hygienist should be aware of the sensory input and motor output of reflexes associated with stimulation to the face and oral cavity. This chapter will discuss reflexes that a hygienist may initiate during oral examinations.

Review Question Box 19-1

1. What is the difference between a reflex and a reflex arc?
2. How is the function of the interneuron and a reflex center similar? How are they different?

BLINKING REFLEX

Blinking is a normal function of the eyelids. The opening and closing of the eyelid spreads the tears across the surface of the eye to keep the cornea moist. The blink reflex protects the eye from an outside stimulus such as touch or bright light.

The **cornea reflex** results in the blinking of the eyelids to touch (Fig. 19–3 and Table 19–1). The sensory fibers of the **ophthalmic nerve (V_1)** carry impulses from stimulated receptors on the cornea to the brain stem. The sensory fibers synapse on neurons within the *spinal nucleus of V*. Fibers from these neurons project to the **facial nucleus** and then synapse on the motor neurons. The motor fibers course through the facial nerve to the **orbicularis oculi muscle**, causing the muscle to contract, which closes the eyelids.

Reflex blinking to light takes an alternate pathway (Fig. 19–4 and Table 19–1). Intense light stimulates receptors of the **retina**. Impulses are carried by the optic nerve and synapse with neurons in the **superior colliculus**. The superior colliculus coordinates reflexes associated with vision. In the light blinking pathway, fibers project and synapse on the motor neurons of the *facial nucleus*. Motor fibers in the facial nerve cause the *orbicularis oculi muscle* to contract and close the eyelids.

TEARING REFLEX

Tears secreted from the **lacrimal gland** are necessary to keep the cornea moist. The constant cleansing of the eye also prevents the sticking of bacteria to the surface of the cornea, which helps prevent infection. Tearing can be stimulated by cold wind, dust, and other particles that touch the cornea. The *ophthalmic nerve (V_1)* carries stimuli from corneal receptors to synapse on neurons in the spinal nucleus of V (Table 19–1). Recall that the lacrimal gland is innervated by the parasympathetic nervous system. Thus, fibers from the spinal nucleus of V synapse on preganglionic parasympathetic neurons in the **superior salivatory nucleus** (controls secretion of the lacrimal, submandibular, and sublingual glands) of VII (Fig. 19–5). Nerve impulses follow the parasympathetic pathway to the lacrimal gland (Table 19–1).

Review Question Box 19-2

1. What component of the blinking and tearing reflex is the same?
2. What is the difference in the afferent nerve of the blink-to-light reflex compared to the blink-to-touch and the tear reflexes?
3. What serves as the interneuron for the blink-to-light reflex?
4. What is the motor nucleus for the tear reflex?
5. What is the effector for the blink reflexes?

COUGH REFLEX

A **cough** is a sudden, noisy expulsion of air from the lungs to help clear respiratory passageways of mucus, dust, and other offensive particles. A cough can be initiated by irritation of cough receptors in the *respiratory passages* by inflammatory, mechanical, thermal, and chemical stimuli. *Inflammatory* receptors can be stimulated by postnasal drip from colds and flu or from infection of the airway. Inhalation of particulate matter, which is possible during dental procedures, and compression of the airway by

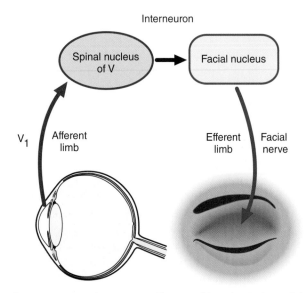

Figure 19–3 In the cornea reflex, touching the surface of the eye causes the eyelid to close. Fibers of the ophthalmic nerve synapse in the spinal nucleus of V, which serves as an interneuron. Fibers from the nucleus synapse with neurons in the facial motor nucleus that innervates the orbicularis oculi muscle, which closes the eyelids.

TABLE 19–1	Reflex Arcs of the Eyes				
	Afferent Limb			Efferent Limb	
Reflex	Receptor	Nerve	Interneuron	Motor nucleus	Effector
Cornea (blink-to-touch)	Cornea	V_1*	Spinal nucleus of V	Facial nucleus	Orbicularis oculi muscle
Blink to light	Retina	Optic nerve	Superior colliculus	Facial nucleus	Orbicularis oculi muscle
Tear	Cornea	V_1*	Spinal nucleus of V	Superior salivatory nucleus of VII	Lacrimal gland

* V_1 = ophthalmic nerve

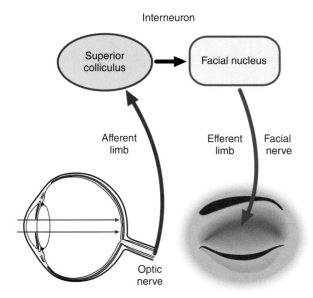

Figure 19–4 In the blink-to-light reflex, bright light strikes the receptors of the retina. The sensory fibers in the optic nerve synapse in the superior colliculus, which functions as the interneuron. Fibers that arise from the colliculus synapse on the motor nucleus of the facial nerve, which cause the lids to close.

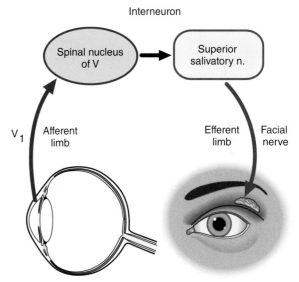

Figure 19–5 The tear reflex can be initiated by cold and debris. The ophthalmic nerve carries sensory information to the spinal nucleus of V, which functions as the interneuron. Fibers from the spinal nucleus synapse on the superior salivatory nucleus of the facial nerve. The nucleus causes the stimulation of the lacrimal gland through the parasympathetic pathway.

Clinical Correlation Box 19-1

Blepharospasm (in Greek, *blephuro* means "eyelid") is the frequent involuntary closure of the eyelid. The eye blinks can become a spasm in which the eyelid closes tightly, causing temporary blindness because of the inability to open the eyelid. The condition can be sporadic or chronic. The etiology is unknown but can be initiated by emotional trauma, bright light, fatigue, or dry eyes.

Meige (named after a French physician) **syndrome** is a combination of blepharospasm with spasms of the muscles of the mandible and surrounding the mouth. In addition to involuntary blinking, individuals with this syndrome may have difficulty smiling, may clench their teeth, and may have difficulty opening their mouths.

various tissue growths are examples of *mechanical* stimuli. Inhalation of cold air and drinking something very cold or hot are *thermal stimuli*, whereas cigarette smoke and noxious chemical gases (chlorine and ammonia in cleaning products) are examples of *chemical stimuli*.

The cough cycle occurs in stages. During the first stage, air is inhaled into the lungs. The more air in the lungs, the more forceful the cough. In the second stage, the vestibular folds (false vocal cords) and vocal folds are closed. The vestibular folds are very effective in preventing air from leaving the lungs. This results in an increase of intrathoracic pressure. When the air pressure has significantly increased, the laryngeal folds suddenly open, releasing a forceful rush of air. The explosive nature of the released air produces the sound but, more importantly, has the force to expel foreign material.

The *superior laryngeal branch* of the vagus nerve supplies afferent fibers to the mucosa of the larynx and efferent fibers to the laryngeal muscles. The reflex arc begins with receptors located in the major air passage. Fibers of the superior laryngeal nerve of the vagus nerve (X) synapse with neurons in the cough reflex center in the medulla. Fibers from the reflex center synapse in the *nucleus ambiguus*, which is the origin of the efferent fibers of the vagus (X). The nerve fibers innervate the muscles of the larynx that open and close the vestibular and vocal folds (Fig. 19–6 and Table 19–2).

Review Question Box 19-3

1. What is a cough?
2. What factors can stimulate the cough reflex?
3. What determines the forcefulness of a cough?
4. What cranial nerve is both the sensory and motor nerve for the cough reflex?

GAG REFLEX

The *gag reflex* is an involuntary contraction of the back of the oropharynx to prevent unwanted objects from entering the lower passageways into the stomach. It is associated with swallowing. The gag reflex can be initiated by *touch* receptors on the posterior surface of the pharynx,

the soft palate, and the posterior one-third of the tongue. Also, *psychic stimuli,* such as visual, auditory, olfactory, and emotional stimuli, can initiate the gag reflex.

The *glossopharyngeal nerve (IX)* supplies the sensory fibers to the oropharynx, whereas *the vagus nerve (X)* supplies the motor fibers to the area (Fig. 19–7). Afferent stimuli from touch receptors are carried to a reflex center in the medulla by the pharyngeal (IX) nerve. Nerve fibers from the reflex center synapse in the *nucleus ambiguus*, which contains the motor neurons for the vagus nerve. Motor fibers from the nucleus course through the vagus nerve (X) to muscles that constrict the pharynx and close the epiglottis (Fig. 19–7 and Table 19–2).

Review Question Box 19-4

1. What factor can stimulate the gag reflex?
2. Why can a hygienist scale teeth and touch the gingiva without initiating the gag reflex?
3. What nerve is the afferent limb of the gag reflex, and where does it synapse?
4. What is the location of the reflex center for cough and gag reflexes?
5. What is the motor nucleus for the cough and gag reflexes?

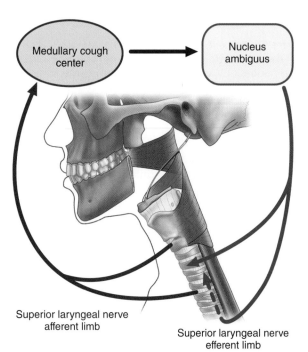

Figure 19–6 The cough reflex is a polysynaptic reflex that includes a reflex center. Sensory fibers of the superior laryngeal nerve carry the stimulus and synapse in a diffuse network of cells that serves as a cough reflex center in the medulla. Fibers from the center synapse in the nucleus ambiguus, which sends motor fibers through superior laryngeal nerve to the muscles of the larynx.

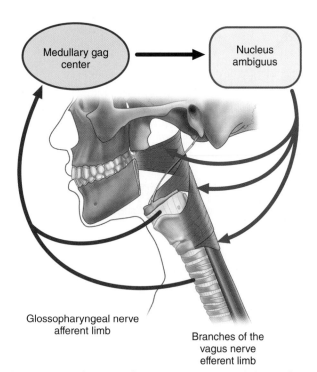

Figure 19–7 The gag reflex prevents unwanted objects from entering the lower passages of the GI tract. The glossopharyngeal nerve carries sensory information to the gag center in the medullary reticular formation. Fibers from the center synapse on the motor neurons in the nucleus ambiguus. Branches of the vagus nerve innervate the muscles of the pharyngeal wall, which causes them to constrict.

TABLE 19–2 | Cough and Gag Reflex Arcs

	Afferent Limb		Efferent Limb		
Reflex	Receptor	Nerve	Reflex center	Motor nucleus	Effector
Cough	Air passages	Superior laryngeal nerve	Medulla	Nucleus ambiguus	Laryngeal muscles
Gag	Pharynx, soft palate, the posterior one-third of the tongue	Pharyngeal nerve	Medulla	Nucleus ambiguus	Muscle that constrict the pharynx and the epiglottis

Box 19-1 Reflex Centers

The *reticular formation* is a network of nuclei located in the central core of the midbrain, the pons, and the medulla. Discrete cardiovascular and respiratory reflex centers have been isolated in the medullary reticular formation. The reflex center for the gag and cough reflex are located in the medulla, but they are probably a more diffuse network of neurons along the lateral surface of the reticular formation.

Clinical Correlation Box 19-2

Learning how to control the *gag reflex* is important to the dental hygienist. Some patients are more hypersensitive to *touch* than others. Patients suffering from chronic sinus problems that cause postnasal drip are very sensitive. The hygienist must be mindful of the placement of instruments in a patient's mouth, particularly while cleaning the molar teeth. Scaling in the more anterior regions of the mouth before cleaning the more sensitive molar regions will help relax the patient. Realize that the accumulation of *saliva* or *water spray* from an ultrasonic scaling device can also stimulate the gag reflex. This can be prevented by tilting the head forward and suctioning the excess fluid. *Psychic stimuli*, such as the unpleasant thought of gagging, can initiate the reflex. A person cannot gag while breathing. Therefore, try to distract the patient from the unpleasant thought of gagging. If necessary, instruct the patient to breathe through the nose, because the first step in gagging is actually the cessation of breathing before the contraction of the pharyngeal muscles.

SUMMARY

A reflex is a predictable involuntary response to a stimulus, and can be protective or follow multiple routine patterns such as swallowing food or fluids. A reflex has sensory and motor components; the combination of these components is called a reflex arc. In the simplest reflex, the afferent limb is composed of a receptor and a sensory nerve, and the motor limb is formed by a motor nerve and its effector—that is, muscle. The central process of the neuron synapses directly onto the motor neuron, and its fiber stimulates the muscle. Other reflexes have an interneuron, which transmits the sensory stimulus to the motor sensory neuron. Some reflexes, such as breathing, require coordination of multiple activities, which take place in reflex centers in the medulla.

Several reflexes, such as blinking and tearing, can be initiated during a dental examination. Eye blinking can be caused by touch or extremely bright light. Touching the retina stimulates the receptors that are innervated by the ophthalmic nerve. The central fibers synapse with neurons in the spinal nucleus of V. These interneurons synapse with the facial nucleus, whose nerve fibers innervate the orbicularis oculi muscle that closes the eyelid. On the other hand, bright light stimulates the receptors in the retina and the stimulus is carried by the optic nerve. Some of the nerve fibers synapse with neurons located in the superior colliculus. Nerve fibers from these neurons synapse with motor neurons of the facial nucleus, which then stimulates the orbicularis oculi muscle. Tearing can be caused by dust or debris that touches the cornea. The sensory fibers of the ophthalmic nerve synapse in the spinal nucleus of V, but in this case, their fibers synapse in the superior salivatory nucleus of VII. The motor limb is the parasympathetic pathway to the lacrimal gland.

The cough and gag reflexes can be initiated to prevent foreign objects from entering the respiratory system and lower passageways that lead to the stomach. These reflexes include multiple responses that are generated from reflex centers. The cough reflex results from stimulation of receptors in the larynx. The sensory and motor limbs are formed by branches of the superior laryngeal nerve. The gag reflex is caused by the stimulation of sensory receptors in the back of the pharynx, the tongue, and the soft palate that are innervated by the glossopharyngeal nerve. The motor limb includes the nucleus ambiguus and motor fibers of the vagus nerve that innervate the muscles of the pharynx, which constrict the pharynx and close the epiglottis.

Learning Activity 19-1

Putting It Together

While studying the various topics within the chapters of this book, you learned about individual bones, muscles, nerves, and blood vessels. Although memorization is one of the first steps in learning, the final goal is to understand how these structures integrate to perform a task and how they can be used to solve a problem. In this activity, you will learn how to integrate what you have studied using the orofacial reflexes as examples.

Example 1: The Cornea Reflex

Let's examine each component of the reflex arc for the *cornea reflex*, which results in the closing of the eyelid after the cornea is touched (Table 19–1).

The *afferent limb* begins with the receptors on the surface of the *cornea* of the eye. We know that receptors are specific to various sensations—that is, specific receptors on the tongue can perceive taste, but the same receptor cannot feel pain. Receptors on the cornea discriminate among pain, temperature, and touch. Once the receptor is stimulated, the information is carried to the central nervous system by sensory nerve fibers. The cell bodies of these fibers are located in the trigeminal ganglion (Chapter 17). So what division of the trigeminal ganglion innervates the eyelids and the cornea? If your answer was the *ophthalmic division*, you are correct. Now, can you specify the branches? As a hint, the nerves that exit along the superior rim of the orbit supply the eyelid and the cornea. Starting medially, these include the *infratrochlear, supratrochlear, supraorbital*, and *lacrimal nerves*. Recall that the ophthalmic nerve divides into three major branches. The infratrochlear nerve is a terminal branch of the nasociliary nerve; the supratrochlear and supraorbital nerves are terminal branches of the frontal nerve; and the lacrimal nerve terminates along the eyelid after supplying the lacrimal gland. After the stimulus is carried by one or more of these nerves, the afferent fibers synapse in the *spinal nucleus of V*. Neurons of this nucleus connect the afferent limb to the efferent limb. Nerve fibers of the spinal nucleus synapse in the *facial nucleus*, which supplies the muscles of facial expression (Chapter 16). The nerve fibers exit the brain stem at the pontomedullary junction as the facial nerve, which enters into the internal acoustic meatus. The nerve exits the stylomastoid foramen, courses through the parotid gland, and divides into five branches. Motor fibers in the *temporal* and *zygomatic nerves* innervate the *orbicularis oculi muscle*. This circle-shaped muscle originates from the orbital rim and inserts into the skin of the eyelids (Chapter 5). Contraction and relaxation of this muscle causes a blink.

Example 2: The Tear Reflex

The afferent limb is the same for the cornea reflex; however, the *efferent limb* is more complex because it includes the *parasympathetic nervous system* (Table 19–1), which requires two neurons to reach the target organ. What is the location of the *preganglionic parasympathetic neurons* that control the secretion of the lacrimal gland? If your answer was the *superior salivatory nucleus* of the facial nerve, you are correct. Let's see what you remember from Chapter 16. The preganglionic parasympathetic fibers enter the internal acoustic meatus and turn anteriorly as the greater petrosal nerve. This nerve joins postganglionic sympathetic fibers from the internal carotid plexus to form the nerve of the pterygoid canal. The fibers synapse on the *postganglionic parasympathetic neurons* in the *pterygopalatine ganglion*. The postganglionic parasympathetic fibers join the *zygomatic branch* of the maxillary nerve (V_2) to reach the orbit. Within the orbit, the postganglionic fibers enter a communicating branch that joins the *lacrimal nerve* of V_1. The fibers enter the gland, causing the release of tears.

The purpose of this activity was not to see how many details you remembered. The head and neck, and for that matter the entire body, do not comprise just a list of bones, muscles, nerves, and vessels, but an integrated unit. When one of its components is not functioning properly, it may affect the others. The dental hygienist needs to know what is normal to recognize what is abnormal and help restore the balance as it pertains to the oral cavity.

Glossary

A

Abducens nerve: Cranial nerve number VI; motor innervation of the superior oblique muscle.

Accessory nerve: Cranial nerve XI; motor innervation of the sternocleidomastoid and trapezius muscles.

Accessory root canal: An aberrant opening on the lateral surface of the root of a tooth.

Afferent: Going toward a structure.

Afferent fibers: Sensory fibers; fibers going toward the central nervous system.

Ala: Wing.

Alar fascia: A loose connective tissue that fills the potential space between the pharynx and the bodies of the cervical vertebrae.

Alpha motor euron: A cell of the ventral horn of the spinal cord that innervates skeletal muscle.

Alveolar bone proper: A portion of the alveolar process that forms the socket of the tooth.

Alveolar mucosa: Nonkeratinized epithelium and connective tissue that covers a portion of the alveolar process.

Alveolar process: A portion of the jaw that contains the teeth.

Alveolingual sulcus: A groove of the floor of the mouth formed by the reflection of the mucosa of the alveolar bone to the under surface of the tongue.

Alveolus: A small sac-like structure; the socket of the tooth.

Anatomical crown: A portion of the tooth covered by enamel and dentin.

Anatomical position: The position in which an individual is standing erect with head, eyes, and toes directed forward and upper limbs hanging at the sides with the palms facing forward.

Aneurysm: A sac formed by the dilation of the wall of a blood vessel.

Angle: The posterior junction between the body and ramus of the mandible.

Angular artery: A terminal branch of the facial artery that ends at the medial commissure of the eye.

Ansa cervicalis: A loop of nerves in the neck that supplies many of the infrahyoid muscles.

Anterior: Toward the abdomen; ventral.

Anterior arch: The anterior curvature of the atlas.

Anterior belly of the digastric muscle: Suprahyoid muscle that assists in depressing the mandible, and raises and steadies the hyoid bone during swallowing and speaking.

Anterior cerebral artery: A branch of the internal carotid artery that contributes to the circle of Willis.

Anterior cervical triangle: One of the two major triangles of the neck that share the sternocleidomastoid muscle as their common border.

Anterior cleft palate: A fissure caused by the improper fusion of the primary palate with the secondary palate.

Anterior communicating artery: A small vessel that forms a bridge between the two anterior cerebral arteries.

Anterior cranial fossa: A depression of the cranial base between the frontal bone and the lesser wing of the sphenoid bone.

Anterior ethmoidal nerve: A branch of the nasociliary nerve that supplies sensory fibers to the paranasal sinuses and the dorsum of the nose.

Anterior horn: An extension of the lateral ventricles into the frontal lobe.

Anterior inferior cerebellar artery: A branch of the basilar artery that supplies a portion of the cerebellum.

Anterior jugular vein: An inconstant vein that drains the submental region.

Anterior scalene muscle: The muscle that elevates the first rib during forceful breathing.

Anterior spinal artery: A branch of the vertebral artery that supplies the ventral surface of the spinal cord.

Anterior superior alveolar artery: A branch of the infraorbital artery that supplies the anterior maxillary teeth.

Anterior superior alveolar nerve: A branch of the infraorbital nerve that supplies the anterior maxillary teeth.

Anterior tonsillar pillars: Folds of mucosa that form the entrance into the fauces; the palatoglossal folds.

Antibody: An immunoglobulin that complexes with antigens.

Antigen: A protein that stimulates the formation of an antibody.

Anulus fibrosus: The outer cartilaginous ring of an intervertebral disc.

Aorta: The outflow vessel of the left ventricle; conducts blood via its branches to all tissues and organs of the body.

Aortic arch: The curved portion of the aorta.

Aperture: A large opening.

Apical foramen: An opening at the apex of the root of a tooth.

Aponeurosis: A flattened sheet of connective tissue that attaches muscle to bone or cartilage; a sheet-like tendon.

Arachnoid granulation: A specialized capillary-like structure that returns cerebral spinal fluid to the venous circulation.

Arachnoid mater: A delicate connective tissue cover of the brain and spinal cord that contains a network of spider-web fibers.

Articular capsule: The connective tissue covering of a synovial joint.

Articular cartilage: The cartilage that covers the surface of bone where it comes in contact with another bone.

Articular disc: A connective tissue partition that divides the temporomandibular joint into upper and lower joint spaces.

Articular eminence: The anterior sloping surface of the mandibular fossa.

Articular tubercle: A projection on the zygomatic process for the attachment of the articular capsule of the temporomandibular joint.

Articulations: The union between bones; joints.

Aryepiglottic fold: A fold of mucosa that connects the epiglottic and arytenoid cartilages of the larynx.

Arytenoid cartilage: A small cartilage of the larynx for the attachment of the vocal cords.

Ascending aorta: The first part of the aorta that courses superiorly before it bends and crosses the median plane.

Ascending pharyngeal artery: A branch of the external carotid artery that supplies the pharynx.

Atlas: The first cervical vertebra.

Atrium: An entrance hall; the chamber of the heart that receives blood.

Attached gingiva: The portion of the gingiva that is directly attached to the alveolar process or the surface of the tooth.

Auditory tubes: Cartilaginous tubes that connect the nasopharynx and the middle ear.

Auriculotemporal nerve: A branch of the mandibular nerve that supplies postganglionic parasympathetic fibers from the otic ganglion to the parotid gland and sensory fibers to the parotid gland, TMJ, and skin anterior to the ear.

Autonomic nervous system: The efferent or motor division of the brain and spinal cord that controls involuntary movement and functions.

Axial plane: A term used by radiologists for a horizontal plane.

Axis: The second cervical vertebra.

Axon: The cytoplasmic process of a neuron that carries a stimulus away from the nerve cell body.

B

Bacteremia: The presence of bacteria in the peripheral blood.

Bartholin's duct: The major duct of the sublingual gland.

Basilar artery: The vessel formed by the fusion of the two vertebral arteries.

Bell's palsy: A paralysis of the muscles of facial expression because of possible viral infection to branches of the facial nerve.

Belly: The portion of a muscle that contains the contractile elements.

Bicuspid valve: A flap that separates the left atrium and ventricle; two cusps; the mitral valve.

Blepharospasm: Frequent involuntary closure of the eyelid.

Body: The central or main mass of a bone.

Body of the hyoid bone: The central mass of the hyoid bone.

Bone: A calcified connective tissue that forms the skeleton.

Bone marrow: The blood-forming tissue found within a bone.

Brachial plexus: A nerve plexus that innervates the upper extremity.

Brachiocephalic trunk or artery: The first of the great vessels to branch off the aorta.

Brachiocephalic vein: A vessel that receives blood from the head and upper extremity via the internal jugular and subclavian veins.

Brain: The cerebrum, diencephalon, brain stem, and cerebellum.

Brain stem: The mass of nuclei and fiber tracts that connects the spinal cord to the diencephalon.

Bridge of the nose: A portion of the external nose formed by the nasal bones.

Broca's aphasia: Difficulty speaking because of injury to the motor speech area of the frontal lobe.

Broca's area: A collection of neurons located on the inferior frontal gyrus on the frontal lobe of the dominant gyrus that controls the ability to form words.

Bruxism: Grinding of the teeth.

Buccal: Referring to the cheek wall.

Buccal artery: A branch of the third part of the maxillary artery that supplies the buccinator muscle and cheek wall.

Buccal nerve: A branch of the facial nerve that supplies motor fibers to the muscles of facial expression around the mouth.

Buccal vestibule: A space between the cheek wall and the teeth.

Buccinator muscle: A muscle of facial expression that presses the cheek against the teeth.

Buccopharyngeal fascia: A layer of connective tissue that covers the posterior surface of the pharynx.

Bulging disc: An intervertebral disc characterized by the inner gelatinous core extending into the cartilaginous outer ring, but does not rupture the cartilage.

C

Calcarine fissure: A cleft on the medial surface of the cerebrum that subdivides the occipital lobe; a cleft that is perpendicular to the lateral fissure.

Calvaria: The brain cap; the portion of the skull that is removed to expose the brain.

Canal: A tubular passageway.

Canine eminence: An elevation of the maxillary bone created by the canine tooth.

Canine fossa: A depression of the maxillary bone posterolateral to the root of the canine tooth.

Capillary: A thin-walled vessel where gas, nutrients, and waste are interchanged from the blood and body tissues.

Cardiovascular system: The heart and vessels that distribute and return blood to the heart.

Carotid canal: A channel through the skull allowing for the passage of the internal carotid artery.

Carotid sheath: A sleeve of connective tissue that surrounds the carotid vessels, internal jugular vein, and vagus nerve in the neck.

Carotid triangle: A subsidiary triangle of the neck that contains the carotid sheath.

Cartilage: A semirigid connective tissue that forms part of the skeletal system.

Cartilaginous: Pertaining to cartilage.

Cauda equina: Literally means "horse's tail"; formed by the motor and sensory rootlets of the inferior segments of the spinal cord.

Caudal: Toward the feet.

Cavernous sinus: A dural sinus located lateral to the pituitary gland.

Cavernous sinus thrombosis: A blood clot in the cavernous sinus.

Central nervous system (CNS):   The brain and spinal cord.

Central sulcus: A deep fissure that separates the frontal and parietal lobes of the cerebrum.

Cerebellum: Literally means "tiny cerebrum"; the portion of the brain that coordinates balance, equilibrium, and smooth movements of skeletal muscle.

Cerebral aqueduct (aqueduct of Sylvius):   A small canal in the midbrain that connects the third ventricle to the fourth ventricle.

Cerebral hemispheres: Two masses of nervous tissue that form the cerebrum.

Cerebral peduncles: The large fiber tracts of the midbrain that arise from neurons in the cerebrum.

Cerebral spinal fluid: The protective fluid that bathes the brain and spinal cord.

Cerebrum: The cerebral hemispheres; the main portion of the brain.

Cervical enlargement: An enlarged area of the spinal cord to accommodate the neurons needed to innervate the upper extremity.

Cervical nerve: A branch of the facial nerve that supplies motor fibers to the platysma muscle.

Cervical plexus: A nerve plexus that innervates muscles and the skin of the neck.

Cervical vertebrae: The bones that form the structure of the neck.

Cervicalis: Pertaining to the neck.

Chiasm: Crossing line.

Chief sensory nucleus of V: The location of sensory neurons that perceive touch and proprioception.

Choana: Literally means "a funnel"; openings between the nasal cavities and the nasopharynx.

Chondrocytes: The cells found within the cartilage matrix.

Chorda tympani nerve: A branch of the facial nerve that carries preganglionic parasympathetic fibers and taste fibers.

Choroid plexus: A specialized capillary-like structure that forms cerebral spinal fluid.

Ciliary ganglion: An aggregation of postganglionic parasympathetic neurons.

Cingulate gyrus: A major component of the limbic lobe.

Circle of Willis: A circle of blood vessels on the inferior surface of the brain formed by branches of the internal carotid and basilar arteries.

Clavicle: The collar bone.

Clinical crown: The exposed portion of the tooth in the oral cavity.

Cochlear nerve: A branch of the vestibulocochlear nerve that carries fibers for the special sense of hearing.

Col: The portion of the gingiva between the contact points of adjacent teeth.

Collateral ganglion: A sympathetic ganglion of the aortic plexus.

Columella nasi: A column-like structure; fleshy portion of the nasal septum.

Common carotid artery: The artery that supplies blood to the head and portions of the neck.

Common facial vein: The vessel formed by the union of the facial vein and the anterior division of the retromandibular vein.

Compact bone: Dense layers of bone that do not contain marrow spaces.

Conducting division: The portion of the respiratory system that cleans, warms, and humidifies the air.

Condylar process: A posterior extension of the ramus of mandible.

Condyle: A round articular process of bone.

Contralateral: Opposite side of the body.

Conus medullaris: The tapering terminal end of the spinal cord.

Cornea reflex: A blinking of the eyelid in response to touching the surface of the eyeball.

Coronal plane: Divides the body into front and back parts.

Coronal pulp: The connective tissue that is located in the crown of a tooth.

Coronal suture: A fibrous joint between the frontal bone and the parietal bones.

Coronary arteries: The vessels that supply oxygenated blood to the cardiac muscles of the heart.

Coronoid process: An anterior extension of the ramus of the mandible.

Corpus callosum: The bundle or body of crossing fibers that connect the two cerebral hemispheres.

Corrugator supercilii muscle: A muscle of facial expression that draws the eyebrows medially and inferiorly, causing vertical wrinkles.

Cortical bone: The outer weight-bearing portion of a gross bone formed by compact bone.

Cortical plate: The outer layer and inner layers of compact bone of the face and skull.

Cough: A sudden noisy expulsion of air from the lungs.

Cranial: Toward the head.

Cranial base: The bone of the floor of the skull on which the brain rests.

Cranial cavity: The space in which the brain is contained.

Cranial fossae: Depressions in the internal surface of the cranial base.

Cranial nerve: A peripheral nerve that arises from the brain or brain stem.

Cranial vault: The bones of the skull that encase the brain.

Craniosacral nervous system: An alternate term for the parasympathetic nervous system.

Cranium: The bones that form the head; skull.

Crests: Ridges on the surface of bone.

Cribriform bone: The sieve-like portion of the alveolar process.

Cribriform plate: The portion of the superior surface of the ethmoid bone that is characterized by numerous small openings for the passage of the olfactory nerves.

Cricoid cartilage :   The ring-shaped cartilage of the larynx.

Crista galli: A median extension of the ethmoid bone for the attachment of the dura mater.

D

Danger space #3:   A potential space between the buccopharyngeal fascia anteriorly and the alar fascia posteriorly; the retropharyngeal space.

Danger space #4:   A potential space between the alar fascia anteriorly and the prevertebral fascia posteriorly.

Deciduous: Falling off or shedding at maturity.

Decussate: Cross over to the other side.

Deep: Away from the surface.

Deep cervical lymph nodes: A chain of lymph nodes that follows the course of the internal jugular vein.

Deep fascia: A layer of connective tissue that covers the muscle.

Deep temporal artery: A branch of the second part of the maxillary artery that supplies the temporalis muscle.

Dendrite: A cytoplasmic process of a neuron that receives a stimulus and carries the information toward the nerve cell body.

Dens: Tooth.

Dentin: The mineralized connective tissue that surrounds the pulp.

Depressor anguli oris muscle: The muscle of facial expression that lowers the corners of the mouth.

Depressor labii inferioris muscle: The muscle of facial expression that lowers the lower lip.

Descending palatine artery: A branch of the maxillary artery that supplies the palate.

Diaphysis: The tubular shaft of long bones.

Diastole: Relaxation of the heart muscles.

Diencephalon: A mass of neural tissue that surrounds the third ventricle and connects the cerebrum to the brain stem.

Digastric: Having two bellies.

Digastric fossa: A depression in the mandible for the attachment of the anterior belly of the digastric muscle.

Diploë: The spongy area between the cortical plates of the flat bones of the skull.

Diplopia: Double vision.

Distal: Far from a fixed point.

Dorsal: Toward the back; posterior.

Dorsal columns: An alternate name of the fasciculus gracilis and cuneatus.

Dorsal funiculus: The white matter between the two dorsal horns.

Dorsal horn: The upper sensory portion of the H-shaped gray matter of the spinal cord.

Dorsal median sulcus: A narrow midline cleft on the dorsal surface of the spinal cord.

Dorsal primary ramus: A branch of a spinal nerve that supplies the skin and muscle of the back.

Dorsal root: A sensory component of the spinal nerve that contains afferent fibers from the dorsal root ganglion.

Dorsal root ganglion (DRG):   A swelling on the dorsal root that contains the sensory pseudounipolar neurons.

Dorsum: The surface of the external nose.

Dura mater: Literally means "hard mother"; the tough outer covering of the brain and spinal cord.

Dural sinuses: Specialized venous structure found within the dura mater.

Dysphagia: Difficulty swallowing.

E

Effectors: Structures that receive motor input.

Efferent: Going away from a structure.

Enamel: The mineralized tissue that covers the anatomical crown of the tooth.

Endothelium: The simple squamous epithelium that lines all blood vessels.

Epicranius muscle: The muscles and connective tissue covering on the top of the head.

Epidural space: The space between the dura mater and bones of the vertebral canal that contains fat and blood vessels.

Epiglottic valleculae: The depressions between the mucosal folds that connect the tongue to the epiglottis.

Epiglottis: The lid-like structure that overhangs the entrance into the larynx.

Epiphysis: The head or distal ends of long bones.

Epistasis: Nosebleed.

Epithalamus: The portion of the diencephalon that contains the pineal gland.

Ethmoid bone: An irregularly shaped bone of the neurocranium that contributes to the formation of the walls of the nasal cavity, orbit, and anterior cranial fossa.

External acoustic meatus: The external opening of the ear.

External carotid artery: A branch of the common carotid artery that distributes blood to structures in the neck, tongue, and face.

External jugular vein: A vessel formed by the anterior division of the retromandibular vein and posterior auricular vein.

External nasal artery: A terminal branch of the facial artery that supplies the nose.

External occipital protuberance: A protrusion of the external surface of the occipital bone.

F

Facial: Regarding the face; toward the face.

Facial artery: A branch of the external carotid artery that supplies the superficial face.

Facial nerve: Cranial nerve VII; supplies taste fibers to the anterior two-thirds of the tongue, motor fibers to skeletal muscle, and preganglionic parasympathetic fibers.

Facial nucleus: The location of the motor neurons for the facial nerve.

Facial palsies: Paralysis of the muscles of facial expression.

Facial skeleton: The bones that form the surface features of the face.

Facial vein: The vessel that drains venous blood from the face.

Falx cerebri: A double fold of dura mater located in the longitudinal fissure that forms a physical barrier between the cerebral hemispheres.

Fascia: Sheets of connective tissue.

Fascial space: A potential space located between the connective tissue covering muscle or other structures.

Fascicle: A bundle of nerve fibers and its surrounding connective tissue sheath.

Fasciculus cuneatus: A tract formed by touch and proprioceptive fibers from the upper trunk and upper extremities.

Fasciculus gracilis: A tract formed by touch and proprioceptive fibers from the lower trunk and lower extremities.

Fauces: A passageway from the oral cavity to the pharynx.

Fibrous: Containing fibers.

Fibrous capsule: A connective tissue covering of a synovial joint.

Filiform papillae: Slender projections on the surface of the tongue.

First-order neuron: The first neuron in a sensory pathway; the pseudounipolar neuron in the dorsal root ganglion.

Fissure: A narrow, cleft-like slit.

Flat bones: The bones of the brain case.

Foliate papilla: A columnar folding of the mucosa on the lateral surface of the tongue that contain taste buds.

Fontanels: The connective tissue membranes between bones of the neurocranium that have not completely formed.

Foramen: A round hole.

Foramen lacerum: A ragged opening lateral to the fossa of the pituitary gland.

Foramen magnum: A large opening in the occipital bone.

Foramen ovale: An opening in the sphenoid bone for the passage of the mandibular nerve.

Foramen rotundum: An opening in the sphenoid bone for the passage of the maxillary nerve.

Foramen spinosum: An opening in the sphenoid bone for the passage of the middle meningeal artery.

Fordyce granules/spots: Sebaceous glands that open into the oral vestibule.

Forehead furrows: Horizontal grooves on the forehead.

Fossa: A trench or channel.

Fourth ventricle: The portion of the ventricular system that lies above the pons and medulla.

Fovea: A pit or depression.

Free gingiva: The non-attached portion of the gingiva that is separated from the tooth by the gingiva sulcus.

Frontal bone: The anterosuperior portion of the skull; the forehead.

Frontal crest: A linear elevation on the internal surface of the frontal bone for the attachment of the dura mater.

Frontal eye fields: The areas of the frontal lobe that controls eye movement.

Frontal lobe: A subdivision of the cerebrum that lies deep to the frontal bone.

Frontal nerve: One of the major orbital branches of the ophthalmic nerve.

Frontal plane: Divides the body into front and back parts.

Frontal process: An extension of the maxillary bone that articulates with the frontal bone.

Frontalis muscle: A muscle of facial expression that raises eyebrows and causes horizontal wrinkling of the forehead.

Functional drift: The tendency of the teeth to move in a mesial direction because of the forces of occlusion; mesial drift.

Fungiform papilla: A mushroom-shaped projection on the surface of the tongue that contains taste buds.

Funiculus: A region of white matter in the spinal cord.

Fusion: Appearance of a tooth with two crowns because of the fusion of two adjacent teeth.

G

Ganglion: An aggregation of neurons located outside of the central nervous system.

Gemination: Splitting of the crown of a tooth primordium resulting in more than one crown.

General sensation: Pain, temperature, and proprioception.

Geniculate ganglion: The location of second-order neurons in the visual pathway.

Genioglossus muscle: The muscle that protrudes the tongue.

Geniohyoid muscle: A suprahyoid muscle that elevates the hyoid bone during swallowing or depresses and retracts the mandible when opening the mouth.

Geographic tongue: Patches of the dorsum of the tongue devoid of papillae.

Gingiva: The mucosa surrounding the teeth; the gums.

Glenoid cavity: A pit or socket.

Gliding movement: The sliding of the articular disc on the articular eminence of the temporomandibular joint.

Glossopharyngeal nerve: Cranial nerve IX; supplies motor fibers to the stylopharyngeus muscles, sensory fibers to the oropharynx, general sensory and taste, to the posterior one-third of the tongue and vallate papillae, and preganglionic parasympathetic fibers that controls the secretion of the parotid gland.

Glottis: The vocal folds and the aperture between them.

Gomphosis: The fibrous connective tissue joint between the teeth and bones of the jaw.

Gray communicating ramus: A branch that connects a spinal ganglion to the spinal nerve and contains postganglionic sympathetic fibers.

Gray matter: The location of the perikarya of neurons in the spinal cord and brain.

Great vessels: The large vessels that enter and exit the heart.

Greater palatine artery: A branch of the descending palatine artery that supplies the secondary palate.

Greater palatine canal: A channel that connects the pterygopalatine fossa to the foramina of the hard palate.

Greater palatine foramina: The openings in the palatine bone for the passage of the greater palatine artery, vein, and nerve.

Greater palatine nerve: A branch of the maxillary nerve that supplies sensory and postganglionic parasympathetic fibers to the secondary palate.

Greater wing of the sphenoid bone: The portion of the bone that contributes to the formation of the middle cranial fossa.

Groove: A shallow linear depression.

Gyrus: A ridge or fold produced by the convolutions of the cerebral hemisphere.

H

Hard palate: A bony partition between the oral and nasal cavities.

Head: The superior extremity of the body that contains the command center that controls the body.

Herniated disc: An intervertebral disc characterized by the inner gelatinous core extending outside of the cartilaginous outer ring.

Hinge movement: Motion in one direction.

Horizontal plane: Divides the body into upper and lower parts.

Horizontal plate: A process of bone in the horizontal plane.

Hydrocephalus: An enlargement of the ventricles by an obstruction of the flow of cerebral spinal fluid.

Hyoglossus muscle: The muscle that lowers the tongue into the floor of the mouth.

Hyoid bone: A bone of the neck that has no articulations with other bones.

Hyperdontia: Possessing extra teeth.

Hypodontia: Less than the normal number of teeth; missing six or less teeth excluding the third molars.

Hypoglossal canal: A small channel in the occipital bone that serves as a passageway for the hypoglossal nerve.

Hypoglossal nerve: Cranial nerve XII; supplies motor fibers to the tongue.

Hypothalamus: Regulates the autonomic nervous system.

I

Incisal: The edge or cutting surface; having the ability of cutting.

Incisive artery: A terminal branch of the inferior alveolar artery that supplies the anterior mandibular teeth.

Incisive canal: A channel in the primary palate for the passage of blood vessels and nerves.

Incisive fossa: A depression of the external surface of the maxillary bone between the roots of the lateral and central incisors.

Incisive nerve: A terminal branch of the inferior alveolar nerve that supplies the roots of the anterior mandibular teeth.

Incisive papilla: A fold of mucosa posterior to the central incisors.

Inferior: Toward the feet.

Inferior alveolar artery: A branch of the first part of the maxillary artery that supplies the mandibular teeth and periodontal tissues.

Inferior alveolar nerve: A branch of the mandibular nerve that supplies sensory innervation to all the mandibular teeth.

Inferior articulating processes: A portion of a vertebra that forms a synovial joint with another vertebra.

Inferior belly of the omohyoid muscle: An infrahyoid muscle that depresses the hyoid bone while swallowing and speaking.

Inferior colliculus: A collection of neurons in the midbrain that is involved in auditory reflexes.

Inferior constrictor muscle: One of the three muscles that constricts the pharynx.

Inferior longitudinal muscle: An intrinsic muscle of the tongue that curls the tongue.

Inferior nasal concha: A facial bone of the nasal cavity that looks like a shell.

Inferior orbital fissure: A deep orbital cleft between the maxillary bone and the greater wing of the sphenoid bone.

Inferior pharyngeal constrictor muscle: One of three muscles that move food through the pharynx by sequential contraction of the muscles.

Inferior rectus muscle: The muscle that lowers and adducts the eye.

Inferior thyroid artery: A branch of the subclavian artery that supplies the thyroid gland.

Inferior vena cava: A large venous vessel that receives blood from the trunk.

Infiltration anesthesia: A technique to block pain by diffusion of an anesthetic through the cortical bone of the maxilla.

Infraorbital artery: A continuation of the maxillary artery in the orbit.

Infraorbital foramen: An opening in the maxillary bone inferior to the orbital rim for the passage of blood vessels and nerves.

Infraorbital nerve: A continuation of the maxillary nerve in the orbit.

Infratemporal crest: A linear elevation of the sphenoid bone for the attachment of the lateral pterygoid muscle.

Infratemporal fossa: A space located below the zygomatic arch and medial to the ramus of the mandible.

Infratrochlear nerve: Terminal branch of the nasociliary nerve that supplies general sensation to the skin in the medial corner of the eye.

Infundibulum: A stalk of neuronal tissue that attaches the pituitary gland to the hypothalamus.

Inner cortical plate: The inner layer of compact bone of the alveolar process.

Insertion: The moveable attachment of a muscle.

Interatrial septum: A partition between the right and left atria of the heart.

Interdental papilla: The tent-shaped gingiva between the teeth.

Interdental septum: The bone that separates the teeth.

Intermediolateral cell column (IMLCC):   The location of the cell bodies of the preganglionic sympathetic neurons in the spinal cord.

Internal acoustic meatus: An opening on the medial surface of the petrous portion of the temporal bone that leads into the tympanic cavity.

Internal carotid artery: A branch of the common carotid artery that supplies the brain.

Internal carotid plexus: Postganglionic sympathetic fibers that course along the surface of the internal carotid artery.

Internal jugular vein: A vessel that collects venous blood from the brain and portions of the head and neck.

Interneuron: A neuron in the reflex arc that connects the sensory nerve to the motor nerve.

Interpeduncular fossa: A depression between the cerebral peduncles on the inferior surface of the midbrain.

Interradicular septum: The bone in between the roots of a tooth.

Interventricular foramen: An opening in the lateral ventricles that allows the flow of cerebral spinal fluid into the third ventricle of the midbrain.

Interventricular septum: A partition between the right and left ventricles of the heart.

Intervertebral disc: The cartilage between the bodies of adjacent vertebrae.

Intervertebral foramen: An opening between two adjacent vertebrae through which the motor and sensory roots of a spinal nerve leave the spinal cord.

Intrinsic: Within.

Investing fascia: A layer of connective tissue that envelops the neck.

Ipsilateral: Same side of the body.

Irregular bones: Bones that vary in shape.

Isthmus of the fauces: Entranceway into the throat.

J

Joints: The place of union or junction of two or more bones; an articulation.

Jugular foramen: A large opening at the junction of the occipital and temporal bones.

K

Kiesselbach's area: The anteroinferior portion of the nasal septum where nosebleeds commonly occur.

L

Labial artery: A branch of the facial artery that supplies the upper and lower lip.

Labial commissures: The corners of the mouth where the lower and upper lips unite.

Labial frenulum: A fold of the mucosa that attaches the lip to the alveolar bone.

Labial glands: The small intrinsic salivary glands of the lips.

Labial tubercle: A fleshy protuberance of the upper lip.

Labial vestibule: A space between the lips and the teeth.

Labiomental groove: A depression that lies between the lower lip and the chin.

Lacrimal bones: Small facial bones located in the anteromedial orbital wall.

Lacrimal gland: A gland in the orbit that secretes tears.

Lacrimal nerve: A branch of the ophthalmic nerve that contains sensory fibers and post-ganglionic parasympathetic fibers from the pterygopalatine ganglion.

Lambdoid suture: A fibrous joint between the occipital and parietal bones.

Lamellae: Layers.

Lamina: A flat plate.

Laryngeal pharynx: The inferior portion of the pharynx that lies posterior to the larynx.

Laryngeal protuberance: A projection in the anterior portion of the neck caused by the fusion of the laryngeal cartilages; the Adam's apple.

Larynx: The voice box.

Lateral: Away from the median plane.

Lateral corticospinal tract: The path of the crossed fibers of the upper motor neurons of the cerebrum to the lower motor neurons of the spinal cord.

Lateral fissure: A deep crevice between the parietal and temporal lobes of the cerebrum.

Lateral funiculus: The white matter between the dorsal and ventral horns of the spinal cord.

Lateral ganglion: A ganglion of the sympathetic trunk; a vertebral ganglion.

Lateral glossoepiglottic folds: Folds of mucosa that attach the tongue to the epiglottis.

Lateral horn: An extension of the lateral ventricles into the temporal lobe.

Lateral masses: The segments of the atlas to which the anterior and posterior arches are attached.

Lateral pharyngeal space: A conical connective tissue space bordered medially by the wall of the pharynx and laterally by the medial pterygoid muscle.

Lateral pterygoid muscle: The muscle of mastication that pulls the articular disc forward over the articular eminence while opening the mouth.

Lateral pterygoid plate: One of two sheets of bone that form the pterygoid process of the sphenoid bone.

Lateral rectus muscle: The muscle that abducts the eye; moves the eye away from the nose.

Lateral spinothalamic tract: The sensory pathway for pain and temperature from the spinal cord.

Lateral temporomandibular ligament: A thickening of the articular capsule.

Lateral ventricle: The fluid-filled cavity inside of the cerebral hemisphere.

Le Fort fractures: The predicted fracture patterns of the skull caused by trauma or by surgical repair.

Left atrium: The chamber of the heart that receives oxygenated blood from the lungs.

Left common carotid artery: A direct branch of the aortic arch that supplies structures of the head and neck.

Left subclavian artery: A direct branch of the aortic arch that supplies the upper extremity.

Lesser palatine artery: A branch of the descending palatine artery that supplies the soft palate.

Lesser palatine foramina: Small openings in the palatine bones for the passage of the lesser palatine artery, vein, and nerve.

Lesser palatine nerve: A branch of the maxillary nerve that contains sensory fibers and postganglionic parasympathetic fibers to the soft palate.

Lesser wing of sphenoid bone: A portion of the anterior cranial fossa of the cranial base.

Levator anguli oris muscle: The muscle of facial expression that elevates the corner of the lips.

Levator labii superioris alaeque nasi muscle: The muscle of facial expression that elevates the upper lip and the wing of the nose.

Levator labii superioris muscle: The muscle of facial expression that elevates the upper lip.

Levator scapulae muscle: The muscle that elevates the scapula.

Levator veli palatini muscle: The muscle that elevates the soft palate during swallowing.

Limbic lobe: The portion of the medial surface of the cerebrum located superior to the corpus callosum; the cingulate gyrus; controls emotions.

Linea alba: A white line of keratinization on the mucosa of the cheek wall.

Lines: Linear elevations on the surface of bones.

Lingual: Regarding the tongue; toward the tongue.

Lingual artery: A branch of the external carotid artery that supplies the tongue.

Lingual frenulum: A fold of mucosa that attaches the tongue to the floor of the mouth.

Lingual nerve: A branch of the mandibular nerve that supplies sensory fibers to the tongue, carries preganglionic parasympathetic fibers to the submandibular ganglion, and carries taste fibers to the anterior two-thirds of the tongue.

Lingual tonsils: The nodules of lymphatic tissue on the root of the tongue.

Long bone: The elongated tubular-shaped bones of the extremities.

Long buccal nerve: A sensory branch of the mandibular nerve that supplies the cheek wall and buccal gingiva of the mandibular molar teeth.

Long ciliary nerve: A sensory branch of the long ciliary nerve.

Long root of the ciliary ganglion: The sensory root of the ciliary ganglion.

Longitudinal fissure: A deep depression or crevice that separates the two cerebral hemispheres.

Lower motor neurons: The neurons of the cranial and spinal nerves that innervate skeletal muscle.

Ludwig's angina: A potentially fatal condition caused by an odontogenic infection spreading from the fascial spaces of the mouth to the fascial spaces of the neck.

Lumbar cistern: An enlarged area of the subarachnoid space at the inferior termination of the spinal cord.

Lumbosacral enlargement: An enlarged area of the spinal cord that accommodates the neurons needed to innervate the lower extremities.

Lymph: A clear-to-white proteinaceous fluid.

Lymph node: An organ that filters the lymph and is the site of antibody production.

Lymphatic capillary: A blind-end vessel that collects fluid and proteins that have escaped the circulation.

Lymphatic system: Collects and returns fluid that escapes from the cardiovascular system.

Lymphatic trunk: A large vessel that returns lymph to the venous circulation.

Lymphatic vessel: A vessel that carries lymph; a vessel that connects chains of lymph nodes.

Lymphocyte: A specialized white blood cell that initiates the immune response.

M

Macrostomia: Large mouth.

Mammillary bodies: A collection of neurons that is related to the memory of smell.

Mandible: The lower jaw.

Mandibular canal: A channel in the body of the mandible for the passage of blood vessels and nerves.

Mandibular condyle: The oval projection of the mandible that articulates with the temporal bone.

Mandibular division/nerve: V_3; supplies sensory fibers to the mandibular teeth, the skin covering most of the mandible, and the temporomandibular joint, as well as motor fibers to muscles of mastication and some accessory muscles of mastication.

Mandibular foramen: An opening on the medial surface of the mandible.

Mandibular fossa: A depression in the temporal bone for the articulation of the mandibular condyle.

Mandibular notch: A depression between the coronoid process and mandibular process of the ramus of the mandible.

Marginal mandibular nerve: A branch of the facial nerve that supplies muscles of mastication along the margin of the body of mandible.

Masseter muscle: The muscle of mastication that closes and retrudes the mandible.

Masseteric artery: A branch of the maxillary artery that supplies blood to the masseter muscle.

Masticator space: The area in which the muscles of mastication and the ramus of the mandible are enclosed by fascia.

Mastoid process: A posterior bugle of the temporal bone that contains the mastoid air cells.

Maxilla: The upper jaw.

Maxillary artery: A terminal branch of the external carotid artery that supplies the meninges, mandibular and maxillary teeth, muscles of mastication, nasal cavity, orbit, scalp, and palate.

Maxillary division: V_2; supplies sensory fibers to the maxillary teeth, nasal cavity, orbit, and skin over the zygomatic arch and anterior scalp.

Maxillary sinus: An extension of the nasal cavity into the maxillary bone.

Maxillary tuberosity: The protuberance of the maxilla that is posterior to the location of the third molars.

Maxillary vein: The vessel that drains the deep face.

Meatus: A tubular passageway that widens at the surface.

Medial: Toward the median plane.

Medial pterygoid muscle: The muscle of mastication that closes and protrudes the mandible.

Medial pterygoid plate: One of two sheets of bone that form the pterygoid process of the sphenoid bone.

Medial rectus muscle: The muscle that adducts eye; moves eye toward the nose.

Median cricothyroid ligament: A membrane of connective tissue that connects the anterior surfaces of the cricoid and thyroid cartilages.

Median glossoepiglottic fold: A fold of mucosa that attaches the tongue to the epiglottis.

Median plane: Divides the body into equal right and left halves.

Median sulcus: Midline groove that bisects the anterior two-thirds of the tongue.

Mediastinitis: Inflammation of the tissue in the mediastinum.

Mediastinum: A region of the thorax bordered laterally by the lungs, anteriorly by the sternum, and posteriorly by bodies of the thoracic vertebrae; location of the heart and its coverings.

Medulla oblongata: The caudal portion of the brain stem; contains the respiratory and cardiac centers.

Medullary region: The central region of bone that is made of spongy bone and bone marrow.

Meige syndrome: The frequent involuntary closure of the eyelids combined with spasms of the muscles of the mandible and the muscles of facial expression that surround the mouth.

Meningeal ramus: A branch of a spinal nerve that innervates the three connective tissue covers of the spinal cord.

Meninges: Plural of *meninx*; connective tissue coverings of the brain and spinal cord.

Meningitis: Inflammation of the spinal cord caused by a virus or bacterium.

Mental artery: The terminal branch of the inferior alveolar artery that supplies the skin of the chin and the lip.

Mental foramen: The small opening on the outer surface of the mandible in the vicinity of the root of the first premolar tooth.

Mental nerve: A terminal branch of the inferior alveolar nerve that supplies sensory innervation to the skin and mucosa of the lower lip.

Mental protuberance: An eminence on the anterior surface of the mandible inferior to the anterior teeth.

Mental spine: A pointed projection on the medial surface of the mandible for the attachment of muscles.

Mentalis muscle: A muscle of facial expression that protrudes the lower lip and wrinkles the skin of the chin.

Mentum: The chin.

Mesial: Toward the median plane.

Mesial drift: The movement of a tooth toward the median plane because of the forces of mastication.

Microstomia: Small mouth.

Midbrain: The portion of the brain stem located between the diencephalon and the pons; the relay area for visual and auditory reflexes.

Middle cerebral artery: A branch of the internal carotid artery that supplies a large area of the cerebrum.

Middle cranial fossa: The depression in the cranial base between the lesser wing of the sphenoid bone and the petrous ridge of the temporal bone.

Middle meningeal artery: A branch of the first part of the maxillary artery that supplies the dura mater.

Middle nasal conchae: One of the shell-shaped extensions of the ethmoid bone.

Middle pharyngeal constrictor muscle: One of three muscles that move food through the pharynx by sequential contraction of the muscles.

Middle scalene muscle: The muscle that elevates the first rib during forceful breathing.

Middle superior alveolar artery: A branch of the infraorbital artery that supplies the maxillary premolar teeth.

Middle superior alveolar nerve: An inconstant branch of the infraorbital nerve that supplies sensory fibers to the mesiobuccal root of the first molar and the roots of the premolar teeth.

Midline raphe: The attachment point of muscles located in the median plane.

Minor: Small.

Mitral valve: A flap that separates the left atrium and ventricle of the heart; two cusps; the bicuspid valve.

Monosynaptic: A reflex arc in which there is only one synapse.

Motor: Information that is carried from the central nervous system to the peripheral structures.

Motor limb: The motor nerve and effector of a reflex arc.

Motor neuron: A neuron that supplies efferent fibers to an effector.

Motor root: The motor component of the spinal nerve that contains efferent fibers from the ventral horn of the spinal cord.

Motor speech area: The location of the motor neurons that control the muscles that form words.

Mucobuccal fold: The reflection of the mucosa of the lip onto the surface of the alveolar process of the jaws.

Mucocele: A swelling of a minor intrinsic salivary gland caused by the blockage of a duct.

Mucogingival line: The junctional line between the alveolar mucosa and the gingiva.

Mucosa: The epithelium and connective tissue layer lining the inside of a hollow organ; the mucous membrane.

Multipolar: Describes a neuron with numerous cell processes.

Mumps: A viral infection of the parotid gland.

Murmur: A sound produced by blood flowing through partially closed valves.

Muscle fascia: The connective tissue that surrounds muscle.

Muscular compartment: The area of the neck that contains the muscles that elevate and depress the hyoid bone while swallowing and speaking.

Muscular triangle: One of the subsidiary triangles of the neck that contains the infrahyoid or strap muscles.

Musculofascial collar: A tubular sheath of connective tissue and muscles that encircles the neck.

Myelinated: Surrounded by a myelin sheath.

Mylohyoid line: A ridge on the medial surface of the body of the mandible for the attachment of the mylohyoid muscle.

Mylohyoid muscle: A suprahyoid muscle that elevates the floor of the mouth and hyoid bone, as well as assists in the depression of the mandible.

Mylohyoid nerve: A motor branch of the inferior alveolar nerve.

N

Nasal ala: The wing of the nose.

Nasal bones: The facial bones that form the bridge of the nose.

Nasal cavity: A space within the nose that is surrounded by structures that cleanse and humidify the air.

Nasal septum: A partition of bone and cartilage that separates the nasal cavities.

Nasalis muscle: A muscle of facial expression that dilates the nostrils.

Nasociliary nerve: A sensory branch of the ophthalmic nerve that supplies the eyes, paranasal sinuses, and the dorsum of the nose.

Nasolabial groove: A depression between the nose and the corner of the mouth.

Nasolacrimal duct: A small canal that drains tears from the eyes into the nasal cavity.

Nasopalatine nerve: A branch of the maxillary nerve that supplies sensory fibers to the mucosa of the primary palate and the gingiva of the anterior teeth and contains post-ganglionic parasympathetic fibers that innervate glands of the nasal mucosa.

Nasopharynx: A portion of the pharynx that is continuous with the nasal cavities.

Neck: A constriction; joins the head and trunk.

Nerve: Fascicles of nerve fibers and its surrounding connective tissue sheath.

Nerve blocks: Procedures to anesthetize nerve trunks creating anesthesia over a large area.

Nerve fiber: An axon.

Nervous system: The structures that coordinate and regulate bodily activities.

Neural (vertebral) arch: A portion of the vertebra that surrounds and protects the spinal cord.

Neurocranium: The portion of the skull that surrounds the brain.

Neuron: The cell that is the basic unit of structure and function of the nervous system.

Neurovascular compartment: The area of the neck that contains the major arteries, veins, and nerves of the neck.

Nose: The specialized structure of the face that contains receptors for the sense of smell and serves as a portal to the respiratory system.

Nostrils: External openings of the nose.

Nucleus pulposus: The central gelatinous portion of an intervertebral disc.

O

Occipital artery: A branch of the external carotid artery that supplies the posterior neck.

Occipital bone: The posteroinferior portion of the cranium.

Occipital condyles: The knuckle-shaped elevations on the external surface of the occipital bone for the articulation with the first cervical vertebra.

Occipital lobe: The subdivision of the cerebrum that lies deep to the occipital bone.

Occipital lymph nodes: The regional group of nodes located in the back of head.

Occipital triangle: One of the subsidiary triangles of the neck that is crossed by the accessory nerve.

Occipitalis muscle: A muscle of facial expression that retracts the scalp.

Occipitofrontalis muscle: The combined frontalis and occipitalis muscles with their connecting aponeurosis.

Occlusal: Referring to the contact point between the maxillary and mandibular teeth.

Oculomotor nerve: Cranial nerve III; controls movement of the eye and opens the upper eyelid.

Odontogenic: Pertaining to the tooth.

Odontoid process: A tooth-like projection of the second cervical vertebra.

Olfactory bulb: An aggregation of second-order neurons in the pathway for the sense of smell.

Olfactory nerve: Cranial nerve I; an afferent nerve carrying the special sense of smell.

Olfactory tract: A collection of fibers carrying sensory stimuli from the olfactory bulb to the cerebrum.

Oligodontia: Less than the normal number of teeth; missing six or more teeth excluding the third molars.

Ophthalmic division: V_1; one of the three divisions of the trigeminal nerve that supply the orbit and skin of scalp.

Ophthalmic nerve: An alternate term for the ophthalmic division of the trigeminal nerve.

Optic canal: A channel through the sphenoid bone for the passage of the optic nerves.

Optic chiasm: The structure in which the nasal fibers of the retina cross.

Optic nerve: Cranial nerve II; an afferent nerve that carries the special sense of vision.

Optic tract: A collection of ipsilateral temporal and contralateral nasal fibers after the crossing of the optic nerves.

Oral cavity: The space between the teeth, tongue, and hard palate.

Oral vestibule: The space between the lips, cheek wall, and the teeth.

Orbicularis oculi muscle: The muscle of facial expression that surrounds the orbit and closes the eyelids.

Orbicularis oris muscle: The muscle of facial expression around the mouth that closes and protrudes the lip, and purses the lips.

Orbit: The cavity in the skull that contains the eyes.

Orbital plate: A portion of the frontal bone that forms the roof of the orbit.

Origin: The nonmovable attachment of muscles.

Oropharynx: The portion of the pharynx that is continuous with the oral cavity.

Ostium: An opening.

Otic ganglion: The collection of postganglionic parasympathetic neurons that innervates the parotid gland.

Outer cortical plate: Outer layer of compact bone of the alveolar process.

P

Palatal: Pertaining to the palate.

Palatine aponeurosis: A sheet of connective tissue for the attachment of the muscles of the soft palate to the hard palate.

Palatine bones: Facial bones that contribute to the formation of the hard palate and the lateral wall of the nasal cavities.

Palatine process: The extensions of the maxillary bone that form the secondary palate.

Palatine raphe: The depression of the hard palate caused by the fusion of the palatine processes of the maxillary bone.

Palatine shelves: The embryonic processes of the maxillary bone that fuse to form the secondary palate.

Palatine tonsils: An aggregation of lymphatic tissue located in the lateral wall of the fauces.

Palatoglossal fold: The mucosa covering the palatoglossus muscle; the anterior tonsillar pillar.

Palatoglossus muscle: The muscle that pulls the sides of the tongue upward and backward, pulls down on the lateral edges of the soft palate, and narrows the space between the right and left palatoglossal folds.

Palatopharyngeal fold: The mucosa covering the palatopharyngeus muscle; the posterior tonsillar fold.

Palatopharyngeus muscle: The muscle that narrows the fauces; elevates and dilates the pharynx behind the tongue.

Palpebra: Eyelid.

Palpebral commissure: The point of attachment of the upper eyelid to the lower eyelids.

Palpebral fissure: The space between the opened eyelids.

Papillary muscles: The muscles that control the closure of the heart valves.

Paranasal sinus: Four pairs of air-filled spaces within the bones that surround the orbit and are extensions of the nasal cavity.

Parasympathetic nervous system: A subdivision of the peripheral motor system that innervates smooth muscle, cardiac muscle, and glands.

Parietal: Pertaining to the body wall or cavity.

Parietal bones: The roof and a component of the lateral wall of the neurocranium.

Parietal lobe: The subdivision of the cerebrum that lies underneath the parietal bones.

Parieto-occipital fissure: A deep depression on the medial surface of the cerebrum that separates the parietal and occipital lobes.

Parotid gland: The largest of the three extrinsic salivary glands, and is located anterior to the ear.

Parotid papilla: A small projection of the oral mucosa that contains the opening of the parotid gland.

Pathway: The neurons and tracts that a stimulus must travel from the cerebrum to an effector or from a receptor to the cerebrum.

Pedicle: Literally means "a foot"; a vertical column of bone that joins the body of the vertebra to its transverse process.

Perikaryon: The cell body of a neuron that contains the nucleus.

Periodontal ligament: The connective tissue that attaches the tooth to its socket.

Periodontium: A connective tissue apparatus that attaches the tooth to the socket.

Peripheral nerve: A nerve attached to the spinal cord or brain that innervates structures of the body.

Peripheral nervous system (PNS):   The cranial and spinal nerves that innervate peripheral structures such as skin, muscle, and glands.

Peristalsis: Waves of contraction of smooth muscle.

Perpendicular plate: A vertical process of bone.

Petrous portion: A rock-shaped elevation of the temporal bone that forms part of the cranial base and contains the tympanic cavity.

Pharyngeal raphe: The connective tissue attachment of the constrictor muscles.

Pharyngeal recess: The lateral expansions of the nasopharynx posterior to the choanae.

Pharyngeal tonsils: The aggregation of lymphoid tissue that is located in the roof of the nasopharynx.

Pharynx: A tubular muscular passage between the mouth and nasal cavity and the larynx and esophagus.

Philtrum: Groove in the median portion of the upper lip.

Pia mater: Literally means "tender mother"; the connective tissue cover that is directly applied to the surface of the brain and the spinal cord.

Pineal gland: A small organ of the epithalamus that controls daily rhythms.

Piriform aperture: The anterior bony opening of the nasal cavity.

Piriform recess: The lateral expansions of the laryngeal pharynx.

Pituitary gland: An endocrine gland found in the middle cranial fossa that controls the function of endocrine glands dispersed throughout the body.

Platysma muscle: A muscle of facial expression that lowers the corners of mouth and tenses the skin of the neck.

Pneumatization: The formation of air cavities in bone.

Poliomyelitis: A viral infection of the lower motor neurons.

Polysynaptic: More than one synapse.

Pons: A portion of the brain stem that relays motor commands from the cerebrum to the cerebellum.

Pontine branches: The branches of the basilar artery that supplies the pons.

Postcentral gyrus: The primary sensory area located in the parietal lobe.

Posterior: Toward the back; dorsal.

Posterior arch: The posterior curvature of the atlas.

Posterior auricular artery: A branch of the external carotid artery that supplies the region behind the ear.

Posterior auricular nodes: A group of small lymph nodes located posterior to the ear.

Posterior belly of the digastric muscle: A suprahyoid muscle that assists in the depression of the mandible, and raises and steadies the hyoid bone during swallowing and speaking.

Posterior cerebral artery: One of the two terminal branches of the basilar artery that contributes to the circle of Willis.

Posterior cervical triangle: One of the two major triangles of the neck that share the sternocleidomastoid muscle as a common border.

Posterior cleft palate: An abnormal cleft caused by the improper fusion of the palatine shelves during development.

Posterior communicating artery: A branch of the internal carotid artery that connects the internal carotid artery to the posterior cerebral artery.

Posterior cranial fossa: A depression in the cranial base in the region of the occipital bone.

Posterior ethmoidal nerve: A sensory branch of the nasociliary nerve that supplies the ethmoidal sinuses.

Posterior horn: An extension of the lateral ventricles in the occipital lobe.

Posterior inferior cerebellar artery: A branch of the vertebral artery that supplies the posteroinferior aspect of the cerebellum.

Posterior scalene muscle: A muscle that elevates the second rib during forceful breathing.

Posterior superior alveolar artery: A branch of the third part of the maxillary artery that supplies the maxillary molar teeth.

Posterior superior alveolar foramina: The small openings on the surface of the maxillary bone for the passage of blood vessels and nerve.

Posterior superior alveolar nerve: A branch of the maxillary nerve that supplies the roots of the maxillary molars, with the possible exception of the mesiobuccal root of the first molar tooth when the middle superior alveolar nerve is present.

Posterior tonsillar pillars: The folds of mucosa that cover the palatoglossus muscle; the palatopharyngeal folds.

Postganglionic fibers: The axons of the postganglionic neurons.

Postganglionic neuron: The second neuron in the two-neuron chain of the autonomic nervous system; located in peripheral autonomic ganglia.

Preauricular lymph nodes: The superficial group of lymph nodes anterior to the ear.

Precentral gyrus: The primary motor area that contains motor neurons that control body movements.

Preganglionic fibers: The axons of preganglionic neurons.

Preganglionic neuron: The first neuron in the two-neuron chain of the autonomic nervous system; located in the lateral horn of the spinal cord and some cranial nerve nuclei.

Preganglionic sympathetic neuron: The first neuron of the sympathetic nervous system that is located in the intermediolateral cell column of the spinal cord.

Pretracheal fascia: The connective tissue that surrounds the viscera of the neck.

Prevertebral fascia: A layer of connective tissue that surrounds the intrinsic muscles of the neck.

Prevertebral ganglion: A sympathetic ganglion of the aortic plexus; a collateral ganglion.

Primary motor area: The main motor areas of the frontal lobe.

Primary palate: The anterior portion of the palate that is characterized by rugae on its surface.

Primary sensory area: The main sensory areas of the parietal lobe.

Primary visual cortex: The gyri that surround the calcarine fissure in the occipital lobe.

Procerus muscle: A muscle of facial expression that depresses the medial portion of the eyebrows, causing horizontal wrinkles.

Process: A projection from a structure.

Prone position: The position in which the body is lying with the face downward.

Proprioception: The sense of movement in space.

Protrusion: To move forward.

Protuberance: A prominence.

Proximal: Close to a fixed point.

Pseudounipolar: Describes a neuron that appears to have one cell process that actually has a peripheral and a central process joined at a common stem.

Pterygoid arteries: Branches of the second part of the maxillary artery that supply the medial and lateral pterygoid muscles.

Pterygoid fossa: A depression between the medial and lateral pterygoid plates of the sphenoid bone.

Pterygoid hamulus: A spine-like process of the medial pterygoid plate of the sphenoid bone.

Pterygoid plexus: A network of veins in the infratemporal fossa that receives blood from areas that are supplied by the maxillary artery.

Pterygoid process: A wing-like inferior extension of the sphenoid bone.

Pterygoid tuberosity: A roughened surface on the ramus of the mandible created by the attachment of the pterygoid muscles.

Pterygomandibular fold: A fold of mucosa in the oral cavity medial to the ramus of the mandible.

Pterygomandibular raphe: A seam connecting the buccinator muscle and the superior constrictor muscle.

Pterygomaxillary fissure: A space between the posterior surface of the maxillary bone and the pterygoid process of the sphenoid bone.

Pterygopalatine fossa: A pyramidal space bounded by the perpendicular plate of the palatine bone, maxillary bone, and the pterygoid process of the sphenoid bone.

Pterygopalatine ganglion: A collection of postganglionic parasympathetic neurons that control the secretion of glands in the palate, nasopharynx, nasal cavity, maxillary sinus, and lacrimal gland.

Pterygopalatine nerves: Nerve fibers that connect the pterygopalatine ganglion to the maxillary nerve.

Pterygotemporal depression: A fossa between the pterygomandibular raphe and the ramus of the mandible that is a site for intraoral injections.

Pulmonary arteries: Vessels that carry deoxygenated blood to the lungs.

Pulmonary circulation: The distribution of blood to and from the heart and lungs.

Pulmonary trunk: The outflow vessel of the right ventricle.

Pulp: The connective tissue that contains the dentin-forming cells and provides nutrients to the tooth.

Pulp chamber: A space or cavity in the crown of the tooth.

Pupillary light reflex: The automatic closure of the pupil stimulated by bright light.

R

Radicular pulp: The connective tissue of the root of a tooth.

Ramus: A branch.

Receptors: Structures that receive sensory stimuli.

Reflex: A predicted involuntary response to an outside stimulus.

Reflex arc: The pathway from the sensory receptor to the effector that produces a response.

Reflex center: An aggregation of neurons that serves as an interneuron and coordinates complex responses to a stimulus.

Respiratory division: The portion of the respiratory system where gas exchange takes place.

Respiratory system: All the structures from the nose to the lungs that conduct air and exchange oxygen and carbon dioxide.

Retina: The portion of the eye that contains visual receptors.

Retrodiscal pad: The area posterior to the articular disc of the temporomandibular joint that contains blood vessels and nerves.

Retromandibular vein: The vein that collects venous blood from the temporal region, infratemporal fossa, nasal cavity, orbit, teeth, and areas supplied by the maxillary artery.

Retropharyngeal space: A potential space between the buccopharyngeal fascia anteriorly and the alar fascia posteriorly; danger space #3.

Retrovisceral space: A connective tissue space located posterior to the pharynx and anterior to the bodies of the cervical vertebrae and bounded by the carotid sheath laterally; divided into danger spaces #3 and #4 by the alar fascia.

Retrusion: To move backward.

Rima glottidis: The aperture between the vocal folds.

Ring of Waldeyer: The tonsils that encircle the entranceways of the pharynx.

Risorius muscle: A muscle of facial expression that pulls the corners of the mouth laterally.

Rivinian ducts: 2–12 minor ducts of the sublingual gland.

Root: Origin; attachment.

Root canal: A space or cavity in the root of the tooth.

Root of the neck: The region posterior to the clavicle.

Rotational movement: Turning on an axis.

Rugae: The horizontal folds of the mucosa on the surface of the primary palate; the transverse palatine folds.

S

Sagittal plane: A vertical plane passing through the body parallel to the median plane, but does not divide the body into equal right and left parts.

Sagittal suture: The fibrous joint between the parietal bones.

Saliva: A watery fluid that cleanses the surface of the mouth and teeth.

Salpingopharyngeal fold: The fold of mucosa covering the salpingopharyngeus muscle.

Salpingopharyngeal muscle: The muscle that elevates the pharynx during swallowing.

Second-order neuron: A neuron in the central nervous system that transfers the stimulus from the first-order neuron to the thalamus.

Secondary palate: Posterior portion of the hard palate formed by the palatine processes of the maxillary bone.

Sella turcica: The fossa in the body of the sphenoid bone that contains the pituitary gland.

Semilunar valve: A flap composed of three crescent-shaped cups that are located in the pulmonary trunk and ascending aorta.

Sensory: Information that is carried to the central nervous system from peripheral receptors.

Sensory limb: The sensory receptor and sensory neuron of the reflex arc.

Sensory neuron: A nerve cell that receives a stimulus from a receptor.

Sepsis: A toxic condition caused by the spread of bacteria from a localization of the infection.

Septal cartilage: The cartilage that forms the anterior portion of the nasal septum.

Septum pellucidum: A partition that separates the two lateral ventricles.

Short bones: The cuboid-shaped bones of the ankle and wrist.

Short ciliary nerves: Branches of the ciliary ganglion.

Sialolith: A stone in the duct of a salivary gland.

Sigmoid sinus: A large dural sinus that contributes to the formation of the internal jugular vein.

Skeletal muscles: The muscles under voluntary control that are attached to the bones and move the body.

Skeletal system: The bones and cartilage that provide the basic shape and support to the body.

Skull: The skeleton of the head; also called the *cranium*.

Soft palate: The fleshy, muscular portion of the palate that separates the oropharynx from the nasopharynx.

Somatic: Pertaining to the body wall.

Somatomotor nervous system: The efferent or motor division of the brain and spinal cord that controls voluntary movement.

Special sensation: Taste, hearing, equilibrium, smell, and vision.

Sphenoethmoidal recess: The space above the superior nasal concha.

Sphenoid bone: A wedge-shaped or butterfly-shaped bone of the neurocranium.

Sphenomandibular ligament: The connective tissue structure that helps stabilize the temporomandibular joint.

Sphenopalatine artery: A branch of the maxillary artery that supplies the walls of the nasal cavity and nasal septum.

Sphenopalatine foramen: An opening in the lateral wall of the nasal cavity for the passage of blood vessels and nerves.

Spinal cord: The portion of the central nervous system that extends from the brain into the vertebral canal.

Spinal nerve: A peripheral extension of the spinal cord that innervates the skin and muscles of the body wall.

Spinal nucleus of V: The location of the second-order neurons for the pain and temperature pathway for the head.

Spine: A small thorn-like projection.

Spinous process: The posterior projection of the vertebrae for the attachment of muscles.

Spiral ganglion: The location of the cell bodies for the first-order neurons for hearing.

Splanchnic: Refers to the visceral organs.

Splanchnic nerve: A branch of the thoracic sympathetic ganglia that contain preganglionic sympathetic fibers that synapse within the ganglia of the aortic plexus.

Spongiosa: The spongy bone of the alveolar process.

Spongy bone: Thin layers of bone surrounded by large spaces containing bone marrow.

Squamous: Flat; scale-like.

Squamous suture: The fibrous joint between the parietal and temporal bones.

Stensen's duct: The excretory duct of the parotid gland.

Sternocleidomastoid muscle: The muscle of the neck that tilts and rotates the head.

Sternohyoid muscle: The infrahyoid muscle that depresses the hyoid bone while swallowing and speaking.

Sternothyroid muscle: The infrahyoid muscle that depresses the hyoid bone while swallowing and speaking.

Stroke: A sudden, severe attack.

Styloglossus muscle: The muscle that elevates and retracts the tongue.

Stylohyoid ligament: A bundle of connective tissue between the styloid process of the temporal bone to the hyoid bone.

Stylohyoid muscle: A suprahyoid muscle that elevates and retracts the hyoid bone.

Styloid process: A spine-like extension of the temporal bone for the attachment of muscles and ligaments.

Stylomandibular ligament: A connective tissue sheath that attaches the styloid process of the temporal bone to the mandible.

Stylomastoid foramen: A small opening between the styloid and mastoid processes of the temporal bones where the facial nerve exits the skull.

Stylopharyngeus muscle: The muscle that elevates the pharynx during swallowing.

Subarachnoid space: A space between the arachnoid and pia mater that contains cerebral spinal fluid.

Subclavian artery: The vessel that supplies the upper extremities and portions of the neck.

Subclavian vein: The vessel that drains venous blood from the upper extremities and portions of the neck.

Subdural space: A potential space between the dura mater and arachnoid mater.

Sublingual caruncle: A nipple-like elevation of the oral mucosa lateral to the lingual frenulum that contains the opening of the ducts of the submandibular and sublingual salivary glands.

Sublingual fold: A fold of mucosa on the surface of the sublingual salivary gland.

Sublingual fossa: A depression on the medial surface of the mandible for the sublingual gland.

Sublingual gland: The smallest of the three extrinsic salivary glands that are located in the floor of the mouth.

Sublingual space: The connective tissue space between the mucosa of the floor of the mouth and the mylohyoid muscle.

Sublingual sulcus: A groove under the surface of the tongue.

Submandibular fossa: A depression on the medial surface of the mandible for the submandibular gland.

Submandibular ganglion: An aggregation of postganglionic sympathetic neurons whose fibers innervate the submandibular and sublingual glands.

Submandibular gland: One of the three major salivary glands found inferior to the body of the mandible.

Submandibular lymph nodes: The regional lymph nodes located deep to the submandibular gland; drain mandibular and maxillary lateral incisors, the canines, the premolars, some of the molars, the lateral surface of the tongue, and the lateral portion of the floor of the mouth.

Submandibular space: The connective tissue space bordered by the inferior surface of the mandible, the two bellies of the digastric muscle, the investing fascia of the neck, and the mylohyoid muscle.

Submandibular triangle: One of the subsidiary triangles of the neck that contains the submandibular gland.

Submental lymph nodes: The small group of nodes located under the chin; drain the tip of the tongue, the anterior floor of the mouth, and the mandibular central incisors.

Submental space: A connective tissue space bordered by the mandible, the two anterior bellies of the digastric muscle, the hyoid bone, the investing fascia of the neck, and the mylohyoid muscle.

Submental triangle: The small subsidiary triangle of the neck enclosed by the anterior bellies of the digastric muscles and the hyoid bone.

Sulcular gingiva: The mucosa lining the space between the teeth and free gingiva.

Sulcus: A shallow depression between gyri of the cerebral hemisphere.

Sulcus terminalis: The v-shaped sulcus that separates the root and body of the tongue; the terminal sulcus.

Superficial: Near the surface.

Superficial cervical lymph nodes: A chain of lymph nodes that follows the course of the external jugular vein.

Superficial face: The surface features formed by the facial bones and their soft tissue coverings.

Superficial fascia: A layer of connective tissue that lies deep to the skin.

Superficial temporal artery: A terminal branch of the external carotid artery that supplies the skin on the side of the head.

Superficial temporal vein: The venous vessel that drains the skin on the side of the head and contributes to the formation of the retromandibular vein.

Superior: Toward the head.

Superior articulating processes: An extension of a vertebra for its attachment to another vertebra.

Superior cerebellar artery: One of two terminal branches of the basilar artery.

Superior colliculus: A collection of neurons in the midbrain that serves as a center for visual reflexes.

Superior dental plexus: A mixing of the sensory fibers that supply the roots of the maxillary teeth.

Superior laryngeal artery: A branch of the superior thyroid artery that supplies blood to the larynx.

Superior longitudinal muscle: An intrinsic muscle of the tongue that curls the tongue.

Superior nasal conchae: The uppermost surface of the ethmoid bone that resembles a shell.

Superior nuchal lines: Linear elevations on the occipital bone for the attachment of muscle.

Superior oblique muscle: The muscle that abducts and lowers the eyeball.

Superior orbital fissure: A cleft between the greater and lesser wings of the sphenoid bone.

Superior pharyngeal constrictor muscle: One of the three circular muscles of the pharynx that moves food by the sequential contraction of the muscle.

Superior rectus muscle: The muscle that elevates and adducts the eyeball.

Superior sagittal sinus: A dural sinus located in the superior border of the falx cerebri.

Superior salivatory nucleus: The location of the preganglionic parasympathetic neurons of the facial nerve.

Superior thyroid artery: A branch of the external carotid artery that supplies the thyroid gland.

Superior vena cava: A large venous vessel that receives blood from the head, neck, and upper extremities; formed by the brachiocephalic veins.

Supernumerary: Extra; more than the normal number.

Supine position: A position in which the body is lying on its back.

Supraciliary ridge: An elevation of bone above the eyebrow.

Supraclavicular triangle: A subsidiary triangle of the neck located superior to the clavicle that contains the subclavian vessels.

Supraorbital nerve: A terminal branch of the frontal nerve that supplies the skin of the anterior scalp.

Supraorbital notch: A shallow indentation on the superior orbital rim for the passage of blood vessels and nerves.

Supraorbital vein: A venous vessel that drains the scalp.

Supraperiosteal injection: The release of anesthesia on the periosteum of the alveolar process above the roots of the maxillary teeth.

Supratrochlear nerve: A terminal branch of the frontal nerve that supplies the skin of the anterior scalp.

Suture: A fibrous union between the bones of the skull.

Sympathetic ganglion: A collection of nerve cell bodies that are located along the sympathetic trunk.

Sympathetic nervous system: The portion of the autonomic nervous system that prepares the body for "fight or flight."

Sympathetic trunk: The sympathetic ganglia and their connecting fibers.

Symphysis: A type of cartilaginous joint that holds bones together and acts as a shock absorber.

Synchondrosis: A cartilaginous junction between two bones.

Synostosis: A bony remnant of a cartilaginous joint; ossification of a cartilaginous joint.

Synovial fluid: A viscous fluid that lubricates the articular surface of a fully moveable joint.

Synovial joint: A fully moveable joint that contains fluid and is held together by a connective tissue capsule.

Synovial membrane: The lining of the articular capsule that forms synovial fluid.

Systemic circulation: Distribution and return of blood from the heart to the body.

Systole: The contraction of the heart muscles.

T

Taste: One of the special senses.

Temporal bones: Form part of the lateral wall of the skull.

Temporal fascia: The connective tissue that covers the external surface of the temporalis muscle.

Temporal fossa: A depression on the side of the skull that contains the fleshy origin of the temporalis muscle.

Temporal lobe: A subdivision of the cerebrum that lies deep to the temporal bones.

Temporal nerve: A branch of the facial nerve that supplies motor fibers to the skeletal muscles around the eye.

Temporal process: An extension of the maxillary bone that contributes to the formation of the zygomatic arch.

Temporalis muscle: The muscle of mastication that closes and retrudes the jaw.

Temporomandibular joint (TMJ):   The articulation between the condyle of the mandible with the mandibular fossa of the temporal bone.

Tendon: The connective tissue that attaches muscle to bone or cartilage.

Tensor veli palatini muscle: The muscle that tenses the soft palate; opens the auditory tube when yawning and swallowing.

Tentorium cerebelli: The tent-like fold of the dura mater that separates the cerebrum from the cerebellum.

Thalamus: A relay nucleus for sensory information en route to the cerebrum.

Third-order neuron: A neuron in the thalamus that relays sensory information to the proper sensory areas of the cerebrum.

Third ventricle: Space within the midbrain that contains cerebral spinal fluid.

Thoracolumbar nervous system: Another name for the sympathetic nervous system.

Thyrohyoid muscle: An infrahyoid muscle that depresses the hyoid bone while swallowing and speaking.

Thyroid cartilage: The shield-shaped cartilage of the larynx.

Tinnitus: A ringing sound in the ear.

Tonsillar bed: The depression in the lateral wall of the oropharynx that contains the palatine tonsil.

Torticollis: Twisted neck.

Torus tubarius: The cartilaginous opening of the auditory tube in the nasopharynx that is covered by mucosa.

Touch: The ability to feel contact.

Trabeculae: Thin layers of bone found in the medullary region of a gross bone.

Tracts: Bundles of nerve fibers within the brain and spinal cord that serve as communication cables.

Translation movement: The sliding of the articular disc on the articular eminence of the temporomandibular joint.

Transverse foramen: An opening in the transverse process of the vertebrae for the passage of blood vessels.

Transverse muscle: An intrinsic muscle of the tongue that flattens the tongue.

Transverse palatine folds: The horizontal folds on the surface of the primary palate; the rugae.

Transverse plane: Divides the body into upper and lower parts.

Transverse process: A lateral extension of the vertebrae for the attachment of muscles.

Trapezius muscle: A large triangular-shaped muscle of the back that moves the scapula and supports the arm.

Tricuspid valve: A flap that separates the right atrium and ventricle; three cups.

Trigeminal ganglion: An aggregation of cell bodies of the first-order neurons of the trigeminal nerve.

Trigeminal nerve: Cranial nerve V; major sensory nerve of the head; motor fibers to the muscles of mastication; branches serve as a highway for carrying fibers from other cranial nerves to their targets.

Trochlear nerve: Cranial nerve IV; motor innervation to the superior oblique muscle.

Tubercle: A small rounded eminence.

Tumor: Uncontrolled growth of tissue.

Tunica adventitia: The outer connective tissue layer surrounding a blood vessel.

Tunica intima: The inner epithelial lining of a blood vessel.

Tunica media: The middle muscular layer of a blood vessel.

Tympanic cavity: The cavity in the skull that contains the organs for hearing and equilibrium.

Tympanic portion: The part of the temporal bone that is characterized by the external acoustic meatus.

U

Uncinate: Shaped like a hook.

Unmyelinated: Surrounded by a single membranous layer.

Upper motor neurons: The cells of the gray matter of the cerebrum that initiate movement.

Uvula: A fleshy mass.

Uvular muscle: The muscle that shortens and broaden the uvula.

V

Vagus nerve: Cranial nerve X; supplies preganglionic parasympathetic fibers to the viscera of the thorax and abdomen, and motor fibers to the muscles of the larynx and pharynx; contains general sensory and taste fibers.

Vallate papilla: The cup-shaped projection on the surface of the tongue that contains taste buds.

Varicose: Swollen, dilated.

Ventral: Toward the abdomen; anterior.

Ventral corticospinal tract: The path of the uncrossed fibers of the upper motor neurons of the cerebrum to the lower motor neurons of the spinal cord.

Ventral funiculus: The white matter between the ventral horn and the anterior median fissure of the spinal cord.

Ventral horn: The lower motor portion the H-shaped gray matter of the spinal cord.

Ventral median fissure: A deep midline cleft on the anterior surface of the spinal cord.

Ventral primary ramus: A branch of a spinal nerve that supplies the skin and muscle of the anterior body wall, anterior neck, legs, and arms.

Ventral root: The motor fibers that are attached to the ventral horn of the spinal cord and contribute to the formation of a spinal nerve.

Ventricle: A chamber of the heart that pumps blood.

Vertebral artery: A branch of the subclavian artery that supplies the brain.

Vertebral canal: An opening in the vertebral canal that contains the spinal cord.

Vertebral compartment: The area of the neck that contains the intrinsic muscles of the neck.

Vertebral foramen: A large opening between the neural arch and body of a vertebra.

Vertebral ganglion: A ganglion of the sympathetic trunk; a lateral ganglion.

Vertebral vein: A venous channel located in the transverse foramen.

Vertical muscle: An intrinsic muscle of the tongue that narrows the shape of the tongue.

Vestibular folds: The false vocal cords.

Vestibular fornix: The v-shaped sulcus formed by the reflection of the labial mucosa onto the alveolar process.

Vestibular ganglion: The location of the cell bodies for the first-order neurons for equilibrium.

Vestibular nerve: The division of the vestibulocochlear nerve that carries the special sense of equilibrium.

Vestibulocochlear nerve: Cranial nerve VIII; receives stimuli for the special sensation of hearing and equilibrium.

Visceral: Pertaining to the organs.

Visceral compartment: The area of the neck that contains organs of the respiratory, digestive, and endocrine systems.

Visceral nerve: The branch of the thoracic sympathetic ganglion that innervates the thoracic viscera; postganglionic sympathetic fibers.

Viscerocranium: The bones that form the facial skeleton.

Vocal folds: The superior folds of mucosa of the larynx that produce sound; the vocal cords.

Vomer: Literally means "part of a plow that cuts a furrow; plowshare"; a small facial bone that contributes to the structure of the nasal septum.

W

Wernicke's aphasia: The difficulty in understanding language with possible difficulty in reading and writing.

Wernicke's area: A portion of the temporal lobe associated with language and comprehension.

Wharton's duct: The excretory duct of the submandibular gland.

White communicating ramus: A branch that connects a spinal ganglion to the spinal nerve and contains preganglionic sympathetic fibers.

White matter: The location of the fiber tracts in the spinal cord and brain.

X

Xerostomia: Dry mouth.

Z

Zygomatic arch: A curved, bony elevation on the side of the face.

Zygomatic bones: The facial bones that form the lateral border of the orbit and the cheek.

Zygomatic eminence: The protrusion of the zygomatic bone on the surface of the face.

Zygomatic nerve: A branch of the maxillary nerve that carries postganglionic parasympathetic fibers destined to the lacrimal gland and sensory fibers to the skin on the cheek bone and temporal region.

Zygomatic process: The extension of the temporal bone that contributes to the formation of the zygomatic arch.

Zygomaticofacial nerve: A branch of the zygomatic nerve that supplies sensory fibers to the skin over the cheek bone.

Zygomaticotemporal nerve: A branch of the zygomatic nerve that supplies sensory fibers to the skin in the temporal region.

Zygomaticus major muscle: A muscle of facial expression that elevates the corner of the mouth.

Zygomaticus minor muscle: A muscle of facial expression that draws the upper lip upward and outward.

Learning Lab
Appendix

Self-Test Activity

Test yourself by correctly labeling the following illustrations. For an additional challenge, use colored pencils or pens to shade in the anatomical structures. These sheets are perforated for your convenience and may be copied for self-study.

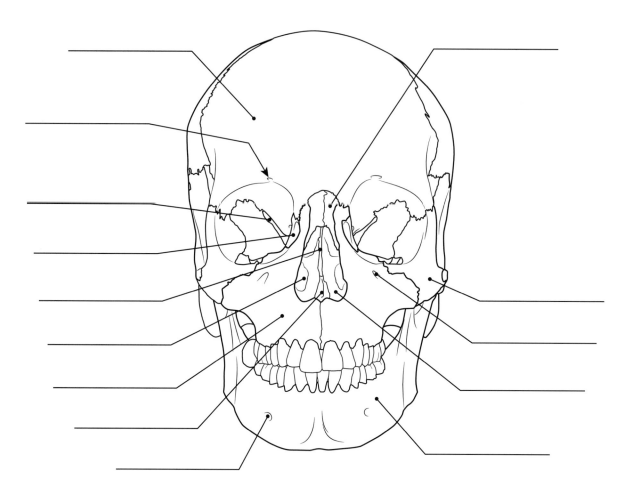

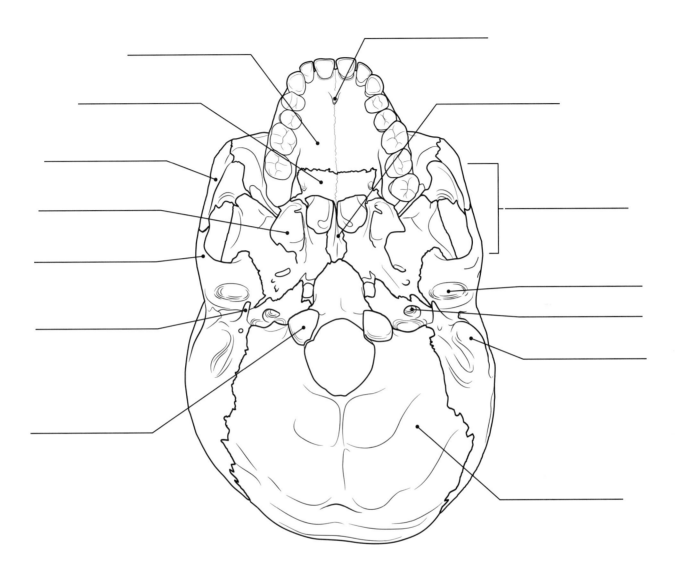

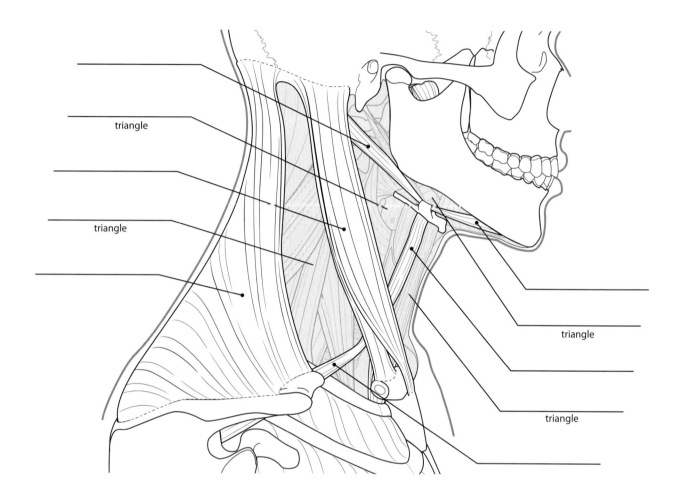

triangle

triangle

triangle

triangle

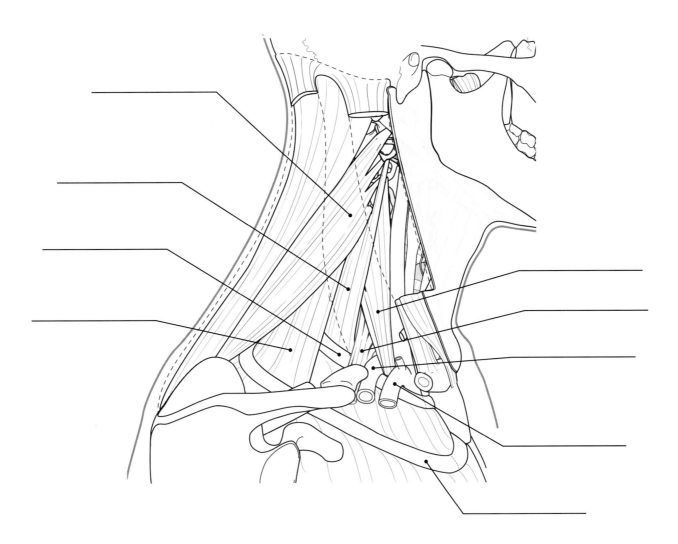

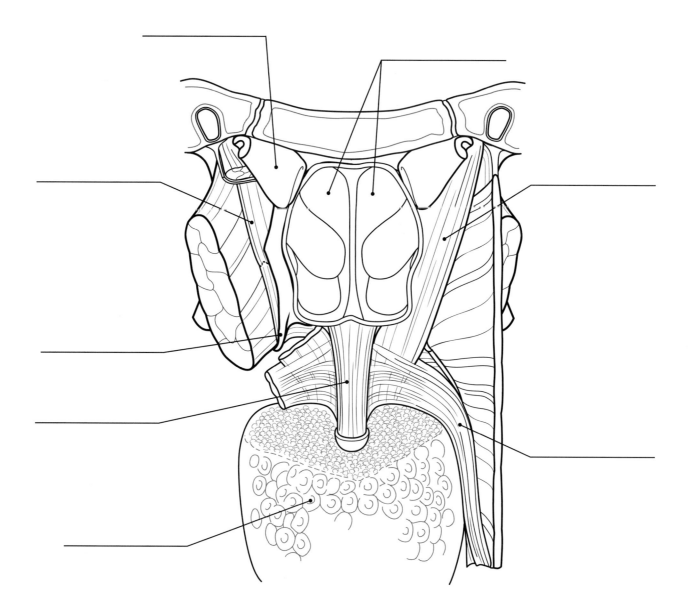

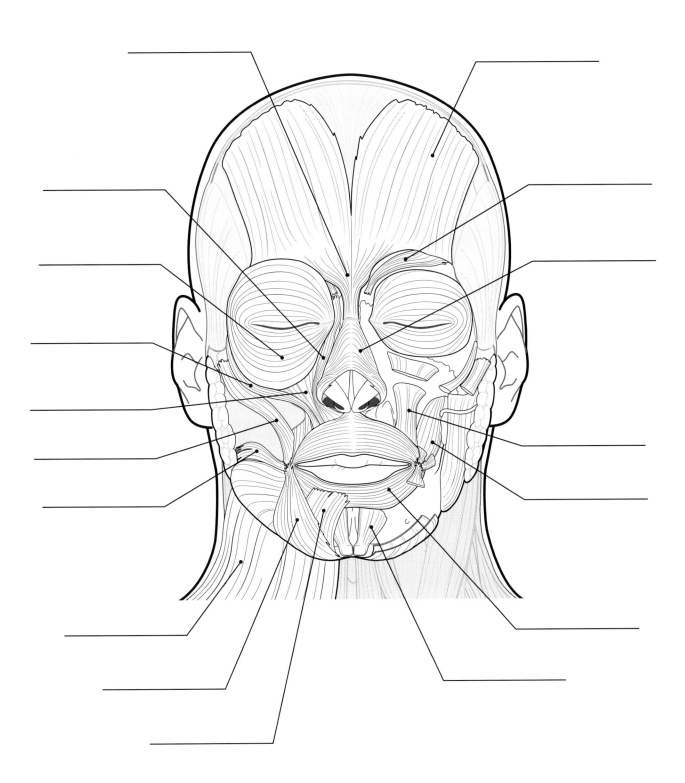

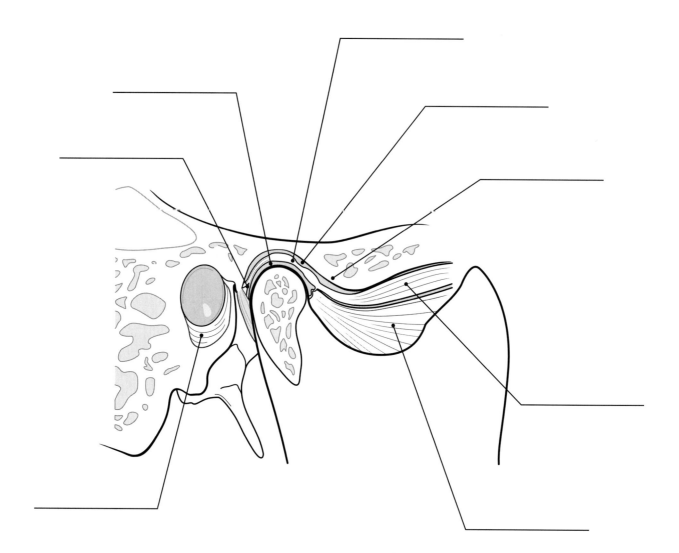

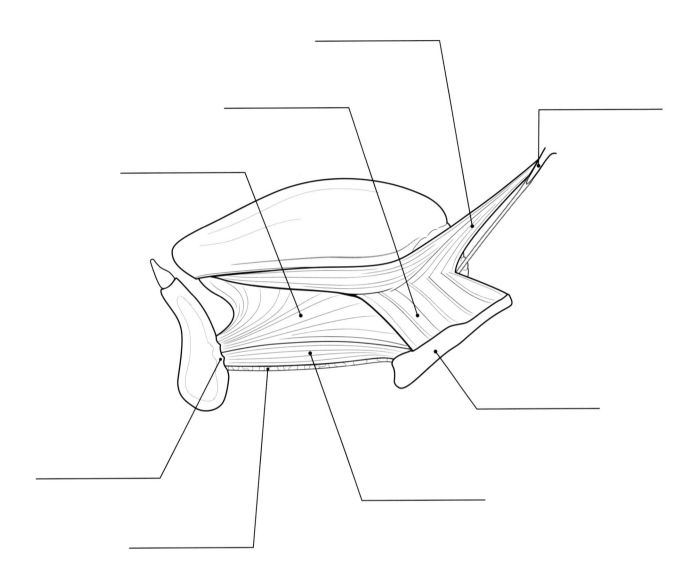

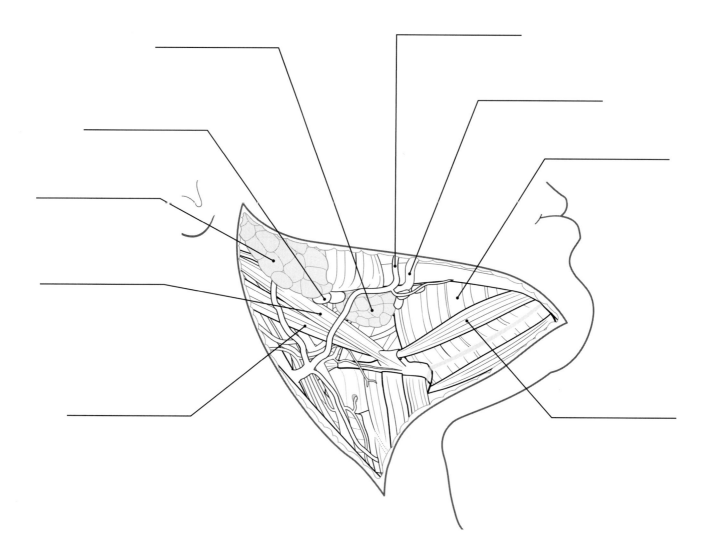

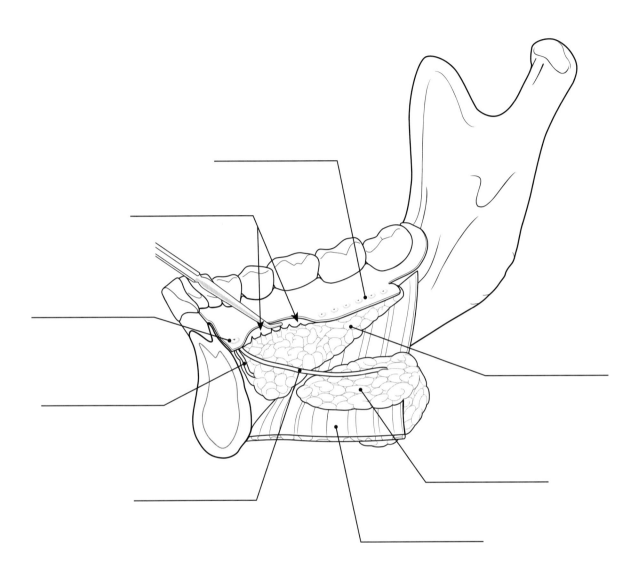

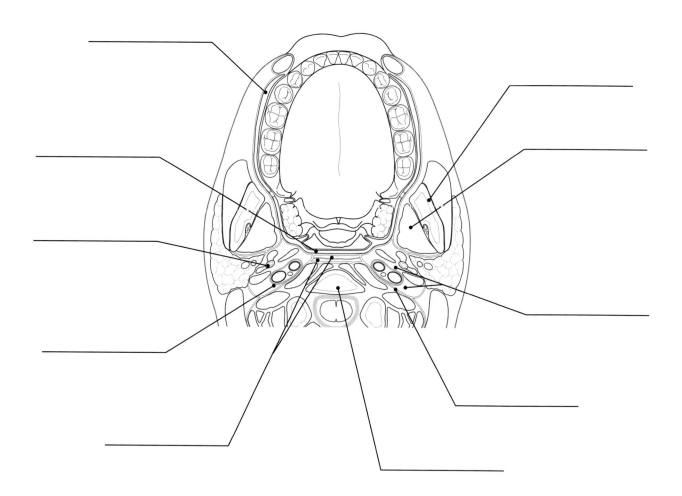

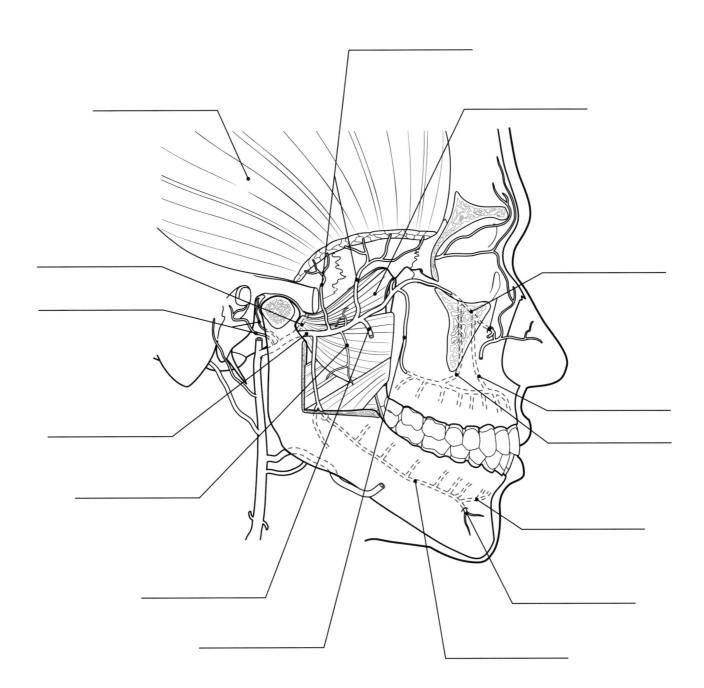

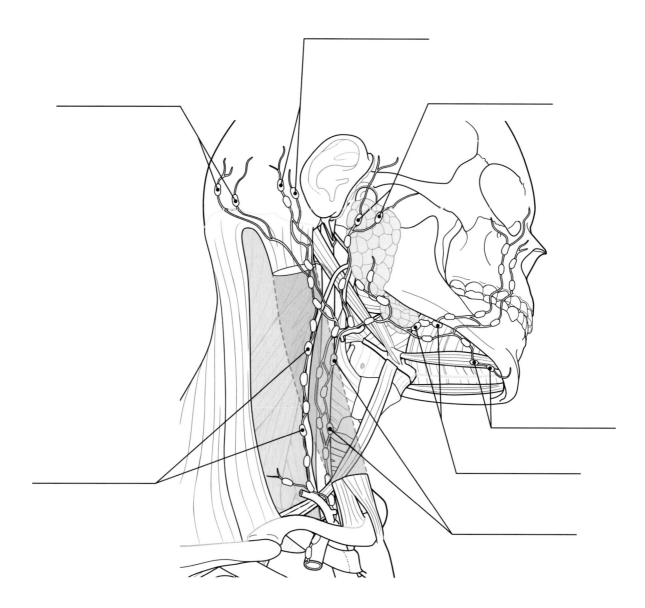

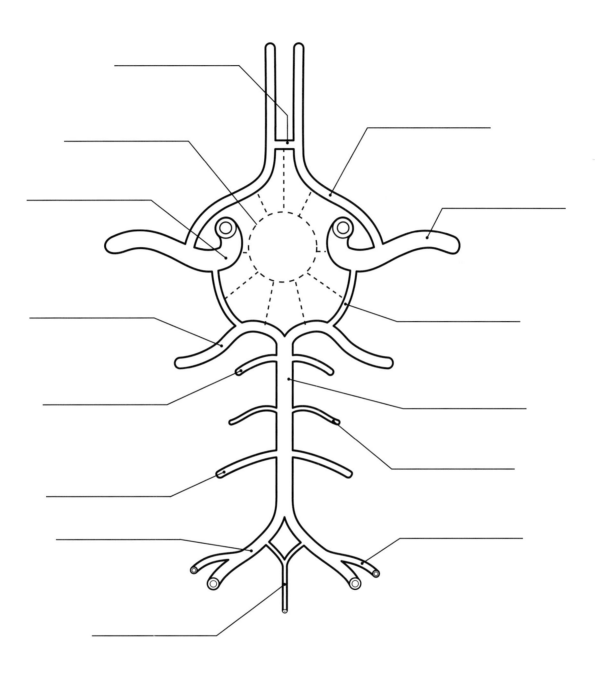

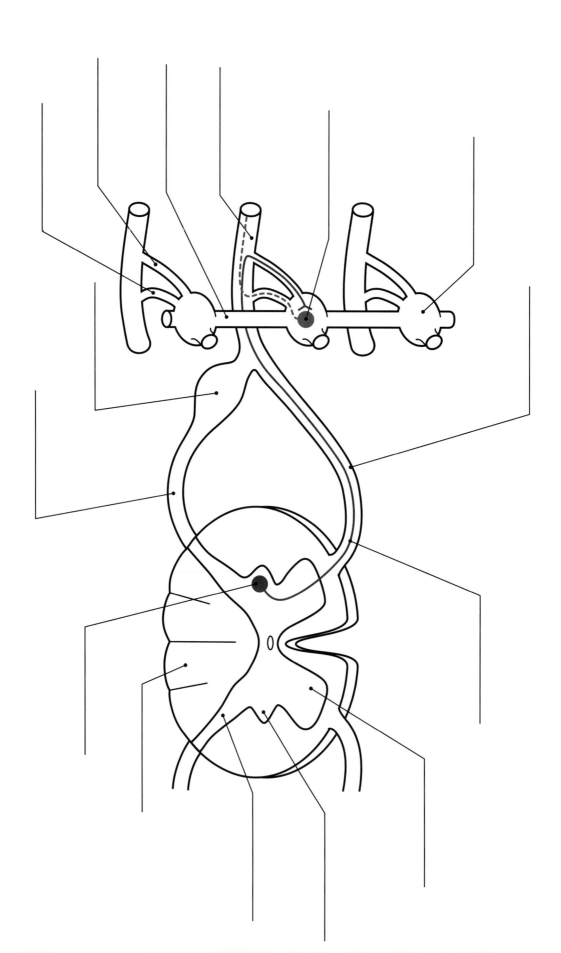

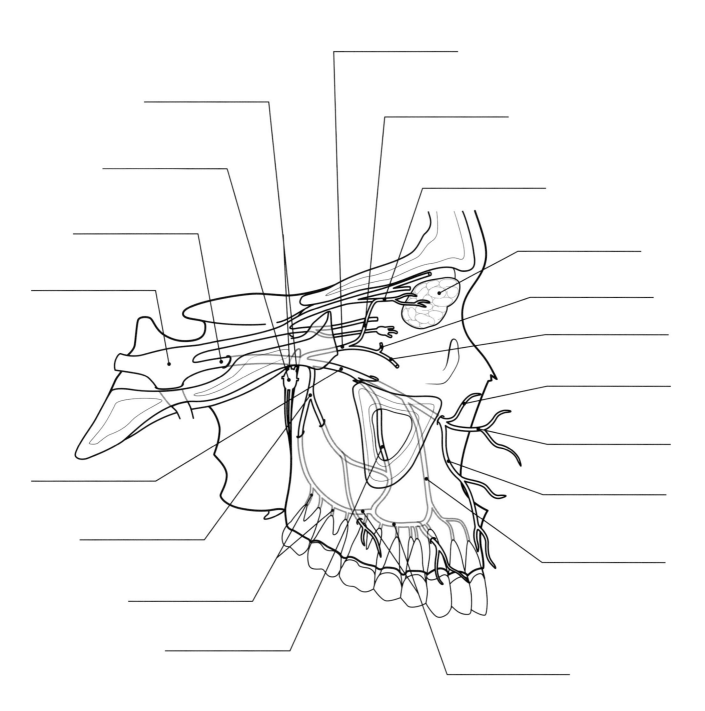

INDEX